THE ECONOMICS OF HEALTH RECONSIDERED

Third Edition

THE ECONOMICS OF HEALTH RECONSIDERED

Third Edition

Thomas Rice
and
Lynn Unruh

Health Administration Press, Chicago
Association of University Programs in Health Administration, Arlington, Virginia

Your board, staff, or clients may also benefit from this book's insight. For more information on quantity discounts, contact the Health Administration Press Marketing Manager at (312) 424-9470.

13   12   11   10   09   5   4   3   2   1

Library of Congress Cataloging-in-Publication Data
Rice, Thomas H.
 The economics of health reconsidered / Thomas Rice and Lynn Unruh.—3rd ed.
    p. ; cm.
 Includes bibliographical references and index.
 ISBN 978-1-56793-328-4 (alk. paper)
 1. Medical economics—Mathematical models. 2. Medical care—Cost effectiveness.
I. Unruh, Lynn. II. Title.
 [DNLM: 1. Economics, Medical—United States. 2. Cost-Benefit Analysis—United States. 3. Models, Economic—United States. W 74 AA1 R497e 2009]
 RA410.R53 2009
 338.4'33621—dc22

                                                                      2009001073

The paper used in this publication meets the minimum requirements of American National Standard for Information Sciences—Permanence of Paper for Printed Library Materials, ANSI Z39.48-1984. ⊗ ™

Acquisitions editor: Janet Davis; Project manager: Dojna Shearer; Text design: BookComp Inc.; Cover design: Trisha Lartz

Found an error or typo? We want to know! Please e-mail it to hap1@ache.org, and put "Book Error" in the subject line.

Health Administration Press
A division of the Foundation of the
   American College of Healthcare Executives
1 North Franklin Street, Suite 1700
Chicago, IL 60606-3529
(312) 424-2800

Association of University Programs in
   Health Administration
2000 N. 14th Street
Suite 780
Arlington, VA 22201
(703) 894-0940

To Clara, Danny, and Kate, and to Dorothy Rice and the late Jim Rice
—TR

To my family, my friends, and Pablo
—LU

BRIEF CONTENTS

DETAILED CONTENTS

ACKNOWLEDGMENTS

We would like to express our deep appreciation to a number of people who provided comments on the research itself or on the individual chapters, not only in this edition but in the previous two as well. Special thanks to those who reviewed the new material in this third edition: Janet Cummings, who commented on chapters 4 through 10; Jack Needleman, who commented on chapters 6 through 8; Brian Elbel, who commented on Chapter 4; and Sally Stearns, who commented on Chapter 8. Thanks also to Yaniv Hanoch, who collaborated on the ideas presented in Section 5.3, on whether there can be "too much choice." In addition, several people reviewed individual sections in the appendix: Susan Giaimo, Parick Hassenteufel, Jeremiah Hurley, Ayano Kunimitsu, Gavin Mooney, Adam Oliver, Richard Saltman, Erik Schut, Stephanie Stock, and Peter Zweifel.

Material in the first and second editions was read and commented on by Henry Aaron, Ronald Andersen, Gerard Anderson, William Comanor, Katherine Desmond, Robert Evans, Rashi Fein, Paul Feldstein, Susan Haber, Diana Hilberman, Miriam Laugesen, Donald Light, Harold Luft, David Mechanic, Glenn Melnick, Gavin Mooney, Joseph Newhouse, Mark Peterson, Uwe Reinhardt, John Roemer, Sally Stearns, Greg Stoddart, Deborah Stone, Pete Welch, Joseph White, and Miriam Wiley. Reviewers of the materials on the individual countries in the appendix of the second edition (not listed above) included John Creighton Campbell, Finn Diderichsen, Eddy Van Doorslaer, Kieke Okma, Valérie Paris, Kristina Bränd Persson, Lise Rochaix-Ranson, Björn Smedby, Clive H. Smee, and Paul Talcott.

Finally, we would also like to express our appreciation to Miriam Laugesen for preparing most of the material in the appendix on the healthcare systems of various countries. She wishes to acknowledge Nell Marshall for her able research assistance.

It goes without saying that all conclusions, and any errors, are entirely our own and are not the responsibility of any of the reviewers.

PREFACE TO THE THIRD EDITION

The new edition of *The Economics of Health Reconsidered* greatly expands on the previous versions. In response to comments from users, we have re-conceived the book to better meet the needs of health economics professors and students. It covers much more material, making it possible for instructors to use it as a stand-alone text in health economics courses. Instructors should further note that password-protected instructor's resources that provide (among other things) a list of concepts, discussion questions, and further readings for each of the main chapters in the book are available. For access to the instructor's resources, e-mail hap1@ache.org.

In addition to substantial revision of and updates to existing chapters, three chapters are entirely new:

- Chapter 2 attempts to synthesize the relevant microeconomic theory necessary in a health economics class, thereby obviating the need to purchase a separate microeconomics textbook.
- Chapter 7 discusses for-profit versus nonprofit organizations in healthcare, including specialty hospitals and the nursing home and pharmaceutical industries.
- Chapter 8 employs labor economics theory as applied to healthcare workforce issues—in particular, the markets for physicians and nurses.

Another change in this edition is a second author: Lynn Unruh. Dr. Unruh is trained as an economist and as a nurse. Her research has focused on the market for nurses and on hospital and nursing home organization and financing. While both authors were substantially involved in all aspects of the book, Dr. Unruh focused on the three chapters related to healthcare supply.

Despite these changes, the basic theme of the book remains consistent with the first edition, published more than ten years ago. It attempts to show that, despite assertions to the contrary, neither economic theory nor evidence shows that reliance on market forces leads to superior healthcare systems. Government has a critical role to play in making the healthcare sector not only more equitable but more efficient as well.

Tom Rice
Lynn Unruh

INTRODUCTION

As the book's title indicates, the economics of health needs to be reconsidered. While health economists recognize the need for government involvement in the marketplace, they still tend to advocate reliance on market forces in healthcare system reform. This book questions the wisdom of this mindset, using theory and empirical evidence.

To understand the advisability of alternative reform methods, one must first understand the traditional competitive model. After providing a context for the book in Chapter 1—where we make the case that health economic theory needs to be reconsidered—we present a detailed summary of microeconomic theory in Chapter 2. That chapter explains the key tools of the trade: demand, supply, competition, monopoly, and social welfare. The remainder of the book examines the assumptions underlying the competitive model, whether they are met in the healthcare realm, and the advisability of alternative ways of reforming healthcare markets.

Chapter 3 lists 14 assumptions that need to be met to ensure socially optimal results from the use of market forces. Later chapters examine whether each of these assumptions is met; we provide evidence that they are not. This does not mean government intervention is necessarily superior, however. One must evaluate empirically where markets succeed and fail. Indeed, just as markets fail, so can government. Of course, all countries use markets and governments in varying degrees, so it is not an either/or choice but a matter of emphasizing the appropriate policy tools in a specific proposed reform. One of the book's key points is that because so few of the assumptions of competitive markets are met in healthcare, one cannot presume that pro-competitive policies will be superior.

WHY SHOULD THE ECONOMICS OF HEALTH BE RECONSIDERED?

1.1 Context

Recent years have seen a surge of interest in reforming the organization and delivery of health systems by replacing government regulation with reliance on market forces. Although much of the impetus has come from the United States, the phenomenon is worldwide. Spurred by ever-increasing costs coupled with competing priorities such as education, welfare, and—much more recently—environmental concerns, analysts and policymakers have embraced the competitive market as the means of choice for reforming medical care systems. To a great extent, this belief stems from economic theory, which purports to show the superiority of markets over heavy government involvement.

In the United States during the middle and latter part of the 1990s, increased competition in the healthcare sector helped control the rate of increase in costs. The main manifestation of this competition was the increase in managed care enrollment and concomitant decline in fee-for-service. Between 1993 and 2001, for example, the percentage of workers covered by conventional fee-for-service insurance declined from 49 percent to just 7 percent (Jensen et al. 1997; Gabel et al. 2001). The second half of the 1990s also saw less use of hospital care and much lower inflation in health costs than in previous decades. Average per capita health expenditures rose only 5 percent annually, approximately the same increase as the economy as a whole, and far less than in previous years (Centers for Disease Control and Prevention 2001). Studies showed that the geographic areas with the highest managed care penetration experienced the smallest increases in health costs (Zwanziger and Melnick 1996; Bamezai et al. 1999). Whether this meant the market was operating more efficiently was less clear, however, as improved efficiency depends not only on costs but also on access to care and quality of care received.[1] Access has been declining; the number of uninsured Americans increases nearly every year. Definitive conclusions about trends in quality are harder to make (Miller and Luft 1997).

But heavy-handed managed care had severe side effects. Talk of a backlash began as early as 1997 (Blendon et al. 1998) and a special issue of a leading health policy journal, the *Journal of Health Politics, Policy and Law*, was devoted to the topic in 1999. Since that time, softer forms, sometimes dubbed "managed care light," have become more prominent. Preferred provider organization (PPO) enrollment has increased, and health maintenance organization (HMO) enrollment has decreased, and within HMOs, access to specialists is less restricted.

A resurgence of rising costs accompanied the managed care backlash. These pressures are now primarily being addressed not through regulation, but through higher prices—a classic market (as opposed to regulatory) response. Annual growth in premiums for job-based health insurance coverage increased at rates well into the double digits from 2001 to 2004, although the rate began to decline in 2005 and continued to do so through 2007 (Claxton et al. 2007). One reason the pressure on premiums has lessened is the substantial growth in patient cost-sharing requirements, such as deductibles and copayments. Between 2001 and 2006, average PPO deductibles rose by 60 percent, and copayments for preferred, brand-name drugs, by 50 percent (Claxton et al. 2006). Consumer prices in the economy as a whole rose by only 14 percent during this five-year period (Bureau of Labor Statistics 2008). This underlies a larger change: the movement toward health insurance policies with high deductibles in general and consumer-directed health plans in particular.

Three strategies exist for confronting growing costs: government regulation (e.g., limiting reimbursements or resources), private regulation (e.g., managed care restrictions), and the price mechanism. The United States has moved from the first to the second, and now moves toward the third.

The perceived success of this increasingly competitive marketplace in healthcare sectors is part of a broader trend in the United States, in which markets are viewed as efficient and government is viewed as inefficient. As Robert Kuttner (1997) wrote, "America . . . is in one of its cyclical romances with a utopian view of laissez-faire." The relevance of this statement persists more than a decade later because the cycle has not yet ended. This does not imply, either in the health sector or in the economy as a whole, that policymakers have eschewed government involvement. Our concern is that healthcare markets are moving in this direction, and that economic theory is used—inappropriately, we will argue—in support of market-based health policies.

Practically all health economists—even those favoring a more competitive marketplace—recognize the need for government to play a significant role in the health system. Much of the work in this area is based on the writings of Alain Enthoven (1978a, 1978b, 1988, 2003; Enthoven and Kronick 1989a, 1989b), who advocates reliance on consumer choice and competition to improve the efficiency of healthcare markets. Nevertheless, he still believes that government has two key roles: ensuring that competition is based on price rather than selection of the healthiest patients, and providing subsidies to low-income persons.

The corollary to this viewpoint is that government should confine itself to these two roles. Health services policy should be based on competition, with government ensuring that markets operate fairly and helping disadvantaged people. A careful review of economic theory as applied to health, however, does not permit government such a limited role.

This book contends that one of the main justifications for the superiority of market-based systems stems from a misapplication of economic theory to health. As we will show, this application is based on a large set of assumptions that are not met and cannot be met in the healthcare sector. This is not to say that competitive approaches in this key sector of the economy are inappropriate; rather, their efficacy depends on the policy being considered and the environment in which it is to be implemented. Stated more colloquially, it works well in some instances but not in others. There is, however, no reason to believe market-based systems will operate more efficiently or provide a higher level of social welfare than alternative systems based on governmental financing and regulation. This argument is further bolstered by the deviation of many other developed countries from market-based health systems.

Although economists know that claims about the superiority of competitive approaches are based on fulfillment of assumptions, the healthcare literature rarely mentions the large number of such assumptions or their importance. One should not put undue blame on health economists, however; this problem pervades the entire economic discipline. In this regard, Lester Thurow (1983) has written that "every economist knows the dozens of restrictive assumptions . . . that are necessary to 'prove' that a free market is the best possible economic game, but they tend to be forgotten in the play of events." Chapter 3 provides the authors' list of these assumptions, and in subsequent chapters we show their implications in the fields of health economics and health policy.

The book thus centers on a description, analysis, and application of the assumptions upon which the superiority of competition is based—and in particular, what happens in markets for health services if they are not met.

1.2 Purpose of the Book

The purpose of this book is to reconsider the economics of health. It does so by examining the assumptions on which the superiority of competitive approaches is based, and how failure to meet those assumptions affects health policy choices.

Although each chapter provides applications, the book is also about theory—its use and its misuse. The book will attempt to show that economic theory does not support the belief that competition in the health services sector will necessarily lead to superior social outcomes.

If economic theory does not demonstrate the superiority of market forces in health, questions must be answered empirically. To a large extent, that is exactly what health economists and health services researchers are trying to do. The authors have few reservations about the kinds of research studies being conducted. Our concern is that the work will suffer if researchers approach it with preconceived notions of what the results ought to be.

Some readers will be disappointed to see that although the book critiques the competitive model, it does not explicitly offer a theoretical alternative. It does, however, compare the health systems of countries that use varying ratios of government and markets. Unfortunately, there is little useful data for drawing conclusions about the success of alternative systems, although this is improving. Ultimately, readers must draw their own conclusions about the most desirable system using theory and the extant empirical literature. We hope this book can help them do so.

Unlike the two previous editions, the third is designed to serve as a stand-alone text for courses in health economics. Chapter 2 provides the microeconomics basis necessary for understanding the rest of the book, and we have included several topics not addressed in the previous editions—specifically, material on workforce (e.g., physicians and nurses), institutions (e.g., not-for-profit organizations), and products (e.g., pharmaceuticals). Needless to say, supplemental material, especially articles in professional journals, is always helpful to round out one's understanding of an issue.

The book is also addressed to non-economics professions. Because students and practitioners in these disciplines obviously tend to be less schooled in the details of economic analysis, they often have to take health economists at their word when the latter speak about the policy implications of economic analysis in general, and the superiority of markets in particular. (In this regard, Joan Robinson has been quoted as advising, "Study economics to avoid being deceived by economists" [Kuttner 1984].) We hope this book will help put those in disciplines other than economics on a more level playing field when it comes to discussions of health policy.

1.3 Outline of the Book

The book is divided into ten chapters and a conclusion. Chapter 2 covers nearly all of the major topics a course in microeconomic theory would cover. A few remaining topics (e.g., externalities, labor economics) are discussed later in the book. Those who are already familiar with intermediate microeconomic theory can proceed directly to the other chapters. Others may want to refer back to Chapter 2 when reading the subsequent material.

Chapter 3 provides a list of the assumptions upon which the superiority of market competition is based, as well as an overview of the role of government. We critique those assumptions in the chapters that follow.

The next five chapters provide the core of the book. Chapter 4 focuses on the theory of demand, and Chapter 5 applies the theory of demand to health, insurance, and particular health services. Chapters 6 through 8 focus on supply: issues of competition and market power in healthcare supply and demand, for-profit medicine, and workforce issues, respectively. Chapter 9 explores equity and redistribution, a topic of tremendous importance to policy but one that has received insufficient attention from health economists. Chapter 10 discusses different ways developed countries can and have organized their healthcare systems, and includes cross-national empirical evidence on outcomes and costs and tentative lessons from this evidence. The conclusion offers some final thoughts concerning the role of competition in health services. The appendix, the writing of which was led by Miriam Laugesen, provides a brief overview of the health services systems in ten developed countries, to support the material in Chapter 10.

Note

1. Alain Enthoven (1988) makes this point nicely, writing, "An efficient allocation of healthcare resources to and within the healthcare sector is one that minimizes the social cost of illness, including its treatment. This is achieved when the marginal dollar spent on healthcare produces the same value to society as the marginal dollar spent on education, defense, personal consumption, and other uses. Relevant costs include the suffering and inconvenience of patients, as well as the resources used in producing healthcare. This goal should not be confused with minimizing or containing healthcare expenditures. Policymakers focus much attention on the total amount of spending on healthcare services, often as a share of gross national product (GNP). But a lower percentage of GNP spent on healthcare does not necessarily mean greater efficiency. If the reduced share of GNP is achieved by denial or postponement of services that consumers would value at more than their marginal cost, then efficiency is not achieved or enhanced by the cut in spending" (11).

THE TRADITIONAL COMPETITIVE MODEL

The field of microeconomics is devoted to the study of competition—mainly its virtues, but also some of its pitfalls. Although many of the techniques economists use are fairly new, the emphasis on competition dates back more than 200 years, to the writings of Adam Smith (1776 [1994]). Smith believed that people driven by their own economic interest in the marketplace are guided by an "invisible hand" to act in the manner that most benefits society at large. The concept that societal outcomes are optimal when individuals and firms act in what one might view as a completely selfish manner is a key insight of economic theory. As we will explain later in this chapter, the word "optimal" has a specific economic meaning that differs from the word's common definition.

The notion of competition is intuitively appealing. In a competitive market, people are allowed but not compelled to trade their wealth, including their labor, if they find it beneficial to do so. Theoretically, if everyone stops trading when doing so stops being beneficial, the market is in *equilibrium*. Such an outcome is desirable in two senses: (1) People are making their own choices and (2) by not engaging in any more trades, people reveal themselves to be as satisfied as possible with their economic lot, given the resources with which they began. Analogously, firms can enter and exit the market at will, and produce as much or as little as they wish. To beat the competition, however, they will endeavor to produce only what people demand, using the fewest possible resources in order to obtain the highest profits. This leaves more resources available to fulfill demand for other products and services.

This chapter outlines the economic theory of competition and what competition can and cannot achieve. It is divided into five subsections: utility and demand; production, cost, and supply; equilibrium in a competitive market; equilibrium for a monopolist; and the economy as a whole. A few other microeconomic issues, particularly externalities (Chapter 5) and labor supply (Chapter 8) are discussed in subsequent chapters where the topic naturally arises.

It is necessary to understand the basics of microeconomic theory to appreciate the book's critiques of its application to health. Those familiar with the standard theory can proceed immediately to Chapter 3, while those seeking more detail may wish to consult a microeconomics textbook.[1]

2.1 Utility and Demand

Utility

We begin with the notion of *utility*. Perhaps the easiest way to think about this term is through some synonyms, such as "happiness," "satisfaction," or even "physical and mental well-being." One of the key concepts of microeconomic theory is that consumers attempt to maximize their utility.

The utility obtained from the consumption of one more unit of a good is its *marginal utility*. Economists generally believe that the marginal utility a person receives from a particular good declines as he or she obtains more of the good. For example, having one automobile might give you a lot of utility, and having a second might give you more—but not as much extra as the first one did. This is called *diminishing marginal utility*.

Some early theorists, collectively known as the *classical utilitarians*, believed that one could compute how well off an entire society was by adding up each person's utility. But to do this, we would need to assign a quantitative value to the utility possessed by each person in a society. This naturally led to the question of whether it was possible to quantify such measures. A leading early advocate of classical utilitarianism, Jeremy Bentham, thought it was possible to measure utility through its manifestations of pleasure and pain. In rather colorful language, he wrote:

> Nature has pleased mankind under the governance of two sovereign masters, *pain* and *pleasure*. It is for them alone to point out what we ought to do, as well as to determine what we shall do. On the one hand the standard of right and wrong, on the other the chain of causes and effects, are fastened to their throne. They govern us in all we do, in all we say, in all we think: every effort we can make to throw off our subjection, will serve but to demonstrate and confirm it. (Bentham 1968)

Economics is rarely viewed as a left-wing social science—how could it be if it is based on an axiom of self-interest? But if, as the classical utilitarians claimed, everyone has the same capacity to experience pleasure and pain, and if we assume the existence of diminishing marginal utility, then social welfare is maximized when everyone has the same income. It is easy to see why this is the case. Suppose one person has $10,000 in income and another has $5,000. If an additional dollar is spent by the former person, it will bring less utility than if the same dollar were spent by the latter. Only if everyone has the same income will total welfare be maximized.

Although some radical utilitarians were comfortable with this, others—some of whom presumably would have lost a great deal through the equalization of incomes—were not. And it was not hard to poke holes in the theory. Classical utilitarianism is based on two key assumptions: (1) Utility can be quantified and (2) it is possible to add utilities across different individuals. That is, everyone has a common quantitative metric, whereby three units of utility (or *utiles*) for you is equivalent to the same number of utiles for me.

Modern economists eschew these assumptions in favor of a milder form of utilitarian principles. Microeconomics now proceeds under the *Pareto principle*, where a policy is considered desirable if it makes someone better off without making anyone worse off. But to go further—say, to advocate one public program or tax over another as better for society as a whole, when there will be winners and losers—requires explicit value judgments. Despite occasional claims to the contrary, economic theory almost never implies that one policy is better than another, since this would involve weighing the benefits that accrue to one group against the losses incurred by the other. The most theory can do is demonstrate the advantages and disadvantages of each alternative.

Indifference Curves

Recall that economic theory assumes that people seek to maximize their utility. Utility, the outcome, is on the left side of Equation 2.1, and the determinants of utility, an example of which is the goods and services people consume, are on the right side.

Let:

$$U = f(X, Y, Z, \ldots, n) \tag{2.1}$$

where U is a person's utility. There are n goods or services that person consumes, three of which are labeled X, Y, and Z. The possession of this bundle of goods leads to the person's utility level, U. We further assume that although there is diminishing marginal utility, consumers do not reach a *saturation point*, at which an additional unit of X, Y, or Z actually reduces their utility. In other words, people are happier when they have more stuff—an issue we deal with in chapters 3 and 4.

Chapter 4 revisits another important and somewhat hidden assumption inherent in this theory: People are affected only by the things they possess, and are affected neither positively nor negatively by what others have, or by how their bundle of goods compares to those of others. This only becomes apparent if we explicitly denote that we are dealing with only a representative individual, person i.

$$U_i = f(X_i, Y_i, Z_i, \ldots, n_i) \tag{2.2}$$

Clearly, this person's utility is only affected by what he or she has, not by what others have. We can represent an alternative scenario in which people are affected by both their own possessions and those of others by including another subscript for a representative other individual, j.

$$U_i = f(X_i, X_j, \Upsilon_i, \Upsilon_j, Z_i, Z_j, \ldots, n_i, n_j) \tag{2.3}$$

The conventional theory assumes people seek to maximize their utility, which, as we noted, is determined by the bundle of goods and services they possess. To do so, they purchase their ideal bundle based on their desire or *taste* for the alternative goods and the prices of these alternatives, subject, of course, to how much income they have available to spend.

We will use graphs throughout this chapter, as they are helpful in illustrating these concepts. In doing so, however, we can show at most only two of the many goods and services people wish to have—one on each axis.

Figure 2.1 shows *indifference curves*, which represent alternative combinations of two goods that result in the same level of utility. Curve U_2 conveys a higher utility than U_1 because at each point, the person possesses more of both goods. In theory, a consumer has an infinite number of indifference curves, each corresponding to different combinations of quantities of the two goods.

The typical indifference curve has three characteristics. First, it tends to have a convex-to-the-origin shape because of diminishing marginal utility. Once a person has a great deal of one good and little of another, that person has to receive a lot more of the former in order to give up even a little bit of the latter. The slope of the indifference curve, which of course varies at each point if it is not a straight line, is called the *marginal rate of substitution*. It is equal to the ratio of the marginal utilities of the two goods.[2]

Second, indifference curves don't bend all the way back around. Stated more technically, they never exhibit a positive slope. A given quantity on the x- or y-axis corresponds to only one point on an indifference curve. This implies that consumers do not reach a satiation point—they always get more utility from an additional unit of a good, no matter how much they already have.

Third, two indifference curves cannot intersect. If they did, then all points on *both* curves would confer the same amount of utility. That would imply that having more of both goods would not bring higher utility, which violates the definition of the curve.

To make this less abstract, Figure 2.1 shows two goods that might appear in a consumer's utility function: visits to physicians (MDs) and visits to nurse practitioners (NPs). For expository purposes, it is helpful to assume that all of a person's money is spent on these two services. The quantity of nurse practitioner visits appears on the horizontal axis, and the quantity of physician visits appears on the vertical axis. The consumer is indifferent to all points on a particular curve since by definition all points bring equal levels of satisfaction. Three NP visits and four MD visits (point A) are equal in desirability to five NP visits and three MD visits (point B) on curve U_1. The person would be even happier to have more (for example, point C on curve U_2), but that might involve spending more money than he or she has available.

FIGURE 2.1: Consumer Indifference Curves

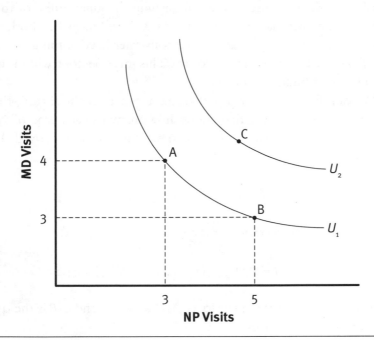

The Budget Constraint

The choice of how much of each type of visit to purchase depends not only on how much the person wants of each visit type, but also on the price of each type. A rational consumer (defined and discussed in chapters 4 and 5) maximizes utility by spending each successive dollar in a way that brings about the most utility. This means that when they have spent their last dollar, consumers will have equalized, across all the goods in their utility function, the ratio of the marginal utilities (MU) with the ratio of the prices (P) of the goods.

It we define P_M as the price ot MD visits, and P_{NP} as the price of NP visits, then, for a consumer who has maximized his or her utility,

$$MU_M/P_M = MU_{NP}/P_{NP} \qquad (2.4)$$

By cross-multiplying and rearranging the terms, we can write it and think of it another way, where the ratios of the marginal utilities are equal to the price ratios of the two goods:

$$MU_M/MU_{NP} = P_M/P_{NP} \qquad (2.5)$$

It is easy to see why a consumer must fulfill Equation 2.4 (and therefore Equation 2.5) to maximize utility. Suppose the equality is not met at a particular combination of MD and NP services purchased (which could be point B in Figure 2.3). In this case, buying more NP visits and fewer MD visits would benefit the consumer. However, the result will be lower marginal utility of NP visits (because of the diminishing marginal utility of the extra NP visits), and higher marginal utility for MD visits. Only when both sides of Equation 2.4 (or 2.5) are equal will the consumer have nothing left to gain from trading one type of visit for another. This must be done within the confines of his or her budget, however.

We can illustrate this concept using another graphical tool, the *budget constraint*. This is a line that shows how many of each type of visit the consumer can purchase with a given income, and it can be derived through equations 2.6 and 2.7.

$$I = (P_M \times M) + (P_{NP} \times NP) \tag{2.6}$$

and solving for *NP* by rearranging the terms,

$$M = I / P_M - [(P_{NP} / P_M) \times NP)], \tag{2.7}$$

where *I* is income, *M* is the quantity of MD services, and *NP* is the quantity of nurse practitioner services.

Figure 2.2 graphs this, using the assumption that all a person's income during a given period is spent on these two goods. The point at which the budget constraint line intersects each axis shows how many of each good or service the consumer could buy by spending all income on that single service. The first term of Equation 2.7 shows the intercept on the vertical axis, and the term $-P_{NP} / P_M$ is the slope.

The consumer can afford to purchase any combination of these two services that is either on the line or in the shaded area below and to the left of the line, but cannot afford any combination above and to the right of it. It is easy to construct a budget constraint for any level of income since the slope of the line, which is the ratio of the prices of the two goods, does not change. For example, a 50 percent increase in income would shift the budget constraint line outward and to the right by this exact amount.

We can also see that the slope of the budget constraint is equal to the price ratio between NP and MD visits.[3]

The Consumer Optimum

How does a consumer decide how many of each good or service will maximize utility? He or she chooses the combination of goods that corresponds to the point of tangency between the budget constraint and the highest indifference curve, as illustrated by point A in Figure 2.3. Recall that the consumer has an infinite number of indifference curves; here we show just two of them.

In contrast to point A, at point B the indifference curve and budget constraint do not have the same slope. This puts the consumer on an indiffer-

FIGURE 2.2: The Budget Constraint

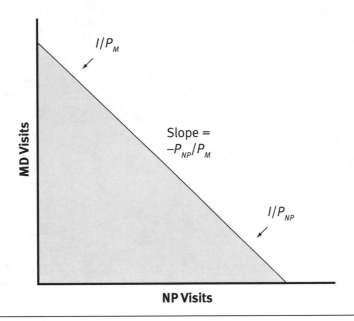

ence curve that conveys less utility, U_0. By trading MD visits for NP visits, it is possible to move down the budget constraint to point A, and increase utility by moving to the higher indifference curve, U_1.

Although much of it may seem obvious, what is remarkable about the theory is that it shows that *everyone* will have the same ratio of marginal utilities between all goods and services. This is certainly clear mathematically. If everyone faces the same prices, equations 2.4 and 2.5 can only hold if everyone has the same ratios. But how can that be the case when people exhibit different tastes for alternative goods? Suppose a person really prefers NP visits and only wants an occasional MD visit. At the prevailing price ratio, that person will purchase far more NP visits. So at the margin—the last visit—the additional utility of that visit will be relatively low. And the person uses so few MD services that the last one has a relatively high utility, even though the consumer prefers seeing the NP.

To illustrate, suppose that the price of MD visits is $100 and the price of NP visits is $50. The ratio of the two is two to one. Anyone trying to optimize purchases would make trades until the ratio of the marginal utility for MD visits to the marginal utility of NP visits equaled two to one. This does not imply that each person necessarily has the same marginal utility for each type of visit at a particular point on his indifference curve. But the ratio of his marginal utilities at the tangency point to the budget constraint will be two to one.

FIGURE 2.3: The Consumer "Optimum"

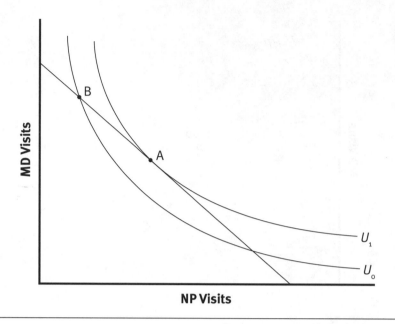

Consumer theory concludes that, taking into account their own preferences and market prices, people will make the choices that will make them best off. When they have done as well as they can do, given their resources, they stop trading, presumably to enjoy the goods that they have acquired. These are strong conclusions; much of chapters 4 and 5 will be devoted to examining and critiquing the assumptions on which they are based.

Demand Curves and Functions

The concept of indifference curves leads naturally to the concept of demand. Here, we develop a demand curve for NP visits. Recall that a consumer has an infinite number of indifference curves, corresponding to the utility received from every possible combination of quantities of the two goods being considered. Figure 2.4 shows three indifference curves for NP and MD visits for a particular consumer. Suppose we vary the price of NP visits from P_{NP} to $P_{NP/2}$ to $P_{NP/4}$—that is, we consider what would happen not only at the original price, but also at half and one-fourth that price—but do not change the price of MD visits (P_M) or income. The result is that the budget constraint pivots outward. Under these three alternative sets of prices, we'll assume the consumer chooses to purchase six, eight, and ten NP visits per year, respectively. These points are then plotted as a *demand curve*, labeled D_1 in Figure 2.5. (Note that, for simplicity, we show demand and supply curves as straight lines, but there is no reason they cannot have a curvilinear shape.)

A demand curve shows how much of a good is purchased at alternative prices. It is drawn under the assumptions that neither the price of other goods

FIGURE 2.4: Derivation of Demand Curve, Step 1

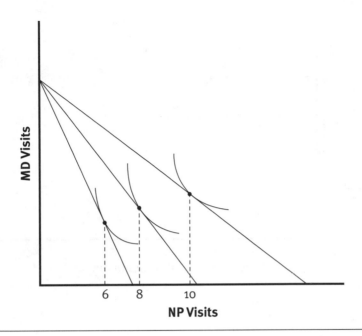

nor the person's income changes. It is further assumed that a person's tastes are unaltered. Thus, in deriving the curve only one thing varies—here, the price of nurse practitioner services.

Demand curves have a further interpretation: They show the marginal utility a consumer derives from the purchase of the good or service. We assume individuals purchase those products whose marginal utility exceeds their price. Note that the downward slope of a demand curve follows the decrease in marginal utility as the quantity of a good consumed rises. This topic will be explored further in Chapter 4, when revealed preference and the concept of consumer surplus are discussed.

Although one needs actual data on consumer behavior to draw an accurate demand curve, in general it will slope downward to the right, indicating that people will demand more when the price is lower.

In functional form:

$$D = f(P, P_a, I, T) \qquad (2.8)$$

where D is demand for a particular good or service, P is its price, P_a is the price of alternatives, I is income, and T is tastes. *Aggregate demand*—how much is demanded by all individuals combined—is simply the sum of the individuals' demands.

Alternative goods, the subscript a, can be categorized two ways: as *complements* or as *substitutes*. Complements are goods that are used in

---

FIGURE 2.5: Derivation of Demand Curve, Step 2

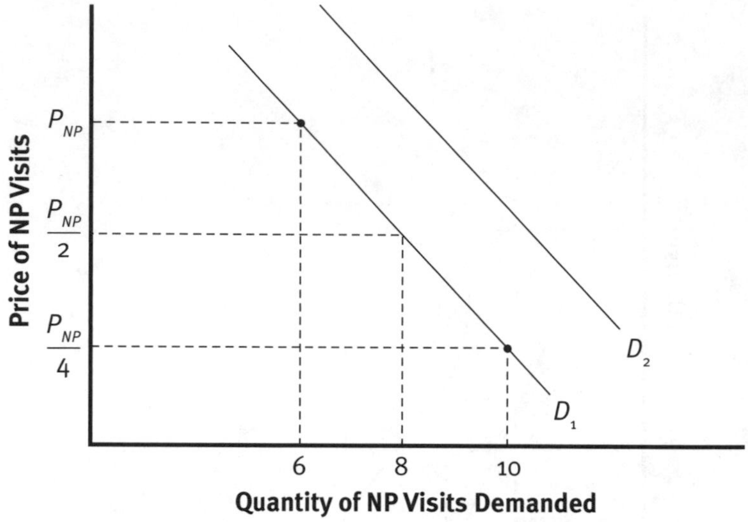

conjunction with the good being studied, and substitutes are those that are used instead. We can therefore refine Equation 2.6 as follows:

$$D = f(P, P_s, P_c, I, T) \qquad (2.9)$$

where P_s is the price of substitutes and P_c is the price of complements.

What is perhaps most noteworthy about these equations is the unobtrusive role of T, tastes. This one variable represents much of what it is to be a human being. Psychology and sociology have studied how individual tastes are formed and the ways in which they are manifested. But economic theory takes the taste variable as predetermined and unaffected by the person's environment.

In the health services area, perhaps the major component of T relates to health status. If people are sick, they are obviously more likely to use medical care than if they are well. In that sense, they have a "taste" for health. This would not be a good way to classify your desire for medical services if, say, you were hit by a truck, but there is no other place for it in Equation 2.8. As a result, the demand for health is sometimes expressed as:

$$D = f(P, P_s, P_c, I, HS, T) \qquad (2.10)$$

where HS is the patient's health status. In Equation 2.10, tastes no longer capture health status, only the non–health related determinants of demand.

As we saw, a single demand curve can illustrate any relationship be-tween the quantity and price of a particular good. We assume, however, that the other determinants of demand—the prices of alternative goods, income, health status, and tastes—remain unchanged. If they do change, the demand curve must also shift. For example, when a person gets sick, his or her de-mand curve is likely to shift outward and to the right—as shown by the de-mand curve labeled D_2 in Figure 2.5—indicating that he or she will demand more medical care at all price levels. Nevertheless, the amount demanded is still expected to depend, in part, on the price of medical care.

The relationships between demand and income and between demand and the price of other goods are more complicated. In general, we would ex-pect the demand curve to shift outward and to the right if income rises. This is true of *normal goods*. But there are goods and services with the opposite re-lationship: When income rises, demand falls, and when income falls, demand rises. These are known as *inferior goods*—although the term does not imply anything pejorative. In the health services area, an example might be visits to emergency rooms (ERs). Those with higher incomes are more likely to have a usual provider of care, and therefore to seek care from an ER less frequently. Thus, if income rises we would expect a person's demand curve for ER visits to shift downward and to the left; at any price, the quantity of ER services demanded will be lower.

The relationship between demand for one good and the price of other goods is even more complicated, and we will explore it further when we discuss elasticities of demand. Two goods are considered substitutes if an increase in the price of one leads to an increase in the demand for the other, and complements if the opposite is true. (A more technical definition, involv-ing cross-price elasticities of demand, is provided later in this chapter.) Most goods and services are substitutes. A classic example is beef and chicken. If the price of beef rises, demand for chicken will increase as people substitute the latter for the former. A classic example of complementary goods is auto-mobiles and tires. If the price of cars rises, demand for cars will decrease, and therefore so will the demand for tires. A health services example of comple-ments is the relationship between inpatient hospital care and outpatient phy-sician services. Although these would seem to be substitutes, there is some evidence to indicate that they are complements: As the price of physician out-patient services rises, the demand for inpatient hospital care falls. (The reason will be explained in Chapter 4.) In summary, if the price of a substitute rises, the demand for the good shifts outward and to the right and the opposite occurs for complements.

Income and Substitution Effects

One of the more challenging concepts in microeconomic theory is income and substitution effects. They are used to illustrate two distinct reasons the quantity of a good or service will tend to rise when the price falls. Suppose the price of MD services falls and the price of nurse practitioner services remains the same. One reason the quantity of MD services demanded will rise is because relative to the price of nurse practitioner services, they are now cheaper. People gravitate toward goods that are relatively cheaper than others; this is the substitution effect. The second reason quantity demanded will tend to rise is that, in effect, the reduction in price means the person is no longer spending all of his or her income. If people use this new-found wealth to purchase more physician services, quantity demanded will rise. This is the income effect. The total change in the quantity of MD services demanded is the sum of these two effects.

Figures 2.6 and 2.7 illustrate the more common case of a normal rather than an inferior good.[4] Figure 2.6 shows the expected increase in quantity demanded, from M_1 to M_2, with a decline in price. Figure 2.7 breaks this down into income and substitution effects.

Figure 2.6 shows two of the consumer's many indifference curves, I_1 and I_2, along with the original, steeper budget constraint and a new, gentler budget constraint corresponding to the reduction in the price of physician services. As the price of physician services falls, the new consumer optimum will shift from point A to point B, corresponding to an increase in the quantity demanded from M_1 to M_2 (illustrated in Figure 2.4).

The key to Figure 2.7 is the broken line. This runs parallel to the new budget constraint, but is closer to the origin. This means the broken line represents the same price ratio as the new budget constraint, since the slope of the budget constraint is equal to the price ratio of the two goods being considered. But note that the broken line is tangent to the original indifference curve, which suggests the consumer is no better off than before the price decrease in MD visits.

Consider consumer optimum point C, where the broken line touches the old indifference curve, and the corresponding quantity purchased, M_3. This represents how many MD services a person would purchase if he or she:

- faced the new price ratio and
- was no better off than before prices fell.

The movement from M_1 to M_3 represents the substitution effect—how much the quantity purchased increased due solely to changes in the price ratio, from the original steep line to the new, more gently sloping one. And the movement from M_3 to M_2 shows the income effect—how much the new-found wealth resulting from the lower price of MD services increased the quantity demanded. Their sum, which is the distance from M_1 to M_2, is the total increase in quantity demanded.

FIGURE 2.6: Derivation of Income and Substitution Effects, Step 1

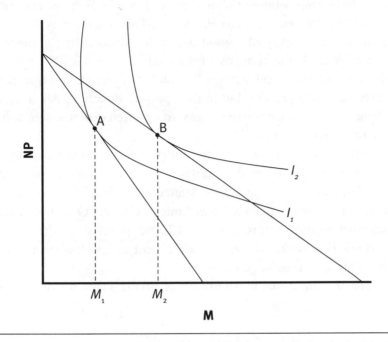

FIGURE 2.7: Derivation of Income and Substitution Effects, Step 2

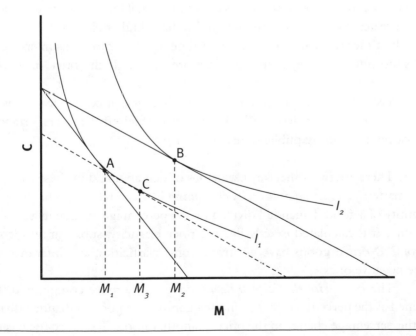

Elasticities of Demand

The exact relationship between the quantity of a good purchased and its price is represented by the *price elasticity of demand*. This is defined as the percentage change in the quantity of a good demanded divided by the percentage change in its price. If the elasticity of demand equals −0.5, this means that when the price of the good changes by, say, 10 percent, the quantity demanded changes by 5 percent, but in the opposite direction. All downward-sloped demand curves have negative signs, so we often drop the sign and refer to its absolute value—here, 0.5.[5]

Health economists have devoted much research to determining various demand elasticities for medical services. By convention, goods and services with elasticities exceeding 1.0 are defined as "elastic," those less than 1.0 as "inelastic," and those equaling 1.0 as "unitary elastic." One should not put too much stock in these terms, however. Chapter 4 will show that, although demand elasticities for health services are almost always less than 1.0, they would certainly appear to be price sensitive.

There are three major determinants of the elasticity of a good or service.

- **The extent to which substitutes are available.** If a consumer can easily switch to another good when the price of the original good rises, then the latter will tend to be more elastic.
- **The proportion of the consumer's income spent on the good.** Naturally, one would be more price sensitive about big budget items, such as housing, than tiny ones, such as chewing gum. Thus, goods that compose a greater share of one's budget tend to have higher elasticities.
- **The time frame in question.** Over time, it's easier for consumers to find substitutes, so long-term elasticities are higher. If the price of gasoline rises, it is hard for consumers to make quick adjustments; gas is price inelastic. Over time, however, persistent high gas prices can lead consumers to lower their demand by buying more fuel-efficient cars, arranging carpools, or using public transportation.

There are two other key elasticities of demand, and in these cases, the sign matters. The *income elasticity of demand* is the percentage change in the quantity of a good demanded divided by the percentage change in a person's income. It is calculated exactly like the price elasticity, substituting income, I, for P. Normal goods have positive income elasticities, and inferior goods have negative ones.

The *cross-price elasticity of demand* is slightly more complicated. It is defined as the percentage change in the quantity of a good demanded divided by the percentage change in the price of another good. To return to an earlier example, we might be interested in the cross-price elasticity of demand between inpatient hospital care and outpatient physician services. Substitutes have positive cross-price elasticities, and complements, negative ones.[6]

2.2 Production, Costs, and Supply

Total Product Curves and Isoquants

In production theory, firms seek to maximize profits in the same way consumers attempt to maximize utility. To do so, they purchase inputs and transform them into outputs through the application of some sort of technology. This process is represented using a *production function*.

We will use one of the goods discussed above, MD visits (Q_{MD}), but this time we will examine how a firm produces the good. Assume that several inputs are used to produce these visits through a production process, f. The production function therefore takes the form

$$Q_{MD} = f(a, b, \ldots, m) \tag{2.11}$$

where m inputs, two of which are indicated by the letters a and b, are used in the production of these visits. The two most important classes of inputs are labor and capital. In the case of MD visits, one would also include supplies (e.g., gloves, dressings, syringes).

The *total product* curve, shown in Figure 2.8, shows the relationship between output (the vertical axis) and increasing use of one input (the horizontal axis). Note that when little of the input is used, output increases at an increasing rate, called *increasing marginal productivity*. This is because the input is being underused given the amount of capital available. Loosely, one can think of this as not taking advantage of economies of scale. (The term "economies of scale" has a specific meaning that relates to the long run, and will be defined later.) For example, a single nurse in a big hospital would not be very productive, but as more nurses are added, each will become more productive as she can specialize in particular tasks. In Figure 2.8, the rate of output increase eventually decreases as the use of input rises further; this is *diminishing marginal productivity*. It occurs because each new input has less capital (e.g., machines, work space) to use and is therefore less productive than those previously employed.

Returning to Equation 2.11, we will restrict ourselves to just two inputs so that these concepts can be represented graphically. Figure 2.9 shows curves known as *isoquants*. Quantities of each of two inputs, nurse practitioners and examination rooms, are represented on the two axes. The isoquant labeled "Visits = 20" shows the different amounts of inputs required to produce 20 visits per day. The other isoquant indicates the inputs necessary to

FIGURE 2.8: Total Product Curve

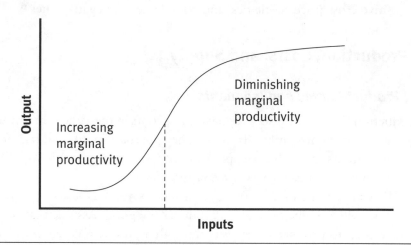

produce 30 visits per day. The slope of an isoquant at each point is called the *marginal rate of technical substitution* and is equal to the ratios of the marginal productivities of each input at that particular point.[7]

As with indifference curves, the reason isoquants are concave is due to diminishing marginal productivity. The *marginal product* is the change in output when a single input is increased by one unit and the other input is held constant. We might expect that a second nurse practitioner would be able to treat more patients. A third nurse practitioner would mean even more patients could be treated—but the increase in number of visits that would result from adding a third nurse would likely be smaller than the increase that resulted from adding a second nurse. This is not because the third nurse practitioner is necessarily less skilled. Rather, the fixed number of examination rooms creates a physical constraint on the number of patients the office can accommodate. The third nurse practitioner might help make the use of the examining rooms more efficient, but only so much can be accomplished. If marginal productivity did not diminish, isoquants would be linear.

Why doesn't the practitioner simply get a bigger office, eliminating the constraint on waiting rooms? He or she can, of course. We distinguish between two periods: the *short run* and the *long run*. Over the short run, we assume firms can alter the use of one input (typically labor) but not the other input (usually capital, such as office space). The long run is defined as the period over which a firm can vary all inputs. How long is the long run? It depends on what is being produced. It may be short in a simple production process, but long for something complicated, like building new jumbo jets or hospitals. We will return to this concept when we discuss cost curves.

At a given level of technology (represented by our production function, f), only a certain number of visits can be produced. The two isoquants

FIGURE 2.9: Producer Isoquants

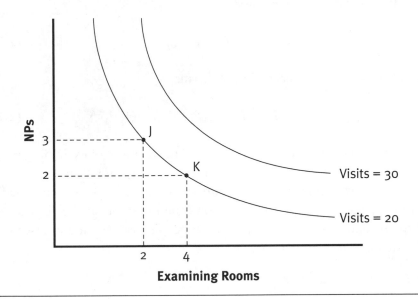

in Figure 2.9 indicate that if the state of technology were more advanced, the same number of inputs could produce more outputs. For now, however, we confine ourselves to the lower curve. Points J and K indicate two different ways the office can produce 20 visits per day: with three nurse practitioners and two examining rooms, or with two nurse practitioners and four examining rooms.

Isocost Lines

Given the state of technology, if a firm produces as much output as possible with a given amount of inputs, production is known to be *technically efficient*. We would expect all firms to strive for this; otherwise they would not be maximizing profits. It would not necessarily mean, however, that production is *economically efficient*. For economic efficiency, a firm must use the mix of inputs that incurs the least costs. This mix will vary depending on the relative prices of the different inputs. To maximize profits, a firm must be technically and economically efficient.

Input prices are indicated by an *isocost line*, as illustrated in Figure 2.10. An isocost line shows how many units of each input the firm can purchase, given their prices and the total amount of money the firm can spend on inputs. It is analogous to the consumer's budget constraint in several ways: (a) Its point of intersection with each axis shows how many units of that single input can be purchased with the available resources; (b) it is linear (we assume that the market for inputs is competitive and a firm can buy as many as it wishes without affecting the market price); (c) parallel lines that are upward and to the right indicate that the firm has more money to spend on inputs; and (d) the slope of the line is significant.

It can be derived as follows:

$$TC_I = (P_E \times Q_E) + (P_{NP} \times Q_{NP}) \qquad (2.12)$$

And solving for Q_P by rearranging the terms,

$$Q_P = TC_I / P_{NP} - [(P_E / P_{NP}) \times Q_E)] \qquad (2.13)$$

where TC_I is the total costs of inputs, Q_E is the quantity of examining rooms used, Q_{NP} is the quantity of nurse practitioners used, and P_E and P_{NP} are the unit prices of examining rooms and nurse practitioners, respectively. The first term of Equation 2.13 (TC_I / P_{NP}) shows the intercept on the vertical axis, and the second term, $-P_E / P_{NP}$, is the slope. The isocost line intersects the horizontal axis at the point TC_I / P_M.

The Producer "Optimum"

As in the case of consumer theory, the firm achieves its goal—here, profit maximization—at point A in Figure 2.11, where the isocost line and isoquant are tangent. At point B, where the lines are not tangent, the production process is economically inefficient: too many examining rooms and too few nurse practitioners are being employed, given the market prices for each of these inputs. Although B is on an isoquant, that isoquant is associated with the production of fewer visits, as indicated by the dashed line.

FIGURE 2.10: Isocost Line

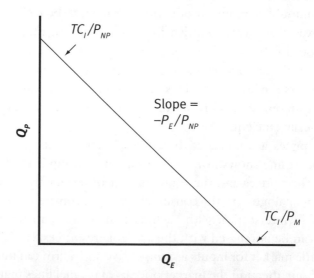

FIGURE 2.11: The Producer Optimum

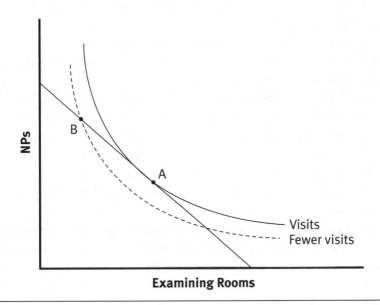

We saw earlier that the slope of the isocost line is the price ratio between examining rooms and nurse practitioners, P_E/P_{NP}. The slope of the isoquant (at a given point) is the ratio of the marginal products of the two inputs. Putting these together, Figure 2.11 indicates that a firm will maximize profits when

$$MP_E/MP_{NP} = P_E/P_{NP} \qquad (2.14)$$

To see why a firm must fulfill Equation 2.14 to maximize profits, imagine that the equality is not met. The marginal productivity of each input equals one, but the price of E is $10 and the price of NP is $5. In such a situation, the firm will benefit from hiring more nurse practitioners and using fewer examination rooms. Eventually, nurse practitioners will become less productive due to diminishing marginal productivity. Only when both sides of Equation 2.14 are equal will the firm have no economic reason to change the ratio of inputs it uses. And since all firms face the same input prices, they will all have the same ratio of marginal productivities if they maximize their profits.

Costs of Production in the Short Run

The economic theory of production costs falls neatly out of the theory of production. Recall our assumption that marginal productivity eventually diminishes in the short run, such that increasing the use of one input while capital stock is fixed will increase output, but at a decreasing rate. It follows, then, that the cost of producing each additional unit of output will rise in the short run.

Costs have two components, *fixed costs* and *variable costs*, and their sum is *total costs*. Fixed costs are costs that are invariant with the amount of a good or service produced. One might view the construction of a new hospital wing as a fixed cost. Variable costs, in contrast, rise as more output is produced. Nurse practitioners would be an example.

Figure 2.12 shows the relationship between fixed (FC), variable (VC), and total (TC) costs of production in the short run. Because fixed costs are constant as output increases, they appear as a horizontal line. Variable costs (and therefore total costs) rise with output. At the beginning, when the input is underused, they rise at a decreasing rate, but eventually they rise at an increasing rate. This is consistent with the notion of diminishing marginal productivity.

We will consider two more types of curves, representing *average costs* and *marginal costs*. Average costs (AC) are simply total costs divided by the number of units of output produced. Average fixed costs (AFC) will always fall as output increases since fixed costs are constant. Average variable costs (AVC) and average total costs (ATC) fall initially, when more use of the input is more economically efficient, but eventually they begin to rise as diminishing marginal productivity sets in.

The other curve in Figure 2.13, *marginal costs* (MC), is key in microeconomic theory. Marginal costs are the change in total costs when one more

FIGURE 2.12: Total, Variable, and Fixed Costs

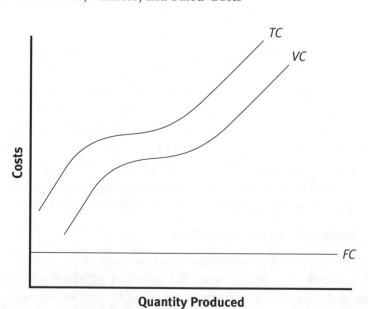

FIGURE 2.13: Average and Marginal Costs in the Short Run

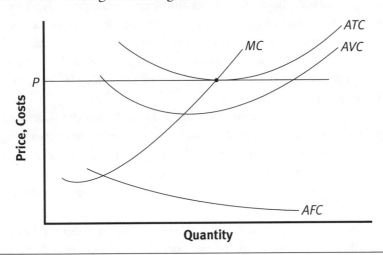

unit of output is produced. Note that marginal costs intersect the minimum points of the average variable costs and average total cost curves. If marginal costs are lower than the average, that last unit produced will pull the average down. If marginal costs are higher than the average, the additional unit produced will pull the average up. But when the marginal and average costs are equal, the last unit produced will not change the average, and average costs will be flat at that point.

A number of factors affect the position of the cost curves. If inputs are more expensive, cost curves will shift upward, reflecting higher total and marginal costs at any given level of output. If a cost-saving technology is developed, the curves will be lower, since it will cost less to produce a given output. Finally, if the quality of output increases, costs will also be affected. In general, it costs more to produce higher quality.

Long-Run Costs and Economies of Scale

Although we will not touch on it again in this chapter, an understanding of the concept of long-run costs is important. Recall that the long run is the period over which a firm can vary all of its inputs. The curve shown in Figure 2.14 represents *long-run average costs* (*LRAC*), the average costs of producing any given level of output over the long run. *Economies of scale* are situations in which output rises at a greater rate than does the increase in the cost of inputs. For example, a firm increases its use of all inputs by 10 percent, and this results in a 15 percent increase in output. The opposite situation would represent a *diseconomy of scale*: in this example, output rising by, say, 5 percent. Situations in which the costs of inputs and outputs rise by the same amount are called *constant returns to scale*. All points to the left of Q^* show areas where a firm experiences economies of scale, and to the right, diseconomies.

Firms can experience economies of scale for several reasons, including specializing, purchasing inputs in greater numbers, and using advertising or labor more efficiently. But why would a firm eventually reach a diseconomy of scale, given that in the long run, more capital can always be purchased? The major cause is managerial issues. Eventually, a firm gets too big and unwieldy to function optimally. A 3,000-bed hospital would probably be far more difficult to manage than one half its size.

The relationship, illustrated in Figure 2.15, between the short-run average cost curve shown in Figure 2.13 and long-run average costs in Figure 2.14 is more complicated. Recall that by definition, in the short run the firm is constrained by a fixed stock of capital. As a result, its costs can never be lower than the firm would face in the long run, when it can vary the use of all inputs.

The long-run average cost curve, shown again in Figure 2.15, is the envelope of all possible short-run average cost curves. In theory, there is one short-run average cost curve that corresponds to the cheapest way to produce a given level of output, given a particular level of capital. $SRAC_1$ shows these costs at a low level of capital, $SRAC_2$ at a middle level, and $SRAC_3$ at a high level. In this case, a firm would be foolish to continue at the low-capital level, since the cheapest average cost at which it could produce is AC_1. At this point, it has so little capital that it cannot take advantage of potential economies of scale. Imagine a hospital with ten beds; it probably could not produce care as cheaply, on average, as a bigger hospital. The opposite is true at the highest level of capital; the facility is just too big. Imagine a hospital with 3,000 beds but only 1,000 patients. At this point, with an average cost of AC_3, it is experiencing diseconomies of scale. Average costs are minimized at AC_2, when the hospital is at the middle size.

FIGURE 2.14: Long-Run Average Costs

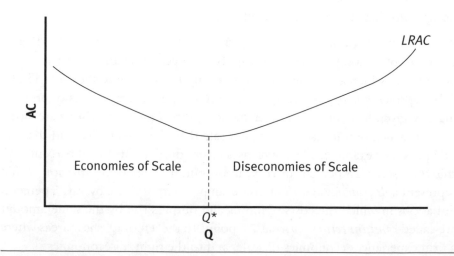

FIGURE 2.15: Relationship Between Short-Run and Long-Run
Average Costs

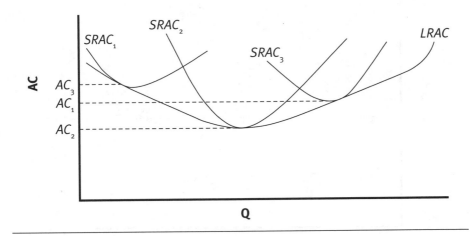

The concept of long-run average costs is more complicated, because one considers it in the planning stages of a production process. A firm has to decide what size capital outlay to make. Once it makes this outlay, it is "stuck" in the short run. If it planned poorly, costs will be higher than necessary until the firm can change its capital stock again. In Figure 2.15, the firm that chose the middle plant size guessed right, because at this point its long-run costs are as low as possible. The firm on the left side of the figure has high costs because its plant is too small to efficiently produce the output demanded. In contrast, the firm that chose the plant that was too big, on the right side of the figure, has high costs because of managerial inefficiencies.

How a Competitive Firm Chooses a Profit-Maximizing Level of Output

We return now to the short run. After choosing the most economically ef-ficient mix of inputs, firms must decide how much to produce and the price for which they will sell their output. In a competitive market, in which the products of alternative firms are indistinguishable, there really is no choice regarding price: A firm will lose all of its market if it charges more than the going price, and it will not maximize profits if it charges less. (We discuss how this market price is determined in Section 2.3.)

A competitive (as opposed to monopolistic) firm chooses the quantity to produce by equating the marginal cost (MC) of production—the cost of producing the last good—to the market price of the good. If it produces less, it is not maximizing profits, because it would make more money by producing more units. If it produces more, it loses money on the last units produced. Point A in Figure 2.16 shows the optimal production amount,

FIGURE 2.16: How Competitive Firms Choose Output Levels

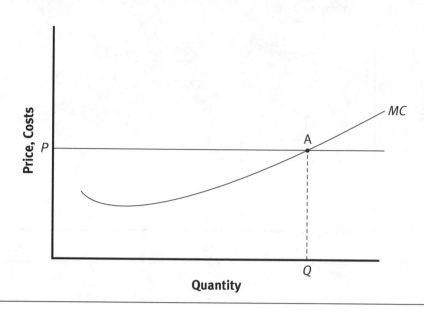

with a corresponding quantity *Q* produced at price *P*. The firm faces a fixed, or horizontal, market price for selling the good, but the marginal cost curve slopes upward, reflecting the likelihood that it will cost more and more to produce successive units of output.

Derivation of the Supply Curve

The *supply curve* shows how much a profit-maximizing firm will produce at different prices. In general, we expect it to slope upward, indicating that firms will produce more if they can receive more from selling their product.

An individual firm's short-run supply curve is its marginal cost curve at all points above average variable costs (*AVC*), as shown in Figure 2.17. All points above and to the right of point B on this curve show how much a profit-maximizing firm would be willing to produce at different price levels. We can clarify this by drawing several horizontal lines that intersect MC, indicating alternative market prices. Each of the intersections represents a profit-maximizing level of output. *Aggregate supply*—the total quantity supplied in a market—is simply the sum of each firm's individual supply.

Imagine a market price that is below and to the left of *AVC*, on the broken portion of the curve. A firm would never produce there because the costs of its labor and supply inputs would exceed the price—it would lose money. A firm *would* be willing to produce at all points above the average total cost curve (*ATC*)—above and to the right of point A—because with prices that high, it would make a profit on each item it produced. As a result, the section of the *MC* curve above *ATC* is the firm's supply curve.

FIGURE 2.17: Derivation of a Firm's Supply Curve

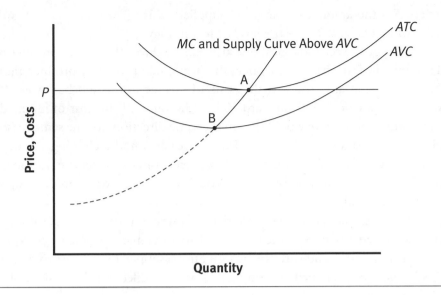

Why would a firm be willing to produce at points on the *MC* curve that are *between AVC* and *ATC* (between points A and B)? The firm would not lose money—the price is high enough to cover labor and supplies, the main components of *AVC*. Thus, the firm would be willing to stay in business, at least in the short run, because proceeds cover expenses. In the long run, however, the price is not sufficient to pay off the firm's fixed costs.

To fully explain these concepts, we must define *economic costs* and *economic profits*. One normally thinks of costs as those expenses associated with production, but in economics, the standard definition includes *opportunity costs* as well. Opportunity costs are usually defined as the value of the next best opportunity. Thus, the value of investing one's resources in something else that would provide a return—for example, the interest rate associated with investments—would be a component of costs. As a result, we include this forgone opportunity as a cost of doing business. Thus, economic costs exceed what an accountant might define as the cost of doing business.

In a competitive market, a firm's profits are *zero*. Certainly, firms wish to make a higher profit, but if profits are to be made, other firms will enter the market, which will lower price and bring profits back to zero. So how can a firm survive on zero economic profits? It goes back to the definition: A zero profit to an economist is a positive profit to an accountant, because economists consider a normal rate of return part of costs. If the normal rate of return is 5 percent per year, then accounting profits of 5 percent would be equivalent to zero economic profits.

The prices of input and technology can cause a supply curve to shift.[8] We can therefore write the firm's supply schedule as:

$$S = f\ (P, P_i, \textit{Tech})\qquad\qquad(2.15)$$

where S is the amount of the good supplied, P is its market price, P_i is the price of inputs, and *Tech* is the level of technology.

Suppose a technological breakthrough reduces the cost of production. This would mean that, at any price, the firm could profitably produce more. Alternatively, at any quantity, the costs of production would be lower. The supply curve would shift outward and to the right. If the cost of inputs declines, the supply curve would shift in the same direction, for the same reason. However, most analysts in the health services area find technology to be, in general, cost increasing rather than cost decreasing (Newhouse 1993b). If this is true, these technologies are probably designed to improve people's health status and/or comfort, not to reduce costs.

Just as there are demand elasticities, there is a *price elasticity of supply*. It is calculated exactly as is the price elasticity of demand, replacing the quantity consumers demand with the quantity firms supply. In contrast to demand elasticites, supply elasticities tend to be positive, reflecting the positive slope of the supply curve.

In summary, production theory predicts that firms will seek to use their inputs as efficiently as possible and make their output choices in a way that maximizes their profits. Doing so also serves social purposes in that firms are (1) not wasting inputs and (2) only producing those goods and services that consumers demand. The next section describes the interaction of the many consumers and products that make up the economy as a whole.

2.3 Equilibrium in a Competitive Market

Short-Run Equilibrium

The combination of demand and supply determines the price and output levels in a market, but we must also consider aggregate demand and supply—that is, all consumers and firms combined for a particular good or service.

In Figure 2.18, the price, P_{NP}, and quantity, Q_{NP}, for a particular market (here, nurse practitioner services) are in equilibrium, shown as point A, where the demand and supply curves intersect. If the price were lower, say P_2, the quantity demanded at point B would be greater than the quantity supplied at point C. This is defined as a *shortage*. In contrast, if the price were higher than the equilibrium level, at P_3, then supply at point D would exceed demand at point E, a situation defined as a *surplus*. Only at the equilibrium price P_{NP} is there no shortage or surplus.

In the short run, a variety of factors can disturb this equilibrium. One example is an increase in demand, shown in Figure 2.19, caused perhaps by an increase in income. If we assume nurse practitioner services are a normal good (that is, more is demanded when income is higher), this would cause

FIGURE 2.18: Short-Run Equilibrium in a Competitive Market

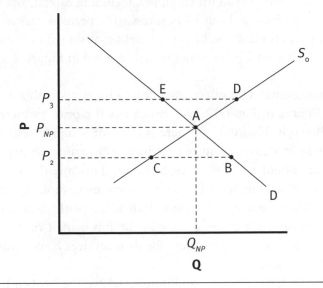

an upward shift to the right in the demand curve, as shown by the broken demand curve, D_2. The new equilibrium would be at point B, which corresponds to both a higher price and a higher quantity, where the new (broken) demand curve intersects the old (solid) supply curve. Supply can also shift in the short run. For example, this would occur if the cost of an important input rose.

FIGURE 2.19: Shifts in Demand and Supply in the Short Run

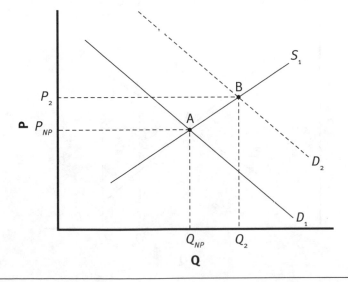

Long-Run Equilibrium

In the long run, firms can adjust all inputs, including capital. Because of this, new firms can go into and out of business. It is perhaps easiest to think of three sequential periods. Period 1 is the baseline, as shown by the equilibrium in Figure 2.18. Period 2 is the short run, illustrated in Figure 2.19. Period 3 is the long run.

Suppose demand for nurse practitioners increases as shown by the broken demand curve in Figure 2.19. This causes the price to increase. In the long run, shown in Figure 2.20, there is time for a supply response. In this case, we would expect more nurse practitioners to enter the market because the profession would become more lucrative. This might seem farfetched, since it takes a long time to train more of these professionals, but it is actually feasible. There may also be many individuals with such training who, for whatever reason, are currently not in the job market or are working in another profession. The higher prices for their services could stimulate them to reenter the market.

In Figure 2.20, the new equilibrium, where the broken demand and supply curves intersect, point C, is at the original price, but at a much higher quantity than before, Q_3. The logic is straightforward. The original price in Figure 2.18 was disturbed by an increase in demand, shown in Figure 2.19. Because the quantity demanded exceeded the amount supplied, the price rose to P_2. But this increase in price stimulated an increase in supply, as shown in Figure 2.20. Because nurse practitioners were less scarce, firms were able to pay a lower price. In reality, the price in Figure 2.20 might be a little higher or

FIGURE 2.20: Shifts in Demand and Supply in the Long Run

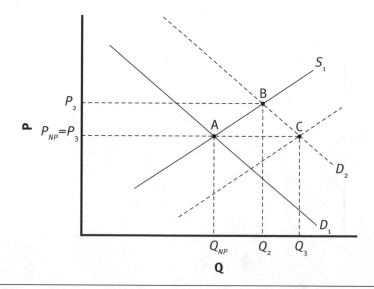

lower than that in Figure 2.18. This would depend largely on whether there were increasing or decreasing economies of scale in the production of nurse practitioner services.

2.4 Equilibrium for a Monopolist

Strictly speaking, a *monopoly* exists when one firm supplies all of the goods or services in a market. (A *monopsony*, in contrast, occurs when there is a single purchaser rather than producer.) There are milder firms of monopoly as well: a *duopoly* exists when there are two firms supplying an entire market, and an *oligopoly* when there are just a few. We will focus on monopoly.

Sometimes we speak of a firm having "monopoly power." This does not mean there is only one firm in the market. Rather, it means the firm has some ability to raise its price without losing its entire market. That may seem odd, if you recall that a competitive firm faces a horizontal demand curve for its product—if it charged more, it would no longer have any customers. Graphically, monopoly power means the demand curve a firm faces has a somewhat downward slope.[9] Most firms do have some monopoly power, and retaining this power is one of the main purposes of advertising. Take Cheerios, for example. There are many substitutes, but if the price of Cheerios goes up, some people will still buy them, albeit fewer than before. This concept will come into play again in Chapter 8, when we discuss the market for physician services.

Monopolists Charging a Single Price

There are two classes of monopolists: those that charge everyone the same price, and those that can charge different prices to different customers. It is difficult to find an example of the former in the health sector, as most monopolists—for example, prescription drug companies—are able to charge different prices to different customers, as they often make (secret) deals with health insurance and managed care companies. Nevertheless, the logic is important to understand.

Consider the concept of *marginal revenue*, which is the amount of money brought in by the sale of the last unit of a good. In a competitive market, a marginal revenue curve (with quantity on the horizontal axis and marginal revenue on the vertical axis) is flat, and is equal to the price. (This, in turn, is equal to the demand curve facing the firm.) No matter how many units a particular firm sells, it receives the same market price or marginal revenue for each one. This is because each firm is assumed to be such a small part of the market that its sales have no effect on overall market price. An example might be a soybean farmer.

This is not the case for a monopolist, however. Since a monopolist *is* the entire market, the demand curve it faces is not horizontal, but downward sloping. If it charges more, demand will decrease.

Recall that demand represents how much people will pay for a product at a particular price. In a competitive market, price, demand, and marginal revenue are all equal. If the market price of a good is $20, that is the demand the firm faces, or how much buyers are willing to pay. If the firm sells an extra unit, it receives an extra $20 in marginal revenue. This is not the case with a monopolist. True, if it sells another unit of a good, it receives more money. However, as we are considering a monopolist that charges a single price, it must lower the price for all units sold to sell an extra unit. As a result, marginal revenue is lower than demand because the extra money it receives from the last unit is reduced by the lower price on all previously sold units.

As a result, the marginal revenue curve will always be lower than the demand curve, as illustrated in Figure 2.21. Consider the marginal revenue for the eleventh unit sold. If 10 units are sold, the monopolist can charge $6 each, but if it wants to sell 11, it can only charge $5. Therefore, the total revenue for 10 units is $60, and for 11 units, $55. The marginal revenue is just $5—well below the demand curve, which is $10. This means that a monopolist's marginal revenue curve must be lower than its demand curve.

Figure 2.22 shows how much a monopolist charges and produces to maximize its profits. The rule of thumb is that it produces where its marginal costs and marginal revenue are equal, at point A, corresponding to a quantity of Q_M. It then chooses the highest price it can charge for this quantity, which is found by locating the point on the demand curve corresponding to this quantity, P_M. What a competitive firm would produce and charge is superimposed on the graph, at Q_C and P_C (the intersection of demand and supply).

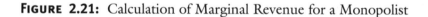

FIGURE 2.21: Calculation of Marginal Revenue for a Monopolist

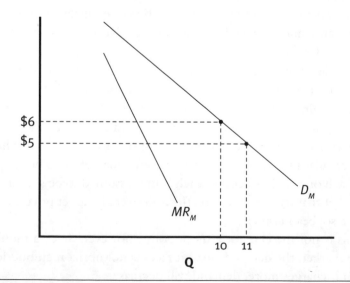

FIGURE 2.22: Equilibrium for a Monopolist Charging a Single Price

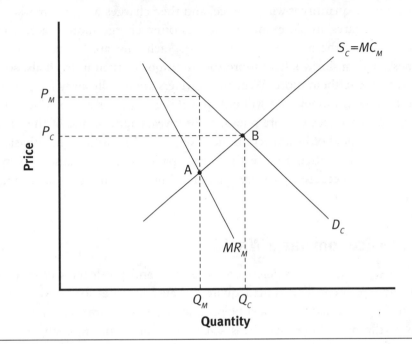

The monopolist charges more and produces less than the competitive firm. This is because to maximize its profits, a monopolist can charge more than a competitive firm. But by charging more, there is insufficient demand to sell as many units as in a competitive market.

A monopolistic market is disadvantageous to society in two respects: Customers pay more, and less is produced for society. As a result, there are *antitrust* laws aimed at preventing the formation and continuation of some monopolies. There are, however, certain situations in which the market will not support more than one firm, necessitating a monopoly. Transportation systems, such as bus, subway, or freeway systems, are possible examples. In such a case, which we refer to as a *natural monopoly*, government may either take over the market or regulate it to ensure that the private-firm monopolist doesn't charge more than is necessary. Traditionally in the United States, utilities such as electricity have been regulated in this way.

Price-Discriminating Monopolist

A price-discriminating monopolist can charge different prices to different customers. Although one can draw a graph illustrating this, it is easier to understand through a description.

By charging different prices to different customers, a monopolist can make even higher profits. It does this by segmenting its market. It charges customers who are more price sensitive—that is, who have a higher price elasticity of demand—less, and those who are less price sensitive more. The monopolist equates marginal revenue and marginal cost in each submarket to determine the quantity it will produce, and then charges what the market will bear. Airline fares are an example. Airlines often charge more if a customer does not spend the night or the weekend. Such trips are typically done for business, and businesses have more spending power than individuals, so airlines can charge them more. Weekend travelers are usually away for pleasure, using their own money, and will not be willing to pay as much. The market for physician services is more relevant. Fifty years ago, in one of the earliest articles in the field of health economics, Kessel (1958) argued that physicians charged wealthy patients more than poor patients, not because they were charitable, but because they were price-discriminating monopolists trying to maximize their profits.

2.5 The Economy as a Whole

Until now, we have considered the consumer and producer sectors of the economy separately. This is inadequate, because in order for goods and services to be consumed, they must be produced, and consumers must purchase them at the price for which firms sell them. Furthermore, changes in the market for a particular good or service may affect other markets. Viewing the consumption or production of a single good or service is called *partial equilibrium analysis*, while considering the economy as a whole is known as *general equilibrium analysis*.

Production Possibilities and Distributional Issues

Figure 2.23 illustrates a *production possibility frontier* (PPF), which shows the amount that can be produced of each of two goods (NP visits and MD visits), given the amount of inputs available to the economy. Producing more MD visits will use scarce inputs that then cannot be used to produce NP visits. Hence, fewer NP visits will be produced. The slope of the PPF (at a given point) is called the *marginal rate of transformation*; it indicates how much of one good or service must be sacrificed to produce an extra unit of the other. The concave-to-the-origin shape indicates that costs increase as we shift production from MD to NP visits or vice versa. (The idea is that it may be costly for society to continue producing more and more of one good or service. In some cases, there may not be major additional costs, and the curve will be less convex, or straighter.) We will assume that our competitive market produces at point A on the PPF, that is, ten NP visits and eight MD visits.

Figure 2.24 uses the same information to produce an *Edgeworth Box*, named for economist Francis Edgeworth. It shows how the output at point A can be divided between two consumers, Paul and Jane. Paul's allotment of both types of visits is shown in the normal fashion: At point A, he has about six (of the ten) NP visits and five (of the eight) MD visits. Jane's allotment,

FIGURE 2.23: Production Possibility Frontier

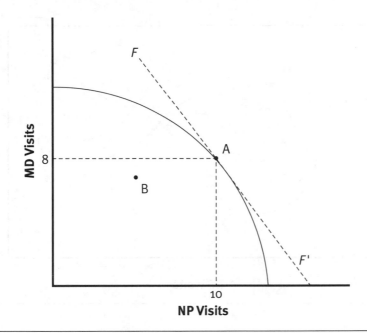

on the other hand, is oriented in the opposite direction (downward for MD visits and from right to left for NP visits). Or more colloquially, imagine she is standing on her head. Either way, she gets the remaining four NP visits and three MD visits.

The figure also includes various sets of indifference curves for each of the two consumers. We saw earlier that equilibrium can occur only when consumers have the same marginal rate of substitution. This occurs where their indifference curves are tangent, along the *contract curve*, which starts at the origin (*O*) and goes up and through point A.

General equilibrium analysis shows that for production and exchange to be efficient, consumers' marginal rates of substitution must be equal to the economy's marginal rate of transformation. That is, the slope of the consumers' indifference curves at equilibrium, indicated by the line $I-I'$, must be equal to the slope of the PPF at point A, indicated by the line $F-F'$ in Figure 2.23.

Why must this be the case? Suppose the marginal rate of substitution between NP and MD visits is one, but the marginal rate of transformation is two. If Jane reduces her consumption of MD visits by one, she needs to get one more NP visit to be indifferent. But by producing one less MD visit, the economy would be able to produce two more NP visits. That leaves an extra NP visit available that could be given to Paul or to Jane. Thus, if the marginal rates of substitution and transformation are not equal, the economy is not

FIGURE 2.24: Edgeworth Box

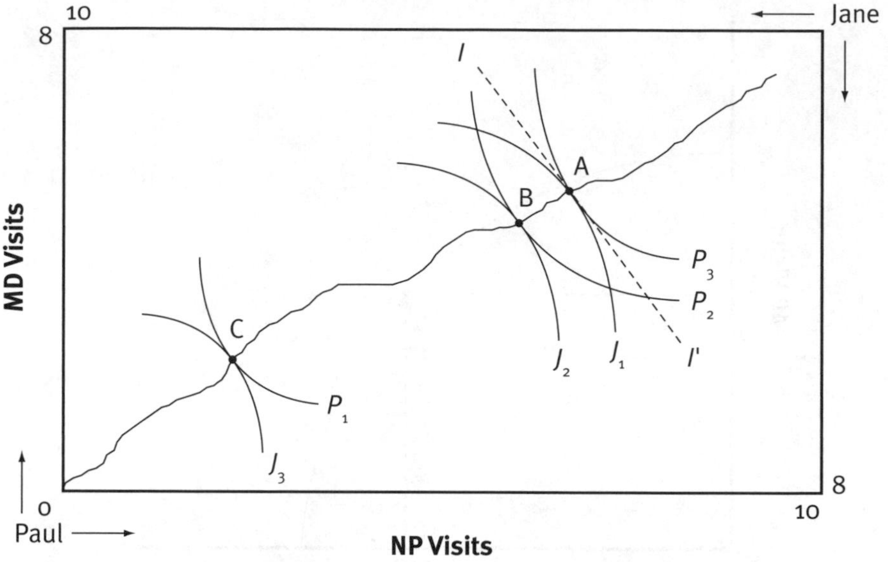

in equilibrium, because it is possible to make one person better off without making another worse off.

It is important to consider the bigger picture here. All points on the contract curve are considered equally efficient, but some might be viewed as inequitable. At points on the contract curve near the top right of Figure 2.24, Paul has almost everything and Jane, nothing. Near the origin the opposite is true.

Although many economists have given considerable thought to the issues of equity and the redistribution of wealth, these issues play only a small part in the traditional microeconomic model. Rather than concerning itself with how people come into possession of their initial stock of wealth, the traditional model devotes nearly all its attention to how they allocate the resources they already have (Young 1994).

Pareto Optimality, Equity, and Social Welfare

When the consumption and production markets are in equilibrium, and when consumers' rates of indifference are equal to the economy's ability to transform one good into the others, the economy is in a position called *Pareto optimality*, named after economist Vilfredo Pareto. In a Pareto-optimal state, it is impossible to make someone better off (that is, increase that person's welfare) without making someone else worse off. Under such a situation, the economy has reached a state of *allocative efficiency*, although this rests on a number of assumptions, as we will show in the next chapter.

How does an economy reach Pareto optimality? Economists have shown that if certain conditions are met, a free or competitive market operating on its own will reach a *competitive equilibrium* that is Pareto optimal.

The concept of Pareto optimality, although useful from a theoretical standpoint, is rather weak from a policy standpoint. It provides little guidance. This is because of the difficulty of imagining even a single public policy that would make some people better off without making other people worse off. Suppose, for example, that the government chooses to subsidize immunizations against chicken pox. Although seemingly benign, such a policy would make worse off a taxpayer with no children who has already had the disease; there would be costs to this person but no benefits.[10]

If there are winners and losers associated with all policies, then deciding which policies to enact involves a value judgment—who should benefit and who should lose. Making such a determination is beyond the realm of economic analysis.

Consequently, over the years, economists have tried to develop tools to make it easier to make policy recommendations that are not value laden. None have been particularly well accepted. Indeed, market competition in general, and Pareto optimality in particular, fails to address issues of equity or the desirability of the distribution of income that results from the workings of a competitive economy. Thus, a competitive equilibrium can occur in which one person has nearly all of the output and another has almost none. In fact, this can easily occur if the first person begins with the vast majority of initial wealth or inputs. Amartya Sen (1970) makes this point graphically:

> An economy can be [Pareto] optimal . . . even when some people are rolling in luxury and others are near starvation as long as the starvers cannot be made better off without cutting into the pleasures of the rich. If preventing the burning of Rome would have made Emperor Nero feel worse off, then letting him burn Rome would have been Pareto-optimal. In short, a society or an economy can be Pareto-optimal and still be perfectly disgusting.

Although it might seem desirable to transfer wealth from the rich person to the poor person, doing so cannot be viewed as improving the economy from a Pareto optimality viewpoint because the change will make the rich person worse off. Under the traditional economic model, competition is designed to enhance efficiency; it does not necessarily improve equity.

This point is critical because members of society do care about equity. Many countries share a social ethic prescribing healthcare to everyone who needs it, even if they do not have the resources. This means that a Pareto-optimal competitive equilibrium does not necessarily make society best off. In fact, a society may be better off with an inefficient use of resources (that is, at point B inside the PPF in Figure 2.23) and a more equitable distribution of income than it would be with an unequal income distribution (at point A).

Thus, it is natural to ask whether some Pareto-optimal points (i.e., points on the contract curve 0—A in Figure 2.24) are socially more desirable than others. In finding the answer, value judgments about how each person's utility affects society's total welfare are inevitable. This is often illustrated by a *social welfare function*, shown in Equation 2.16,

$$W = W(U_1, U_2, \ldots, U_n) \tag{2.16}$$

where W is society's total welfare, U indicates individual utility levels, and the subscripts represent each person in the population.

Determining society's social welfare function is no easy task. It could be imposed by a dictator, of course, but if one prefers more democratic means, a problem arises. The problem, which is proved in Kenneth Arrow's (1963a) *possibility theorem*, is that any method of aggregating individual preferences into a social welfare function violates at least one reasonable and desirable ethical condition. Thus, it is hard to reach a desirable consensus on how to confront distributional issues, a topic to which we will return in Chapter 9.

Notes

1. There are many good introductory microeconomic textbooks; Parkin (2007) is one example.
2. This can be demonstrated as follows. Along an indifference curve, the consumer's level of utility is constant. Thus, any movement along the curve represents a change only in how the consumer achieves a given level of utility. If he or she has more of Y and less of X, the gain in utility from the former must equal the loss in utility from the latter. Specifically,

$$(\Delta Y) \times (MU_Y) = (\Delta X) \times (MU_X),$$

where Y is the quantity of the good consumed on the vertical axis, X is the quantity of the good on the horizontal axis, MU is the marginal utility of each of the goods that is subscripted, and Δ represents the change in a term.

   Rearranging these terms, we find that the slope of the indifference curve $(\Delta Y/\Delta X)$ at a particular point equals the ratio of the marginal utilities of goods X and Y at that point.
3. To see this, suppose a person has $1,000 in income, and the price of physician visits is $100 and the price of nurse practitioner visits is $50. Thus, this income could buy 10 of the former or 20 of the latter, implying that the budget constraint would intersect the vertical axis at 10 and the horizontal axis at 20. Clearly, then, the slope of the budget constraint would be 1/2—which is the ratio of the price of nurse practitioner visits ($50) to the price of physician visits ($100).
4. With most inferior goods, a price reduction will still result in an increase in

quantity demanded—the demand curve will still slope downward. There is one situation—perhaps a hypothetical one—where inferior goods actually have upward-sloping demand curves. These are known as Giffen Goods, and the phenomenon is called Giffen's Paradox (named after a British economist). Suppose a country is very poor and its citizens rely on one particular crop for their sustenance. For example, imagine that in nineteenth-century Ireland, before the potato famine, the price of potatoes fell due to particularly good weather conditions that led to a bounteous crop. Normally we would expect the quantity demanded to rise, and indeed, there will be an increase in demand due to the substitution effect as potatoes are now cheaper relative to other goods. But this could be overcome by a very large negative income effect. As people's incomes rise, they can afford to purchase other foodstuff—fish, for instance—and they would not need so many potatoes in their diet. So overall quantity demanded might fall as the price of potatoes fell.

All Giffen Goods are inferior goods, but only some (if any) inferior goods are Giffen goods. Whether Giffen goods truly exist is not important. The concept still provides a deeper understanding of income and substitution effects.

5. This is a generic formula for calculating the price elasticity of demand (E_d); Q is quantity demand, P is price, and Δ represents the change in a term:

$$E_d = \%\Delta Q / \%\Delta P$$
$$= (\Delta Q / Q) / (\Delta P / P),$$

and re-arranging the terms,

$$= (\Delta Q / \Delta P) \times (P/Q)$$

Notice that the first term of the last equation is the slope of the demand curve, which shows that although the elasticity is related to the slope, it is not equal to it. Moreover, the elasticity will be different at every point on a linear demand curve since the ratio of P to Q varies as one moves along the curve. In fact, the elasticity declines as one moves downward and to the right.

It is often convenient to calculate a single estimate of the elasticity, and this is typically done at the midpoint of a particular range of prices and quantities (sometimes called the *arc elasticity*). Suppose that price rises from P_1 to P_2, with a corresponding reduction in quantity from Q_1 to Q_2. We might like to obtain the same estimate of the value of the elasticity, whether price has risen or fallen. To do that, we can calculate the price elasticity at the midpoint, as follows:

$$E_d = \%\Delta Q / \%\Delta P$$
$$= (\Delta Q / \Delta P) \times (P/Q)$$
$$= (\Delta Q / \Delta P) \times \{[(P_1 + P_2)/2] / [(Q_1 + Q_2)/2]\},$$

and multiplying each side by 2,

$$= (\Delta Q / \Delta P) \times \{[(P_1 + P_2) / (Q_1 + Q_2)]\}$$

6. Here is a generic formula for calculating the cross price elasticity of demand ($E_{X,Y}$) between the quantity demand of good Y and the price of good X:

$$E_{X,Y} = \%\Delta Q_Y / \%\Delta P_X$$
$$= (\Delta Q_Y / Q_Y) / (\Delta P_X / P_X),$$

and rearranging the terms,

$$= (\Delta Q_Y / \Delta P_X) \times (P_X / Q_Y)$$

We can calculate this at the midpoint of prices and quantities in time periods 1 and 2 as follows:

$$= (\Delta Q_Y / \Delta P_X) \times [(P_{X1} + P_{X2}) / (Q_{Y1} + Q_{Y2}]$$

7. This can be demonstrated as follows. Along an isoquant, the output level is constant. Thus, any movement along the curve represents a change only in the way in which the inputs are combined to achieve a given level of output. If a firm uses more of input a and less of input b in producing MD visits, the total number of visits produced cannot change along the isoquant. Specifically,

$$(\Delta a) \times (MP_a) = (\Delta b) \times (MP_b),$$

where MP is the marginal product (i.e., the amount produced) from the last unit of that input. Rearranging these terms, we find that the slope of the isoquant curve ($\Delta b / \Delta a$) at a particular point equals the ratio of the marginal products of the two inputs at that particular point.

8. Other factors sometimes listed as shifting supply curves include expectations about future market price levels and taxes.

9. One of the more confusing concepts in microeconomics is that the demand curve facing an individual firm is horizontal, while the demand curve for the entire market is downward sloping. How can that be? Each firm is assumed to be an infinitesimally small part of the overall market. Thus, each may have a demand curve that is every-so-slightly downward sloping. The sum of these—the total market—therefore can have a more pronounced downward slope.

10. Of course, if this person were altruistic, he or she might find the policy to be desirable. This issue is taken up in Chapter 5, when we consider positive externalities of consumption.

ASSUMPTIONS UNDERLYING THE COMPETITIVE MODEL AND THE ROLE OF GOVERNMENT

As the title suggests, the purpose of this book is to reconsider the economics of health. It does so by examining the assumptions on which the superiority of competitive approaches is based, and how a failure to meet these assumptions affects health policy choices.

As we saw in Chapter 2, standard microeconomic theory suggests that if certain assumptions are met, allowing markets to function without government interference will result in *allocative efficiency*. This means a society's resources are used in the most productive way: Consumers' demands are being satisfied through the most frugal use of resources.

But markets *do* fail, and government can sometimes ameliorate such failure. However, market failure is not the only justification for government intervention. Economists have posited three situations in which government intervention is in society's best interest (Musgrave and Musgrave 1989):

- When markets fail (the focus here and in most of the remainder of the book)
- When markets produce a distribution of resources that society finds unacceptable (the focus of Chapter 9)
- When the economy is unstable (not covered here, but covered in macroeconomics courses)

3.1 The Assumptions of the Competitive Model

The conclusion that reliance on markets is necessarily desirable is based on certain assumptions. No generally accepted list of such assumptions exists, although various economists have come up with different versions. The list presented in Table 3.1 was drawn largely from Graaff (1971), Henderson and Quandt (1980), Mishan (1969a, 1969b), Nath (1969), Ng (1979), Rowley and Peacock (1975), and Sen (1982).

The book thus centers on description, analysis, and application of these assumptions—in particular, what happens if they are not met in healthcare markets. Table 3.1 lists the specific assumptions examined, along with the chapters in which each is analyzed.[1]

TABLE 3.1: Assumptions of Market Competition and Their Further Treatment in the Remaining Chapters

Chapter 4: Demand for Health, Insurance, and Services
1. A person is the best judge of his or her own welfare.
2. Consumers have sufficient information to make good choices.
3. Consumers can accurately predict the results of their consumption decisions.
4. Individuals are rational.
5. Social welfare is solely the sum of individual utilities.

Chapter 5: Special Topics in Demand: Externalities of Consumption and the Formation of Preferences
6. There are no negative externalities of consumption.
7. There are no positive externalities of consumption.
8. Consumer tastes are predetermined.

Chapter 6: How Competitive Is the Supply of Healthcare?
9. Supply and demand are independently determined.
10. Firms do not have any monopoly power.
11. There are not increasing returns to scale.

Chapter 7: The Profit Motive in Healthcare
12. Firms maximize profits.
13. Profit maximization results in the most efficient production and the highest consumer welfare.

Chapter 9: Equity and Redistribution
14. The distribution of wealth is approved by society.

This is only a partial list of the assumptions on which the superiority of the competitive model is based. We have left out other assumptions either because they are essentially the same as those noted above, or because, in the authors' opinion, the health economics profession has dealt with them adequately.[2]

Why are assumptions so important? Why not just look at the data to see whether competition or government works better? A subfield of economics called *welfare economics* can answer these questions.

Welfare economics is concerned with how a society can best organize itself to improve the well-being or welfare of its citizenry. It asks questions like, "Should we rely on competitive policies in the health services sector?" Again, why can't we just look at the evidence? The reason is twofold: (1) Sometimes there is no direct evidence because history provides no good examples, and (2) given the same data, different analysts often reach very different conclusions.

If the United States were to adopt a Canadian-style "single-payer" system, health economists would likely disagree about whether the population was better off under the new system or the old one. As the cynical yet apt adage goes, "where you stand depends on where you sit."

Jan de V. Graaff (1971, 2–3, italics added) has written,

> [W]elfare . . . is not an observable quantity like a market price or an item of personal consumption [so] it is exceedingly difficult to test a welfare proposition. . . . The consequence is that, whereas the normal way of testing a theory in positive economics is to test its conclusions, *the normal way of testing a welfare proposition is to test its assumptions*. . . . The result is that our assumptions must be scrutinized with care and thoroughness. Each must stand on its own two feet. We cannot afford to simplify much.

We must get our theory right when applying economics to health, and the key to this is understanding the validity of the assumptions. If we do not, then we blind ourselves to policy options that might enhance social welfare, many of which simply cannot be derived from the conventional economic model.

3.2 Can Government Fail Too?

Markets are problematic in healthcare, with respect not only to providing services equitably, but also to providing them efficiently. This raises the key policy question: Would government do any better? Economist Henry Sidgwick (1887) once stated, "It does not follow that whenever laissez-faire falls short government interference is expedient; since the inevitable drawbacks of the latter may, in any particular case, be worse than the shortcomings of private enterprise."[3] More than 100 years later, Mark Pauly (1997, 470) expressed a similar view, noting that "a government staffed by angels could undoubtedly do a better job than markets run by humans."

Indeed, just as markets may fail, so might government. The field of economics has devoted considerable effort to studying market failure, but less on developing a comparable theory of government failure. This is not terribly surprising. For such analyses to be tractable, simplifying assumptions are necessary. Economists have successfully analyzed consumers by assuming they focus on maximizing utility, and firms by assuming they seek to maximize profits. But a convincing theory of government behavior can hardly be captured by employing a few simplifying assumptions.

Charles Wolf (1979, 1993) conducted some of the pioneering work in the area of government failure. Wolf contended that just as a market may fail, government intervention may fail for similar (though not precisely the same) reasons. Government, according to Wolf, faces a number of challenges, including the difficulty of defining and measuring outputs (e.g., the *quality* of education), the fact that it is monopolistic by nature and doesn't have to adhere to a "bottom line" of profits or losses, and politicians' preference for quick fixes rather than long-term solutions. As a result, government can operate inefficiently and in some cases inequitably, since it is often beholden to special interests.[4]

Some of these criticisms apply to markets. When markets carry out activities that are traditionally government responsibilities (e.g., primary education), they have comparable difficulty defining outcomes. And just as government workers are not subject to profit-and-loss statements, evidence indicates that employees and managers in private industry often serve their own goals rather than those of the shareholders.

Other economists have contributed to one aspect of understanding the potential for government failure, an area called the *economic theory of regulation*. George Stigler (1971) is usually credited as pioneering this field, although it had various antecedents within and outside of the economics literature.[5] Researchers and laypersons alike have taken what Stigler calls a more idealistic view of regulation—that it serves the public interest by improving efficiency (e.g., correcting externalities and controlling the behavior of monopolists) and equity (e.g., redistributing income from the wealthy to the poor) (Feldstein 1996)—or by protecting health or enhancing safety.

Stigler found this *public interest theory* unsatisfactory and proposed instead what is sometimes called *capture theory*—which is quite the opposite of the public interest theory. Rather than serving the public, regulation serves those it is designed to regulate. Viewed this way, regulation is, by its nature, anticompetitive and anticonsumer.

How can regulated industries capture the regulators whose role, purportedly, is to keep them in check? To answer this, Stigler considered the political process. Just as firms attempt to maximize profits and individuals, utility, so politicians attempt to maximize their self-interest. Politicians, he believed, are interested in retaining their power, and for that to occur they need votes and money. Special interest groups can provide this but will do so only if the politician can offer them something in return. That "something" is regulations that, through various means, make members of the group better off. Examples include regulations that prevent or discourage competition, price supports or subsidies, and actions that harm competitors that sell substitute goods.

But why would consumers allow this to happen? Stigler hypothesized that their interests were too disparate; consumers could not possibly be expert enough to keep up with all industries, and even if they could, they would not bother, because cost-increasing regulations for a single product would have little overall effect on their disposable incomes.

We can extend this theory to regulatory agencies. Legislators do not have time to directly oversee all aspects of government, nor do they and their staffs have the necessary expertise. These tasks are delegated to administrative agencies. The employees of these agencies are arguably motivated "by job security and higher salaries [which] . . . are more likely to occur when an agency's budget is expanding" (Feldstein 1996, 30). This, in turn, will happen only if the agency's behavior is in accordance with the legislature's desires.

Over the years various economists have honed the economic theory of regulation. The major contribution was made by Sam Peltzman (1976), who formalized the theory and worked out some of the kinks. Just as the public interest theory ignored the interests of special interest groups, Stigler's theory seemed to put all of the power in the hands of special interests. Under his formulation, this was a single special interest group—the highest bidder for the favors of the regulator.

Peltzman theorized that regulators would not necessarily serve a single special interest group. Rather, they would consider all competing interests, although not equally.[6] By trying to serve a variety of interests, a self-interested politician or regulator would gain more—in a sense, by trying to make everyone happy. But this would not give consumers as much clout as producers. Those groups that are best able to concentrate their resources toward a particular goal tend to be most influential in the regulatory process.

An extensive literature related to the economic theory of regulation, but with a wider scope, is a school of thought called *public choice* or *rational choice* (not to be confused with the *public interest* literature that assumed that regulation benefits society by improving efficiency and the distribution of resources). Public choice theory studies (among other things) how public organizations make decisions (Stanbury 1986). This theory has been characterized "as the economic study of nonmarket decision making, or simply the application of economics to political science" using the assumption "that man is an egoistic, rational, utility maximizer" (Mueller 1989, 1–2). Its proponents have examined such issues as why people vote, the implications of rulemaking by majorities and alternatives to it, the formation of coalitions and political parties, and theories of government and bureaucratic behavior.[7]

The basis of public choice theory is that individuals act in their own interest. Politicians seek election or reelection to retain power, prestige, and sometimes wealth. Government workers seek job security, pleasant working conditions, and higher pay; one way to achieve the latter is to increase the size of their agency or the number of people they supervise. Interest groups form to obtain favors from government. In return, they provide campaign contributions, attempt to sway the public in favor of certain positions or candidates, and perhaps provide useful information about voter preferences.

A number of criticisms have been leveled at public choice theory. On the theoretical side, it is unclear whether public officials act in a solely self-interested manner. For example, the theory predicts that political parties and individual candidates will focus almost entirely on enticing voters by espousing centrist positions, but often this is not the case. Similarly, the theory leaves little room for ideology in politics; rather, it assumes politicians choose the positions most likely to get them elected rather than seeking election so as to implement their vision[8] and that civil servants are similarly driven by factors devoid of ideology. This is not to say the theory is always wrong—it surely describes many actors in the political scene—but it may be unrealistically cynical. In addition, public choice theory has been criticized as being inconsistent with empirical evidence of actual behavior in a number of areas (Green and Shapiro 1994). One area in particular that has received criticism is citizen involvement in public affairs. Public choice theory does a poor job of explaining why people vote in elections (when their chance of influencing an election is almost nil) or vote to raise their own taxes (Mueller 1989).

Despite their shortcomings, these theories have helped raise society's awareness of government's *potential* for self-serving behavior. This alerts the public to areas in which government failure is most likely to be manifested, and consequently, assists the public in averting its manifestations. As noted by Dennis Mueller (1989, 465):

> [F]rom a knowledge of past mistakes we can design institutions that will avoid similar mistakes in the future. Public choice does provide us with this knowledge. Because of this, I remain optimistic . . . even about the possibility that this research may someday help to improve the democratic institutions by which we govern ourselves.

3.3 Market Versus Government: A False Dichotomy

All countries rely on markets and government. Insisting it must be one or the other creates a false dichotomy; rather, societies need to determine *where* each is most appropriate and how best to mix the two. In this regard, one of the leading exponents of the notion of government failure, Charles Wolf (1993, 7), wrote:

> The actual choice is among imperfect markets, imperfect governments, and various combinations of the two. The cardinal economic choice concerns the degree to which markets or governments—each with their respective flaws—should determine the allocation, use, and distribution of resources in the economy.

Indeed, all countries use markets and government, in varying degrees, to determine the allocation of goods and services in healthcare. The choice is not "either/or"; markets and government can and do complement each other. Markets improve on government by helping ensure that consumer demands are met and resources are not squandered. Governments improve on markets by ensuring that poor and sick individuals have access to care and that providers and insurers do not reap unreasonable profits from selecting healthier patients (Morone 2000; Rice et al. 2000). Thus, each country must decide how much government involvement to employ and just where government should intervene in markets. In the following chapters, we argue that the assumptions listed in Table 3.1 have made market solutions seem more effective than they actually are in solving key social problems in healthcare.

Notes

1. The assumptions about externalities will not be self-explanatory to the non-economist reader; see Chapter 5 for clarification.
2. One exception is the Theory of the Second Best. Suppose two or more of the assumptions in Table 3.1 are not met. It might seem reasonable for public policy to focus on trying to improve one of these particular market imperfections. This is not necessarily the case. The Theory of the Second Best states that if multiple factors cause a market to deviate from the assumptions of market competition, then it is not necessarily appropriate to try to make the market more competitive in selected areas (Lipsey and Lancaster 1956–1957).

    A hypothetical example in the healthcare field should help clarify this. Suppose two of the assumptions on which economic competition is based do not hold: There are few firms, which results in monopoly power, and consumer information is poor. The theory shows that more competition in one of these areas will not necessarily bring us any closer to an optimal state and, in fact, may have the opposite effect. If there are a limited number of firms, then better information about price might allow firms to set prices as in a cartel (Fielding and Rice 1993). Or if information were limited, then as the number of physician firms in an area rose, it would become increasingly difficult for consumers to keep track of prices and reputation in the market. As a result, consumers might have to pay higher physician prices than they would other wise (Satterthwaite 1979; Pauly and Satterthwaite 1981). Thus, even within the economic model, increased competition may not always be desirable.

    Because so many of the assumptions of the competitive marketplace are not met in the health area, second-best considerations are pervasive. The most important one, perhaps, is the very existence of health insurance. When consumers have health insurance, the price they pay out-of-pocket for services is less than the cost of providing the services. (In a competitive marketplace, prices and costs are equivalent in the long run.) The Theory of the Second Best tells us that other competitive policies therefore are not necessarily optimal in the presence of health insurance.

    One problem with using second-best considerations to critique competitive economic policies in the health area is that, realistically, none can pass a second-best test. There are nearly always several aspects of a market that do not conform to the assumptions of competition. None of the arguments made in this book rely on second-best considerations. Readers wishing to pursue this topic should examine Robert Kuttner's (1997) book, *Everything for Sale: The Virtue and Limits of Markets*, for a detailed analysis of applying this theory to the health sector and to several other markets.

3. This quote was obtained from Wolf (1993, 17).

4. Wolf's analysis has been critiqued by Le Grand (1992). He posits that government failure is better considered separately with regard to different types of government intervention in a market (e.g., provision, taxation/subsidy, regulation), and goes on to consider such failure in each of these contexts.

5. In the economics literature, see Mancur Olson's book, *The Logic of Collective Action* (1965). To cite one noneconomic example, in the 1960s historian Gabriel Kolko observed, "The dominant fact of American political life at the beginning of this century was that big business led the struggle for the federal regulation of the economy" (High 1991, 1).

6. Regulators, like consumers and firms, are assumed to reach an equilibrium in which the ratio of marginal benefits to marginal costs is equalized—here, across competing interest groups. We can view marginal benefits as the extra political support or contributions regulators receive from a particular interest group, and marginal costs as the loss of support or contributions. If certain groups, such as producers, can marshal their resources better than consumer groups, then under the theory politicians and regulators would focus more of their attention on aiding such groups.

7. For a detailed review of the public choice literature, see Mueller (1989) and for a critique, Green and Shapiro (1994).

8. Some public choice theorists have tried to incorporate ideology into models of competition among political candidates, but this makes it hard to distinguish the theory from more traditional ones used in political science (Green and Shapiro 1994).

DEMAND

Economists use the concept of demand to argue that allowing consumers to choose in a free market, unfettered by government interference, will lead to an optimal society. This conclusion, however, is based on assumptions about (1) consumers' ability to make the best choices and (2) the stability of consumer tastes and preferences and a lack of interdependence among people. Many of the traditional theory's predictions fall when these assumptions are not met.

In chapters 4 and 5 we apply the concept of demand to healthcare markets. We demonstrate that several key predictions of traditional healthcare economics do not necessarily hold. This includes the predictions that society is worse off when its citizenry are well-insured (i.e., have low cost-sharing requirements), that we should charge more for services if their demand is price responsive, that it is better to provide cash than services in helping the poor, and that more consumer choice is necessarily better.

4

DEMAND FOR HEALTH, INSURANCE, AND SERVICES

Demand, which economists often define as how many goods and services are purchased at alternative prices, is the mechanism that drives a competitive economy. Under demand theory, people's demand for a commodity determines how much of it is produced and consumed. Price is also determined, in part, by consumer demand. If people's tastes change, and they want more of one good and less of another, prices will change, prompting firms to adjust production. Assuming the necessary inputs for production are available, in the long run supply adjusts in response to demand.

But traditional demand theory goes beyond this. It forms the basis by which economic theory evaluates social welfare. If people demand a certain bundle of goods and services, this means they prefer that bundle to all the other ways they could spend their money. The things people demand are, by definition, the things that put them at the highest level of welfare. If all people act in this way, then societal welfare will be maximized.[1]

We can better understand this theory if we consider the microeconomics concept of *revealed preference*. In Chapter 2, we introduced indifference curves but did not discuss where they came from. One way to derive them is to ask people which bundle of goods they would prefer. This technique has two problems. First, it is difficult to imagine administering such a population survey given the nearly countless possible bundles of goods from which people can choose. Second, people may not tell the truth, and even if they do, their responses may not predict their behavior.

The concept of revealed preference, pioneered by Paul Samuelson (1938), eliminates these problems. People are simply assumed to prefer the bundle of goods they choose to consume. If they choose to purchase one bundle over another they could afford, we can say they prefer the bundle they purchased. This theory does not rely on an understanding of the psyche of the individual. Rather, as Robert Sugden (1993, 1949) has noted,

> [T]he most significant property of the revealed preference approach . . . is that we do not need to enquire into the reasons why one thing is chosen rather than another. We do not look into the factors that go into the deliberation which leads to a choice; we look only at the results of that process.

To derive indifference curves through the theory of revealed preference, all one has to do is observe consumer behavior over different sets of prices and income. In doing so, economists make an important assumption: The bundle an individual chooses is the bundle he expects to make him best off.

Section 4.1 provides a critique of this traditional economic model by examining some of the assumptions upon which the model is based. In particular, we focus on whether consumers have sufficient information—and proper comprehension of it—to make effective decisions about health, health insurance, and health services. Section 4.2 presents and discusses the demand for health; Section 4.3, the demand for health insurance; and Section 4.4, the demand for health services. Section 4.4 also presents and critiques important theoretical work by Mark Pauly and empirical work from the RAND Health Insurance Experiment. Several policy applications are discussed along the way, with particular emphasis, in Section 4.5, on new health insurance products that rely on increased patient cost sharing, and in particular, so-called consumer-directed health plans.

4.1 A Critique of the Traditional Economic Model

In Voltaire's (1759) *Candide*, the philosopher Dr. Pangloss attempts to prove that the obviously flawed state of nature and society is, nevertheless, the best of all possible worlds. Dr. Pangloss states,

> It is demonstrated that things cannot be otherwise: for, since everything was made for a purpose, everything is necessarily for the best purpose. Note that noses were made to wear spectacles; we therefore have spectacles. Legs were clearly devised to wear breeches, and we have breeches. . . . And since pigs were made to be eaten, we have pork all year round. Therefore, those who have maintained that all is well have been talking nonsense: they should have maintained that all is for the best. (Voltaire 1759, 18)

Although some economists may not recognize it, demand theory in general and revealed preference in particular bear a striking resemblance to Pangloss's philosophy.[2] By choosing a particular bundle of goods, people demonstrate that they prefer it to all others; consequently, it is best for them. And, if all people are in their best position, then society—which is simply the aggregation of all people—is also in its best position. Therefore, allowing people to choose in the marketplace results in the best of all possible economic worlds.

The purpose of this section is to demonstrate that this sort of argument is tenuous at best because it is based on assumptions that are difficult to support, particularly in the healthcare sector. We will question the conventional meaning of the demand curve where it purports to show the marginal utility consumers obtain by purchasing alternative quantities of a good. The arguments presented in this section have profound implications concerning reliance on competitive markets in health system financing and healthcare delivery.

We begin by questioning five of the assumptions of the competitive economic model presented in Chapter 3:

Assumption 1. A person is the best judge of his or her own welfare.

Assumption 2. Consumers have sufficient information to make good choices.

Assumption 3. Consumers can accurately predict the results of their consumption decisions.

Assumption 4. Individuals are rational.

Assumption 5. Social welfare is based solely on individual utilities, which in turn are based solely on the goods and services consumed.

Social Welfare and Consumer Choice: A Syllogism

As we saw in Chapter 2, the typical argument is that an economic system that allows for consumer choice will, subject to some caveats[3], result in Pareto optimality. Pareto optimality is an economic state in which it is impossible to make someone better off without making someone else worse off. This is desirable because under Pareto optimality, firms are producing as much as they can, given resource constraints, of the products customers demand. But there is no guarantee that Pareto optimality will result in a socially desirable distribution of wealth. If society can reach some agreement on what composes optimal social welfare, it can be maximized through redistribution without moving away from a Pareto-optimal economic state.[4]

In this chapter, we assume society agrees upon and implements such a redistribution. (This is not to say redistribution is unimportant. We deal with it again in Chapter 5, and it is the main subject of Chapter 9.) The implicit assumption is that reaching Pareto optimality will ultimately maximize social welfare. This allows us to examine the assumptions under which allowing consumers to choose in the marketplace will be best for society as a whole.

With this assumption in hand, we can form the following syllogism:

If:
    A. Social welfare is maximized when individual utilities are maximized,
and:
    B. Individual utilities are maximized when people are allowed to choose,
then:
    C. Social welfare is maximized when people are allowed to choose.

This is obviously a strong conclusion because it implies that consumer choice brought about by market competition will result, as Dr. Pangloss would say, in the best of all possible worlds. This argument provides strong ammunition for the superiority of competition. But if either proposition does not hold, the conclusion is not warranted.

Are Individual Utilities Maximized When People Are Allowed to Choose?

One of the basic tenets of market competition is that people are best off when they are allowed to make choices. If, instead, an entity such as government makes choices for them, it is unlikely that consumers will fare as well. Each person is different, and an outsider could not appreciate an individual's exact desires. True, sometimes people are poorly informed about a particular good or service and must rely on the advice of an *agent* such as a physician. But even then, they choose to seek that advice, and they choose the particular agent.

Access to good and timely information seems essential, and Internet savvy appears to be a pre-condition for being a good consumer. So it may seem odd that economists often consider an individual consumer—even one without Web access—to be the world's expert in one particular area. That area, of course, is what he or she wants. Friedrich Hayek (1945, 521–22, 534), one of the founders of modern competitive theory, states this viewpoint nicely:

> Today it is almost heresy to suggest that scientific knowledge is not the sum of all knowledge. But a little reflection will show that there is beyond question a body of very important but unorganized knowledge which cannot possibly be called scientific . . . the knowledge of the particular circumstances of time and place. It is with respect to this that practically every individual has some advantage over all others in that he possesses unique information of which beneficial use might be made, but of which use can be made only if the decisions depending on it are left to him or are made with his active cooperation. . . . If we agree that the economic problem of society is mainly one of rapid adaptation to changes in the particular circumstances of time and place, it would seem to follow that the ultimate decisions must be left to the people who are familiar with these circumstances.

This is indeed a persuasive argument. Nevertheless, in this section we will demonstrate that, at least in healthcare, freedom to make their own choices does not necessarily make people best off.

Is a Person the Best Judge of His or Her Own Welfare? The first question to ask when considering whether sovereignty is best for consumers is whether consumers are the foremost authority on what is in their best interest. As Hayek pointed out, in many instances they unquestionably are. Nevertheless, this may not be the case in all areas. If, in some instances, consumers are not the best judge of what is in their best interest, then choices in such areas could perhaps be relegated to some other entity.

This is perhaps the most difficult assumption we question in this chapter because it seems impossible to test empirically. Obviously, no direct source of information on what is best for a particular person exists. Consequently, we have no way of objectively testing who is the better agent for obtaining what is best for the person. We must rely on indirect methods to further our inquiry.

To demonstrate that the individual is not necessarily the best judge, consider how society decides how to allocate particular goods and services. Most societies set rules that are explicitly designed to thwart the sanctity of individual choice.

Below is a list of practices that a libertarian—a person who believes in the sanctity of individual sovereignty—would likely believe should be left to individual choice rather than proscribed by society:

- personal use of narcotic drugs,
- gambling,
- riding a motorcycle without a helmet,
- seeking the services of a prostitute, and
- selling one's own organs.

These are all decisions that mainly affect the individual engaging in the practice rather than other people. Other illegal activities, such as requiring one's child to work rather than go to school, were left out because they have a direct negative effect on someone other than the decision maker.

There are, of course, a variety of reasons such activities are often illegal. All of them, however, share one characteristic: Society views them as bad for the individual in question. The first two, in addition, are potentially addictive. Perhaps most salient, however, is that all but the last provide immediate gratification rather than maximizing long-run utility.

Why would society abridge individual choice when consumer theory indicates that people can make welfare-maximizing choices themselves? Robert Frank (1985) suggests an interesting possibility: People are overly concerned with their status and will make the wrong economic, social, and/or moral decisions to enhance this status. One way young people might do this is to try to "look cool," for instance, by smoking, using drugs, not wearing seat belts or helmets, or spending $200 on a pair of jeans or athletic shoes. Some of these practices are easy to outlaw, although rules against them cannot necessarily be enforced. Even behaviors such as excessive spending on status-building clothing are not beyond society's grip. Many public schools have adopted uniform requirements as a way of reducing the negative manifestations of status seeking.

Even adults might be lured by choices that, in the long run, are bad for them. Frank suggests that this manifests itself in shortsighted decisions to obtain quick income to spend on ostensibly status-enhancing consumables (e.g., trendy clothing or cars or new electronic equipment). People gambling heavily are likely doing it not to make money to save for their children's college education, but rather, to go on a spending spree or pay off debts.

But harmful status seeking does not fully account for laws abridging personal choice. Consider selling one's own organs, the last example on the list. Although people who do this (mainly in poor countries) have heart-wrenching reasons, society usually views it as a bad idea, and wants to protect its citizenry from making such irrevocable decisions. A study by Goyal and colleagues (2002) found that four out of every five people in a region of southern India who had sold a kidney regretted doing so; five out of six reported a decline in health; and on average, family income declined by one-third. Thus, another reason for paternalistic laws that limit individual choice is that some decisions are bad for one's health.

A related reason for paternalism—one that is frequently cited in the health field—is that there are "experts" who know more than consumers and can thus make better choices. In this regard, Tibor Scitovsky (1976, 149–50) has written,

> The economist's traditional picture of the economy resembles nothing so much as a Chinese restaurant with its long menu. Customers choose from what is on the menu and are assumed always to have chosen what most pleases them. That assumption is unrealistic, not only of the economy, but of Chinese restaurants. Most of us are unfamiliar with nine-tenths of the entrees listed; we seem invariably to order either the wrong dishes or the same old ones. Only on occasions when an expert does the ordering do we realize how badly we do on our own and what good things we miss.

It would seem clear, then, that society does not always judge people's decisions to be in their best interests. As a result, it often acts to prevent people from engaging in some activity. Less often do we see situations in which people are told what they must do. This is certainly the case in health. People are told, for example, that they cannot purchase pharmaceutical drugs without a prescription. However, they are not told that they must take such drugs.

To determine whether people are able to make choices that are in their best interest, three other questions must be answered in the affirmative: (1) Do consumers have enough information to make good choices? (2) Do consumers know the results of their consumption decisions? and (3) Are individuals rational?

Do Consumers Have Enough Information to Make Good Choices?

Even if people know what they want and can pursue it in a rational manner, they may face another impediment—insufficient information about various alternatives.

Information plays an important role in economic theory. Consumers need good information to make utility-maximizing product choices, firms need good information to choose a product niche and obtain the necessary inputs to maximize profits, and workers need good information to obtain a job that satisfies their joint desires for professional satisfaction and good wages.

In healthcare, journal articles by economists calling for more information are common. In discussing whether a welfare loss is associated with excess amounts of health insurance, Roger Feldman and Bryan Dowd (1993, 199) state that, "if there is an inefficiently low level of information in medical care markets, the solution is to inform consumers, not to insure them fully." A contrasting viewpoint is offered by Uwe Reinhardt (2001a, 986–87):

> [I]magine a patient beset by chest or stomach pain in Anytown, USA, as he or she attempts to "shop around" for a cost-effective resolution to those problems. Only rarely, in a few locations, do American patients have access to even a rudimentary version of the information infrastructure on which the theory of competitive market and the theory of managed care rest. The prices of health services are jealously guarded proprietary information. . . . Information on the quality of care is generally unavailable or not trustworthy. Not even the infection or complication rates experienced in hospitals are publicly known. Such information on quality as is made available in the media or on Web sites typically consist of mysteriously weighed aggregate indexes that obscure the detailed information patients would need in a competitive market. Much is made now of the ability of Web-enabled healthcare consumers to view physicians as full partners or mere ordering clerks. Perhaps the typical American patient will fit that image one day. In the meantime, the image will remain the stuff of futurist tracts and of conference circuit fantasy.

Noneconomic observers do not always view sympathetically the standard rallying cry for allowing more competition as long as good information is available. Sociologist David Mechanic (1990, 93) has stated,

> To many economists, purchasing healthcare is fundamentally no different than purchasing carrots or cameras, and many of the uncertainties or imperfections of medical care markets can be accounted for by "information costs," the residual category of economic analysis that seemingly explains away many of the core concerns of the other social sciences.

The question we need to consider, then, is whether people have the information they need to make the right choices. This obviously depends on the health service being considered.

An intriguing debate on how much information consumers need was carried out in a now almost legendary 1977 conference sponsored by the U.S. Federal Trade Commission.[5] (The participants we allude to are still active leaders in the field.) Mark Pauly (1978) argued that we need to consider separately three kinds of services:

1. those purchased relatively frequently by the typical household,
2. those provided frequently by a physician but used infrequently by a patient, and
3. those that even a physician provides infrequently.

The first group would include pediatric care, dental care, prescription drugs, and the like; the second would include most surgical procedures; and the third, unusual and experimental procedures. Although Pauly thought the information currently available should be sufficient for consumers to make good choices in the first category, he estimated that three-fourths of expenditures would fall into the second and third.

In another conference paper, Frank Sloan and Roger Feldman (1978, 61) argued that "standard [economic] theory does not require that *everyone* possess perfect information—only that there be a sufficient number of marginal consumers both able to assess output and willing to seek it out at its lowest price." They quote Pauly in this regard:

> I know even less about the works of a movie camera than I know about my own organs; yet I feel fairly confident in purchasing a camera for a given price as long as I know that there are at least a few experts in the market who are keeping sellers reasonably honest.

Uwe Reinhardt (1978, 165) criticized this viewpoint by presenting two "rather bewildering" sets of specifications for stereo amplifiers. He then notes:

> Consider now a consumer without knowledge of electronics, with an only moderately sensitive ear. It can be wondered how our consumer would necessarily be driven to select the right model from these and other models *for his or her particular circumstances* simply because true experts in the market have established reasonable prices for these models, *given these experts' predilections and circumstances.* Chances are that our consumer would rely on expert advice in making the selection; chances are that the *vendor* would offer much advice freely; and chances are that the consumer will take home a model that may not be the most appropriate for his or her particular circumstances, especially if the vendor is overstocked on a particular model or if profit margins differ among models. It could happen even to an economist![6]

Some empirical research has been conducted on how consumers collect information on the alternatives they face in the health market. A number of fairly old studies found little evidence of "consumerism" in the health services area, with one physician observer sardonically noting that consumers "devote more effort selecting their Halloween pumpkin than they do choosing their physician."[7] A more recent study, by Thomas Hoerger and Leslie Howard (1995, 341, italics added), examined how pregnant women search for a prenatal care provider. The sample included women from Florida who gave birth in 1987. Women who believed they had a choice of providers were asked, "Before you selected your actual prenatal care provider, did you seriously consider using another prenatal care provider?" If they answered in the affirmative, they were asked, "Did you actually speak with or have an appointment with another prenatal care provider?" Curiously, only 24 percent of the respondents seriously considered using another provider, and only 14 percent actually had contact with another provider. The authors conclude:

> This amount of search is surprisingly low, given the importance of childbirth, the ample opportunity for choice, and the relative surplus of information about prenatal care providers compared to providers of other physician services. Recall that we expected the choice of prenatal care providers to establish a benchmark or *upper bound* on the extent of search for other physician services.

Experience from previous births did not explain the results. For most women, the birth examined was the first child; furthermore, women with previous births were more likely to search for a provider. Thus, consumers often do not seek out information to choose a physician.

But another, equally important question needs to be addressed: Can consumers successfully use the information that *is* available to them? Hibbard and Weeks (1989a, 1989b) studied the effect of information about physician fees on consumers' knowledge levels and their use of services. Using data from random samples of state government employees and Medicare beneficiaries in Oregon during the mid-1980s, the researchers divided the sample members into experimental and control groups. The experimental group received a directory listing the fees for common procedures among area physicians and a chart summarizing the ranges. Although knowledge among the government employees (but not the Medicare beneficiaries) increased as a result of receiving the directory, the behaviors the authors examined—including asking about the costs of visits, procedures, tests, or medications, or changing physicians or insurance plans—did not change. Receipt of the information had no effect on costs per physician visit, number of visits, or annual health expenditures (Hibbard and Weeks 1989a). Although some of the sample members had multiple insurance policies that would have covered the cost-sharing requirements associated with higher physician charges, the authors found that cost information had no effect, even on those for whom costs were a financial burden (Hibbard and Weeks 1989b).

The increased importance of managed care and capitation brings many challenges for consumers. To make appropriate choices about health plans, consumers need to understand primary care gatekeeping, financial incentives to providers, and other plan characteristics that affect the care patients receive. Unfortunately, there is little evidence that consumers do understand these concepts.

Survey results show that most consumers do not understand the difference between fee-for-service medicine and managed care plans, even at a rudimentary level (Isaacs 1996). Consumers even fail to understand certain key features of their own health plans. One U.S. survey, for example, found that whereas 62 percent of plan members believed their plans had to approve specialty referrals, the actual figure was just 28 percent (Cunningham, Denk, and Sinclair 2001).

One possible explanation for consumers' lack of understanding of their health plans is that most believe that the plan they choose does not determine the quality of care they will receive (Hibbard, Sofaer, and Jewett 1996; Jewett and Hibbard 1996). This belief indicates that consumers are not aware of the many levers health plans have available to them to affect the types and quantity of services provided to plan members.

Consumers need to be skilled at using the information included in *report cards* on their health plans. People may obtain these report cards from their employers and then choose a health plan by weighing such factors as quality, convenience, flexibility, and costs. Currently, no standard report card format is used, although many use elements based on data from the Healthcare Effectiveness Data and Information Set (HEDIS).

Good report cards should be easy to understand. Some items, such as satisfaction ratings, are comprehensible to most people, but other elements are more problematic. Whether consumers know how to make effective use of information on utilization rates for alternative services or whether they understand the relative importance of survival rates from high-incidence versus low-incidence procedures is not clear.

As we noted, most of the current quality measures on report cards are based on HEDIS, sponsored by the National Committee for Quality Assurance. HEDIS includes various measures of health plan performance in such areas as provision of preventive care to members and appropriateness of care for particular problems, as well as patient satisfaction. Consumers typically ignore the data they do not understand, which tend to be the "objective" measures of quality such as various utilization rates. Similarly, they over-interpret simple satisfaction data, the element they best understand. Judith Hibbard and Jacquelyn Jewett (1997, 224–25) report:

> Interestingly, consumers perceive that patient ratings of overall quality give more information about the monitoring and follow-up of a condition than do the HEDIS indicators designed specifically for this purpose (such as rates of eye examinations among diabetic members, asthma hospitalizations, and low-birthweight infants). . . . These findings suggest that consumers are unsure of what many indicators are intended to tell them.

A great deal of research has been conducted in recent years on the impact of report cards, especially those provided to employees as part of their annual open enrollment decisions for health insurance. (A search of the online database PubMed found 144 articles with "report card" in the title during the period from 2000 to 2008.) If one were to analyze the literature in a sound bite, it might go like this: Report cards do have a positive impact on a small percentage of individuals who read and understand them; these consumers tend to choose higher-quality products. But most people are unaffected. In fact, one study that examined how report cards affected the quality of health insurance choice among federal employees found exactly that. It concluded that report card ratings "had a meaningful influence on individuals' choices, particularly for individuals choosing a plan for the first time. Although . . . a very small fraction of individual decisions were materially affected by the information, for those that were affected the implied utility gains are substantial" (Jin and Sorensen 2006).

Findings of interest from other studies of report cards include the following:

- Certain subgroups of the population, particularly those who are more likely to be economically and/or medically vulnerable, tend to be less responsive to report cards than others. As one group of researchers reports,

  The health care system already offers many barriers and obstacles that hamper these groups from obtaining appropriate, effective, and culturally sensitive care. The characteristics that make individuals vulnerable in the health system (poverty, lack of education, inarticulateness, lack of English language) often come together, leading to multiple cumulative problems. This vulnerability, powerlessness, and potential for additional differential disadvantage arising from the proliferation of report cards provide a compelling argument for further policy analysis and action (Davies, Washington, and Bindman 2002, 394).

  These researchers suggest various strategies to help vulnerable populations use report cards. One issue, obviously, is that members of these populations are less likely to use the Internet, where much of the report card information resides. It is hardly surprising, then, that studies have found that report cards are more influential in the choices made by younger, college-educated consumers (Howard and Kaplan 2006).
- The way information is presented in report cards is critical. Researchers have learned how graphical format, wording, and prose can be used most effectively. For example, a common format where different evaluation criteria are evaluated using one, two, or three stars was not found to be

useful (Vaiana and McGlynn 2002). A study that tested seven reporting formats found that fewer than one-half of respondents ages 45–75 could interpret bar graphs, and that the most successful used words such as "better," "average," or "worse" (Gerteis et al. 2007).

- Report cards can have direct and indirect positive effects. A case in point is a system used in New York State, where the mortality rates of patients served by particular hospitals and individual surgeons are calculated and publicized. This provides two incentives to improve quality: (1) Patients should prefer hospitals and surgeons with better rates, and (2) hospitals and surgeons should prefer not to look bad compared to their peers. Although there has been some disagreement over how much of an effect the program has had and why (Epstein 2006), most studies show that it has resulted in a substantial decrease in mortality—as much as 41 percent (Chassin 2002).

Some research indicates that people can do better with *less* information. A huge amount of information could make you less informed than a smaller amount in either of two ways. One is that you don't even begin sifting the information because the task is so daunting. The other is that you do try to understand it, but because it is so complicated you learn very little.

In one study of the working-age population, Hibbard and colleagues (2000) conducted a randomized controlled experiment examining how well people understood healthcare report cards. One of the experimental interventions was providing a subgroup of subjects with additional information designed to help them better understand the content of the report cards, including "instructions on how to use the information and rationales about why the information is important" (139). Curiously, the group that was given more information performed worse: They answered 84 percent of questions about a comparison chart correctly, compared to 91 percent by those who did not get the additional information. They also answered questions about plan features less accurately (84 percent correct versus 94 percent for those given less information).

McCormack and colleagues (2001) conducted a similar randomized controlled experiment among seniors covered by Medicare. Subjects were randomly assigned to three groups. One group was given a standard information book that all program beneficiaries received, called *Medicare and You*. A second group received the book and a detailed report providing report card ratings on the quality of care provided by Medicare managed care plans in their geographic area. A third group received a shorter version of the report (that is, more information than the first group and less than the second). Once again, this study found that the subgroup that received the detailed quality information was less likely to use the information provided and less likely to change health plans in the next open enrollment period than those who did not receive any information beyond the *Medicare and You* handbook.

Marc Rodwin (2001) notes a number of problems with the report cards. One is that they ignore key aspects of health plan operation, such as the stringency of utilization review and the financial incentives providers face. Another is that many of the tasks previously performed by health plans have now devolved to capitated physician groups, whose performance is only occasionally available from report cards. A third is that report cards tend to be aggregated rather than focused on performance for particular medical conditions, even though the management of chronic conditions is perhaps the most important barometer of the success of a health plan.

Not surprisingly, a study of managed care in 15 representative communities during 1995 concluded that, although much competition exists on the basis of price, "in general, there was almost no competition on the basis of measured and reported technical quality process or outcome measures" (Miller 1996, 116). The same could almost certainly be said 15 years later.

Rodwin (1996, 112) concludes that quality care can come about only through a large-scale, organized consumer movement:

> Effective consumer protection requires organized consumer groups that are strong enough to make plans respond to their interests. . . . Consumers need organized groups to ensure the presence of and to monitor traditional government oversight; to help define policies and practices within managed care organizations; to monitor the performance of managed care organizations and private accrediting groups; to marshal political resources; and to form strategic alliances.

Thus far, few systematic efforts of this kind have been undertaken in the healthcare area.[8]

Do Consumers Know the Results of Their Consumption Decisions?

Another concern about whether consumers can make appropriate choices involves a special characteristic in health, the *counterfactual*. Counterfactual questions concern what would have happened if history had been different. For example, some economists have tried to determine how quickly the western United States would have developed without railways (Fogel 1964; Fishlow 1965). Counterfactual questions can never be answered with certainty.

Healthcare poses many counterfactual questions. Suppose a person seeks care from a primary care physician and tries to determine what he or she learned from the experience. It is difficult for the person to determine whether he or she made the right decision in seeking care from that provider, because to do so would involve answering several counterfactual questions, such as:

- Would the problem have gone away if I had left it untreated?
- What would have happened if I had sought the care of a specialist instead of a primary care physician?

- Would the result have been different if I had seen a different primary care physician than the one I sought?

In this regard, Burton Weisbrod (1978, 52) has written,

> For ordinary goods, the buyer has little difficulty in evaluating the counterfactual—that is, what the situation will be if the good is not obtained. Not so for the bulk of health care. . . . Because the human physiological system is itself an adaptive system, it is likely to correct itself and deal effectively with an ailment, even without any medical care services. Thus, a consumer of such services who gets better after the purchase does not know whether the improvement was because of, or even in spite of, the "care" that was received. Or if no health care services are purchased and the individual's problem becomes worse, he is generally not in a strong position to determine whether the results would have been different, and better, if he had purchased certain health care. And the consumer, not being a medical expert, may learn little from experience or from friends' experience . . . because of the difficulty of determining whether the counterfactual to a particular type of health care today is the same as it was the previous time the consumer, or a friend, had "similar" symptoms. The noteworthy point is not simply that it is difficult for the consumer to judge quality before the purchase . . . but that it is difficult even after the purchase.

Weisbrod (1978, 54) concludes that "when buyers have difficult quality-evaluation problems, the theorem of economics that more information . . . is always preferred to less need not hold."

Even good healthcare report cards do little to solve these problems of the counterfactual. Suppose a report card indicates that a particular physician group provides good cardiac care. This still does not tell a consumer whether he or she should seek care in the wake of a particular symptom, whether to return for follow-up visits, or which, if any, elective diagnostic procedure to use.

Are Individuals Rational? Whether consumers act rationally is a different question than whether people are the best judge of their own welfare. Even if people know what will make them best off, their choices will not necessarily be consistent with this knowledge.

Before addressing this, consider the meaning of *rational*. Economists typically use a technical definition, whereby a person is rational if his or her choices are consistent and transitive over time (Mishan 1969a). We can understand *consistency* to mean that, if a person faces the exact same circumstances more than once, he or she will make the same choice each time. *Transitive* means that if a consumer prefers (and therefore chooses) good A over good B, and good B over good C, then he or she would also prefer (and choose) good A over C.

Research has found numerous situations in which people do not act rationally in the economic sense. (See Thaler [1992] for a book full of such anomalies.) Amos Tversky and Daniel Kahneman (1981, 453) provide a health example. In one experiment, they took two groups of people, asking the first,

> Imagine that the U.S. is preparing for the outbreak of an unusual Asian disease, which is expected to kill 600 people. Two alternative programs to combat the disease have been proposed. Assume that the exact scientific estimate of the consequences are as follows: If Program A is adopted, 200 people will be saved. If Program B is adopted, there is a 1/3 probability that 600 people will be saved, and 2/3 probability that no people will be saved. Which of the two programs would you favor?

Under this scenario, 72 percent chose Program A, exhibiting risk-averse behavior—they prefer a certain rather than uncertain future, even one that guarantees 400 people will die.

The second group was asked the same question, but with two changes: "If Program C is adopted 400 people will die. If Program D is adopted there is a 1/3 probability that nobody will die, and 2/3 probability that 600 people will die" (Tversky and Kahneman 1981, 453). Given this scenario, 78 percent chose Program D. The authors conclude,

> The preferences . . . illustrate a common pattern: choices involving gains are often risk averse and choices involving losses are often risk taking. However, it is easy to see that the two problems are effectively identical. The only difference between them is that the outcomes are described in problem 1 by the number of lives saved and in problem 2 by the number of lives lost. The change is accompanied by a pronounced shift from risk aversion to risk taking. We have observed this reversal in several groups of respondents, including university faculty and physicians.

The economic definition of rationality is not terribly useful to us because the term *rationality* means much more than that. True, preferences often are not transitive or consistent over time. But even if they were, people could prefer things an objective observer might find not in their best interest. Clearly, this is at odds with traditional economic theory, where whatever a person demands will, by definition, make her best off.[9]

Economists, in contrast to other social scientists, sometimes suppose consumers must be rational and must therefore act to maximize their utility. But that supposition seems to be false. An opponent of this viewpoint, Harvey Leibenstein (1976), has noted that "the idea of utility maximization must contain the possibility of choice under which utility is not maximized" (8). Similarly, Lester Thurow (1983, 217–18) writes,

Revealed preferences . . . is just a fancy way of saying that individuals do whatever individuals do, and whatever they do, economists will call it "utility maximization." Whether individuals buy good A or good Y they are still rational individual utility maximizers. By definition, there is no such thing as an individual who does not maximize utility. But if a theory can never be wrong, it has no content. It is merely a tautology.

This book is not the appropriate forum for a thorough consideration of the validity of the rationality assumption. Indeed, psychology and sociology lay claim to this issue. We will discuss only one aspect of it here—cognitive dissonance.

The theory of cognitive dissonance concerns a central aspect of human behavior—self-justification or rationalization. Elliot Aronson (1972, 92–93) explained,

Basically, cognitive dissonance is a state of tension that occurs when an individual simultaneously holds two cognitions (ideas, attitudes, beliefs, opinions) that are psychologically inconsistent. . . . Because [its] occurrence . . . is unpleasant, people are motivated to reduce it. . . . To hold two ideas that contradict each other is to flirt with absurdity, and—as Albert Camus, the existentialist philosopher, has observed—man is a creature who spends his entire life in an attempt to convince himself that his existence is not absurd.

Whether we would define a behavior as rational or irrational depends on how difficult it is to change the behavior in question relative to the cognition. Smoking is one of the best examples. Suppose a person smokes but knows that it is dangerous to his health. This causes cognitive dissonance; how can he continue to do something that is so self-destructive? If he is not addicted or has a particularly strong will, he may quit. But an addict or a weaker person will typically find it easier to change the cognition than the behavior, either by attributing more pleasure to smoking than is truly obtained, or by denying that it is dangerous (Aronson 1972). Although this latter behavior has been repeatedly confirmed and is certainly understandable, it is hardly what we would deem "rational."

Economists George Akerlof and William Dickens (1992, 317, italics added) have used cognitive dissonance to explain various economic behaviors. Examples include the choice of risky jobs, technological development, advertising, and crime. Regarding social insurance, they write,

If there are some persons who would simply prefer not to contemplate a time when their earning power is diminished, and if the very fact of saving for old age forces persons into such contemplations, there is an argument for compulsory old age insurance. . . . [They] may find it uncomfortable to contemplate their old age. For that reason they may make the wrong tradeoff, *given their own preferences*, between current consumption and savings for retirement.

People understand that saving more is in their best interest. Nevertheless, they fail to do so, in part because they do not want to face the prospect of diminished abilities in old age. Hence, to ensure that people will have the financial resources to take care of themselves, society makes the decision for them—we override individual choice by taking money out of people's paychecks when they are younger. This happens in nearly all countries. Examples from the United States are the Social Security and Medicare programs.

In summary, when cognitive dissonance is present, there is little reason to suppose people will act in a rational manner by making decisions that truly maximize their utility.

Is Social Welfare Maximized When Individual Utilities Are Maximized?

This section examines proposition A of the syllogism presented earlier, that social welfare is maximized when individuals maximize their own utility. This is another way of stating Assumption 5 from Table 3.1:

Assumption 5: Social welfare is solely the sum of individual utilities.

For the time being, we will assume that society can and does redistribute income (in a manner that society feels will enable it to achieve Pareto optimality). This allows us to explicitly examine the advantages of allowing for consumer choice in the health market without worrying about issues of equity (which is the focus of Chapter 9).

While the proposition that social welfare is based solely on individuals' welfare is a philosophical issue and cannot be proved true or false, two arguments question its validity. The first is from Sen (1982, 1987, 1992), who calls this philosophy "welfarism," which "is the view that the only things of intrinsic value for ethical calculation and evaluation of states of affairs are individual utilities" (1987, 40). Sen's arguments, which span several books, are too lengthy to be properly summarized here. One reason he rejects the welfarist approach is that it does not allow us to distinguish between different *qualities* of utility. He suggests that if my unhappiness gives you pleasure, that counts as much under the welfarist approach as anything else that increases your well-being. In contrast, one might believe a society should devote its resources to meeting somewhat more lofty desires. A second reason is that individual welfare does not seem to rely solely on the goods a person has; other aspects of life, such as freedom (and health), are also important.

Frank (1985) brings up another reason to doubt that social welfare is the sum of individual welfare, noting that much of what individuals seek is status or rank. But this is relative; if my status rises above yours, your status necessarily goes down. This leads to consumption that does not add to the social welfare. For example, if I buy a fancy car, I get utility from the various characteristics of the car and from the fact that I have distinguished myself from you. Once you (and others like us) buy the car, the latter part of my utility is canceled out. Total utility (or social welfare) is thus lower than the sum of our individual utilities. We consider this issue in much greater detail in Chapter 5, when we discuss negative externalities of consumption.

There is strong reason to believe the welfare of a society is more or less than the sum of its individual components. Individual welfare includes aspects a society may consider too base or selfish to want to maximize, such as wishing ill on others, and individuals tend to emphasize status. We will argue in Chapter 5 that even though seeking status is often a good thing, societies may nevertheless wish to deemphasize it.

To conclude this section, we return to the syllogism with which it began. Neither of the two premises of the syllogism—social welfare is maximized when individual utilities are maximized, and individual utilities are maximized when people are allowed to choose—appears to hold true in the healthcare area. Thus, social welfare is not necessarily maximized when people are allowed to choose. In the following sections, we apply this conclusion to the three key areas in demand analysis: health, health insurance, and health services.

4.2 Demand for Health

The bulk of demand-related research in health economics has been devoted to demand for health services rather than demand for health itself. Health is not a commodity, and thus is much harder to conceive of and to measure. The issue has not been ignored, however. In fact, because Michael Grossman gave the subject a thorough treatment three decades ago, many economists probably have not seen a compelling reason to revisit it. Some recent research (not explored here because it goes beyond the scope of this book) has used the concept to investigate an even broader question: What causes some people to be healthier than others (Evans and Stoddart 1990; Heymann et al. 2006)?

Grossman's original ideas are laid out in a journal article (1972a) and a book (1972b). They are based on (but deviate from) another economic concept, *human capital theory*. That branch of economic theory examines the conditions under which people choose to invest in themselves—for example, investing in education or job training to improve their future economic productivity, and thus, their wages (Becker 1964). Just as investment in capital equipment can result in greater production for a firm, so too can investment in oneself provide a parallel result.

In the Grossman model, what people demand is good health. Good health, along with the various non-health goods and services they purchase, conveys utility. To maximize their utility, people need to decide how to produce their own good health, and how much of it to produce. Like any other good, there are diminishing marginal returns, so it is unlikely that a person would spend an unlimited amount (unless doing so would save her life) since that would mean consuming fewer non–health related goods and services.

Health, moreover, deteriorates over time. This is partly due to the aging process, but also to human bodies needing upkeep just like mechanical goods. Grossman posits that there are three ways people can invest in their health, so as to keep up with or even overcome this deterioration. One is through purchasing medical care services, a second is investment of one's time, and a third is investment in one's human capital.

Most of the interest in this model stems from the role of education. In nearly all countries, there is a strong relationship between education and health: Better educated people, on average, are healthier. The U.S. figures are quite dramatic. When comparing adults age 25–64 who did not finish high school to those who attended one or more years of college, 2004 mortality rates in the lower-educated group were 3.3 times higher among males and 2.9 times higher among females than in the better-educated group (Centers for Disease Control and Prevention 2007, Table 34).

The debate continues, however, whether more education leads to better health or if those in better health seek more schooling. Another possibility is "that no causal relationship is implied by the correlation; instead, differences in one or more 'third variables,' such as physical and mental ability and parental characteristics, affect both health and schooling in the same direction" (Grossman 2004). Perhaps, for example, less impulsive people are better at planning for the future and therefore seek more education and engage in more preventive and less risky behavior. Under this scenario, more education does not directly lead to better health. Rather, a third variable, which economists call "time preference," is responsible both for how much education a person gets and how healthy he is.

Grossman (2004) reviews a large body of literature on this topic, concluding that there is strong evidence to indicate that more education *causes* better health. This certainly is plausible, as those who are better educated may make better lifestyle and care decisions and may be better able to deal with complicated health decisions. Although he cites seven studies in his review, we mention just one, by Lleras-Muney (2005). To disentangle issues of causality, she examines the impact of compulsory education laws in the United States between 1915 and 1939 on the death rates (between 1960 and 1980) of those who were 14 years old during this period. Young people do not have the liberty to leave grade or high school early when states require schooling up to a certain age. Since mortality rates are unlikely to affect whether legislators enact mandatory education laws, we can be fairly certain that if people who lived in states with such laws die at older ages (controlling for factors such as race/ethnicity, wages, and per capita educational expenditures), educational attainment causes better health rather than the other way around. Lleras-Muney found that an additional year of schooling lowers mortality by 3.6 percent. In 1960, an additional year of schooling increased the lifespan at age 35 by 1.7 years.

The fact that more education can improve health is certainly encouraging, but it raises serious issues for society. Critical educational decisions—whether to finish high school, take college preparatory classes, study hard enough to get good grades, and so on—are often made when a person is very young. It's surely fair to say that teens have trouble considering the long-term consequences of near-term decisions. The traditional economic model relies on rational individuals making well-considered decisions. If good health later in life depends on decisions a person makes while young, this has implications for whether government should provide help for those who later in life find themselves in poor health—through such programs as government-subsidized care or subsidized health insurance, or more broadly, through income security or housing.

4.3 Demand for Health Insurance

The first part of this section is devoted to the theory of health insurance. It concludes with a discussion of the responsiveness of the demand for insurance with respect to its price.

Theory of the Demand for Health Insurance

Health economists have a theory that explains why people demand health insurance. It provides some useful insights, but we will argue that at least one of them does not reflect people's preferences in the real world.

To understand the theory, we need to define two terms. The first is *risk aversion*. A risk-averse person is someone who prefers "a bird in the hand to two in the bush." We might say he prefers a certain, although not spectacular, future prospect to an uncertain one that may bring riches but could also leave him wanting.

Not surprisingly, there is a more technical—albeit rather pedestrian—definition of risk aversion: A person is risk averse if the marginal utility of additional income declines as income rises. Suppose you earn $30,000 a year. You are defined as risk averse if the money you make between $25,000 and $30,000 brings you more utility than an additional $5,000 (that would make your income $35,000). Why? If this were not true, you would prefer to take a risk to get an extra $5,000 of income, even if what you risked was your last $5,000.

Here is one way to figure out if you are risk averse. Suppose we have a coin and offer you a bet: If it's "heads," we pay you $1,000; if it's "tails," you pay us $1,000. Risk-averse people tend to reject this sort of bet because they get more utility from the last $1,000 of income than from an extra $1,000. (If we changed the bet to $1 rather than $1,000, a risk-averse person might take it—because he or she may derive enough extra utility from the fun of taking the gamble.)

The second definition is *actuarially fair insurance*. This is a hypothetical insurance policy that pays out in benefits exactly what it collects in premiums. As such, there are no *loading costs* (administration, marketing, or profits). Although no insurance company could survive selling actuarially fair insurance, the concept is useful for understanding the material that follows.

The theory goes back 60 years, to the work of Milton Friedman and L. J. Savage (1948). Their work applied to all insurance; health was not singled out. At the time, health insurance was fairly new, whereas other types, such as fire insurance, dated back more than 100 years.

The derivation goes as follows. Borrowing some of the nomenclature used by Paul Feldstein (1998), let

U = a person's utility

W = a person's wealth

L = the monetary size of a loss that would occur if the person becomes sick

p = the probability of getting sick and experiencing a loss of size L

In Figure 4.1, the curved line shows the person's total utility. As wealth rises, utility rises, but at a declining rate that illustrates the notion of diminishing marginal utility.

This curved line shows the utility that would be derived by purchasing actuarially fair insurance. With insurance that covers all costs in the event of a medical loss, the consumer knows with certainty that her wealth will be W minus the amount she must pay in insurance premiums, $p \times L$. If the chance of a loss is 10 percent, and the average size of a loss is $10,000, then the cost of the insurance would be $p \times L = $1,000. That means the consumer's wealth after purchasing actuarially fair insurance would be $9,000. We illustrate this on the horizontal axis as $W - pL$. The utility one derives by purchasing this insurance is shown at point B. It has a corresponding utility of $U_{(WpL)}$.

The more difficult concept, perhaps, is what the person's utility would be if she did not purchase insurance. In such a case, her utility is a weighted average of two alternative states: one in which she becomes sick, and one in which she does not. Her wealth if she does not become ill is W; we do not subtract anything since she did not purchase insurance and therefore pays no premiums. The utility associated with that is $U_{(W)}$. Now suppose instead she

FIGURE 4.1: Demand for Health Insurance

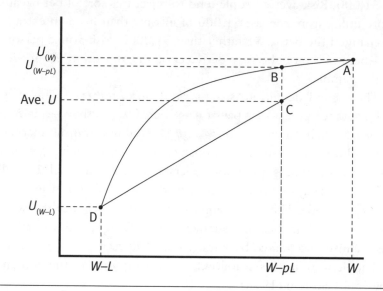

does become sick and experiences a loss of L, so that wealth left over after paying for the illness is $W - L$ and the utility associated with this is $U_{(W-L)}$. All of the weighted averages of these two states are shown on line DA. Point C corresponds to a probability of loss p. Algebraically, the average expected utility of these two states is:

$$\{p \times [U_{(W-L)}]\} + \{(1 - p) \times U_{(W)}\} \tag{4.1}$$

The key result is that the utility at point C, the average when health insurance is not purchased, is lower than the utility at point B, where insurance is purchased. This shows that a risk-averse person will be better off purchasing actuarially fair insurance than not purchasing it.

It is also clear that the more risk averse a person is—that is, the more curved her utility line is with respect to wealth—the more she will benefit from insurance. People who are very risk averse will be willing to pay more (above the actuarially fair premium) for insurance than others will. These insights are borne out by observations of actual behavior in the health insurance market. For example, younger people often engage in more risks, and some may feel that health insurance is not necessary. Their demand for health insurance tends to be lower, even controlling for their incomes.

By manipulating the figure, we can draw other conclusions. Figure 4.2 contrasts the original cost of illness from the previous figure (the loss L) to a situation where the loss is smaller—L' rather than L. Point E is now the utility associated with purchasing insurance, and point F, the average or expected utility when it is not purchased. Even though the purchase of insurance (E) still conveys more utility, the difference is smaller than before (that is, smaller than B—C in Figure 4.2). The implication is straightforward (but, it turns out, probably wrong): The benefits derived from purchasing health insurance are directly proportional to the cost of healthcare—when illness is less expensive, insurance provides less added utility, and when it is more expensive, it adds more.

Although this conclusion may sound reasonable, it is not consistent with empirical studies of the demand for insurance, for it implies that as healthcare costs—and with them, premiums—rise, people will demand more, not less, health insurance. Unlike other goods and services, when insurance gets more expensive, the theory implies that people will buy more of it.[10] This certainly does not correspond to logic or casual experience. People find health insurance increasingly unaffordable as its price goes up; this is supported by findings from the research literature. Studies by Kronick and Gilmer (1999) show a close negative correlation, over a 16-year period, between uninsurance rates and the costs of healthcare (measured by healthcare spending divided by average income). When healthcare costs go up in relation to income, purchase of insurance goes down. Most likely this is because workers have to spend more of their own income on insurance premiums.

This has important policy implications. Healthcare expenditure increases vary year to year, but over time they have risen much faster than inflation and growth in the economy as a whole. Projections of future expenditures suggest that the United States will spend 19.6 percent of gross

FIGURE 4.2: Demand for Health Insurance When Loss from Illness Is Smaller

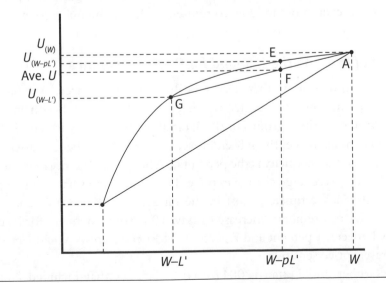

domestic budget on healthcare in 2016, compared to 16.0 percent in 2006 (Poisal et al. 2007). Gilmer and Kronick (2005) project that rising costs will lead to an increase in the number of uninsured from 45 million to 56 million between 2003 and 2013, because individuals and firms can no longer afford insurance. This assumes, of course, that the U.S. government doesn't embark on a policy of universal coverage, discussed further in chapters 9 and 10.

The theory of insurance also implies a relationship between p, the probability that a loss will occur (that is, that a person will get sick and use the policy benefits), and the demand for insurance. The theory predicts that individuals will have less demand for insurance if the chance of experiencing a covered loss is very likely or very unlikely, and more demand for probabilities in between. This seems logical. Coverage for extremely unusual occurrences (sometimes called "Acts of God" in insurance policies) is rare. And for near-certain events, coverage does not seem prudent because it is better to pay out-of-pocket ("self-insuring") than to pay a third party that will likely charge a hefty administrative fee.

But then how do we explain the apparent contradiction of the theory whereby people often *do* have coverage for events that are very likely to occur, such as regular check-ups or, in the dental insurance area, semiannual cleanings? One plausible reason is that people are willing to pay extra to not have to think about the costs of care at the time they are seeking it. Better to know your visit to the dental hygienist is going to be paid in full, than have to think about the benefits versus costs of getting a cleaning every six months.[11]

Though this mind-set is not consistent with the "rationality" predicted by the theory of insurance, in this case it indicates an impressive self-awareness that helps consumers make the right decisions for their health. By analogy, people who are rational in the traditional sense would always ask to see a dessert menu in a restaurant, even if they are on a diet, so that they could make a utility-maximizing decision based on complete information. But perhaps it is equally or even more rational to refuse the dessert menu, recognizing that it might inspire a bad decision on the spur of the moment.

Impact of Price on the Demand for Health Insurance

Nearly all studies show that higher health insurance prices, as reflected in monthly premiums, are negatively related to demand for health insurance. This is true of various groups in the United States: those with employment-based health insurance, the self-employed, and Medicare beneficiaries.

Recall that elasticity is the percentage change in quantity demanded divided by the percentage change in price. Different studies have come up with various elasticity estimates, most in the range of −0.1 to −0.7. That means that as price or premiums increase by, say, 10 percent, demand for insurance falls by between 1 percent and 7 percent. Most economists would view this as moderately price sensitive.

Gruber and Lettau (2004) used a data set that included employer and employee characteristics over the years 1983 and 1985. They calculated two elasticities: The elasticity with respect to the firm offering insurance was −0.25, and the other, with respect to spending on healthcare (by the firm or by the firm and the individual), was −0.7. That is, as price rose by 10 percent, firms were 2.5 percent less likely to offer coverage, and firms' spending on healthcare fell by 7 percent. Gruber and Poterba (1994) examined the self-employed, and found a considerably larger elasticity of −1.8. This is not terribly surprising, since the self-employed are spending their own resources and have to consider the trade-off of spending more money on health insurance versus various other business-related and consumer expenditures.

Researchers have also examined the price sensitivity of Medicare beneficiaries. Atherly, Dowd, and Feldman (2004) used Medicare data from 1998 to see how premiums affected demand for Medicare managed care plans, finding an elasticity of about −0.13. Similarly, Buchmueller (2006), using data from 1997–2002, found demand for alternative health plans among Medicare beneficiaries to be between −0.12 and −0.24. He posits that Medicare beneficiaries are less price sensitive than those with employment-based coverage because they focus more on quality of care and freedom to choose their own doctors and specialists than price, and because they do not like to change plans, in part because it may mean switching away from a provider with whom they are comfortable.

Similar results were found in a study of Canada, which has a universal health insurance system. In Canada, as in many other countries, it is possible to obtain private insurance to cover services not included in the public insurance scheme. In the province of Quebec during the 1990s, a tax break given to employees purchasing such coverage was removed, effectively raising the price of supplemental coverage substantially. Finkelstein (2002) found that this led to a 13 to 14 percent decline in coverage, corresponding to an elasticity of −0.5.

Why should we care about the price elasticity of demand for health insurance? In the U.S. context:

- Some proposals for increasing the number of insured rely on providing subsidies or tax breaks to low- and middle-income workers. The elasticity tells us how likely it is that different proposals will achieve expanded coverage.
- Some conservative observers have suggested that employer-based health insurance should not be tax deductible. If the United States were to remove this tax break, the magnitude of the elasticity would provide information on how many more people would drop their health insurance, as well as the likely reduction in healthcare costs.
- Currently, the Medicare program provides a large subsidy for seniors who join managed care plans (called "Medicare Advantage"). If this subsidy were removed, many of the current enrollees would almost certainly switch to the fee-for-service system. The elasticity can be used to calculate the effect. Such information would be important to the private sector to help plan for the reduction in enrollment.

4.4 Demand for Health Services

If one had to choose the topic that, more than any other, occupies the thoughts of health economists, it would likely be the factors that affect demand for health services. The key relationship in the study of demand is between the quantity demanded of a good or service and its price. While demand has several determinants, economists are particularly interested in the role of prices.

This section is one of the longest in the book, reflecting the central placement of this topic in the field of health economics. The first subsection, on theory, is quite short, however, since this material was covered in Chapter 2. We then examine the design and results of the RAND Health Insurance Experiment and discuss the concept of moral hazard and empirical work on the topic. Next, we backtrack a bit into more theory about moral hazard as we examine whether there is a societal *welfare loss* from "excessive" health insurance, considering the work of Mark Pauly and recent critiques. The chapter ends with an examination of a recent institutional development: health insurance products that rely more on patient cost sharing.

Theory of Demand for Health Services

In Chapter 2, we derived a demand cure for health services (Equation 2.10):

$$D = f(P, P_s, P_c, I, HS, T)$$

where D represents the demand for a particular health good or service, P is its price, P_s is the price of substitute goods, P_c is the price of complementary goods, I is income, HS is health status, and T is tastes.

The field of economics is especially interested in economic factors, so its focus is on prices and incomes. The price elasticity of the demand for services is of particular interest. Other relevant issues include whether certain health services (e.g., hospital stays and physician visits) are complements or substitutes, which relates to the cross-price elasticity of demand, and whether particular medical services are normal or inferior goods, which relates to the income elasticity of demand.

Moral Hazard, Part I: The RAND Health Insurance Experiment

Moral hazard exists when the possession of an insurance policy increases the likelihood of incurring a loss and/or the size of a covered loss. As the term is certainly value-laden, there is confusion about what it means. The term dates back at least 200 years (Dembe and Boden 2000). A common usage in the nineteenth century pertained to the purchase of fire insurance. The owner of a property insured against fire might be more likely to incur a loss—either by deliberately setting a fire (hence, "moral" hazard) or by being less diligent in preventing one. A quotation from an 1877 fire insurance textbook gives some flavor to the term:

We cannot too earnestly impress upon [insurance] agents, everywhere, the necessity of care. The agent who contributes, by over-insurance or in any way, to an incendiary fire, *endangers the common safety and commits a crime against society.** Constant supervision and watchfulness, with a keen judgment of men and values, are necessary. . . . It must be borne in mind that companies sometimes lose as much in consequence of *the indifference of honest men . . . as by the designing villainy of those who do not scruple to apply the match.*

*While over-insurance causes fires, a proper amount of insurance may prevent them by teaching a malicious vagabond that he cannot harm his enemy by burning his property, as the insurance company's interposition restores the loss. (Moore 1877, 18)

In the healthcare area, the existence of a moral hazard implies that people use more services when they are insured or when they are more fully insured. But as Mark Pauly (1968, 535) pointed out in his famous essay on moral hazard, "the response of seeking more medical care with insurance than in its absence is a result not of moral perfidy, but of rational economic behavior." For a fully insured person, the cost of using an additional service will be shared by everyone who pays premiums. Thus, the person is likely to use more services than if he would if he paid the full cost of the additional service. Economists' concern is that with insurance, people will use too many services because they are not bearing the full costs of usage. Costs are therefore being passed on to others.

For purposes of this subsection, though, moral hazard simply means that the demand curve for medical care slopes downward and to the right—people seek more services when their out-of-pocket payments are lower.

Description of the Experiment

The Health Insurance Experiment (HIE) was designed by the RAND Corporation under contract to the U.S. federal government. Although it was conducted long ago—from the late 1970s to the early 1980s—its results are still widely used in health economics and health policy. Its staying power stems from two factors. Unlike most research in the field, it employed a true experimental design, which provides added validity to its findings, and it examined two health economics and policy issues that are as important now as they were then: How do out-of-pocket costs affect the use of different kinds of services? and to what extent does charging for services ultimately affect people's health outcomes?

Answers did not come cheaply: The estimated cost of the experiment was $136 million in 1984 dollars (Manning et al. 1987), which translates to $282 million in 2008. Interestingly, the researchers who conducted the experiment concluded that its value far exceeded its cost, because upon its publication patient cost-sharing rates across the United States increased substantially. This supposedly reduced the "welfare loss" from unnecessarily comprehensive health insurance policies. They write,

[W]e believe that the benefits of this particular experiment greatly exceeded the costs. . . . Between 1982 and 1984, there was a remarkable increase in initial cost-sharing in the United States, at least for hospital services. For example, the number of major companies with first-dollar charges for hospital care rose from 30 to 63 percent in those two years, and the number of such firms with an annual deductible of $200 per person or more rose from 4 to 21 percent. Although it is impossible to know how much of this change can be attributed to the experimental results, the initial findings of the experiment were published . . . and given wide publicity in both the general and trade press. In certain instances a direct link between changes in cost-sharing and the experimental results can be made. (Manning et al. 1987, 272)

Because the experiment showed that increased patient cost sharing reduced medical expenditures—a proportion of which is the purported welfare loss due to excessive health insurance coverage—the researchers estimated that, under the most optimistic scenario, the eight-year experiment could have paid for itself in a week. That is, the publicity surrounding the experiment's findings resulted in employers and other insurers increasing their cost-sharing requirements by enough to exact a large societal savings. This would be true for two reasons. First, if the services forgone due to higher cost sharing are really so wasteful, then reducing their usage frees up these resources for society to use in other ways. Second, and more directly, to the extent that government healthcare programs raised cost-sharing requirements, government spending would fall.

Returning to the experiment's design, the sample of approximately 5,800 people came from six sites in four states. They participated for either three or five years. The main intervention involved random assignment into several experimental groups, all of whom received care through the fee-for-service medicine. (There was also an HMO component, not discussed here.)

The sites chosen for the study were Dayton, Ohio; Seattle, Washington; Fitchburg and Franklin counties, Massachusetts; and Charleston and Georgetown counties, South Carolina. Most people in these areas were eligible for inclusion in the study, including those who previously were uninsured. The main groups excluded were those over age 62 (because they would get Medicare coverage before the experiment ended) and the 3 percent of the population with the highest income, which was $25,000 in 1973 dollars, or the equivalent of $121,000 in 2008 dollars (because it is hard to justify providing insurance benefits to well-off people).

To ensure a representative and unbiased sample, it was necessary that those offered the option of participating in the experiment accept. Researchers were concerned that those who were randomly assigned to the experimental groups with the highest copayments might not want to participate when they found out about their assignments. To prevent this from happening, participants were given cash payments that ensured that their participation could not make them financially worse off. For example, if their previous insurance policy could have resulted in a maximum of $400 in annual expenditures, but they were assigned to an experimental group that could have resulted in $1,000 in spending, they were given $600 to ensure that they could be no worse off. Payments were dispensed monthly throughout participation, so that the money would be treated as normal income and would not bias the study results. If those receiving the payments instead earmarked the money to pay for healthcare, some of the results would be biased.[12]

There were ten primary experimental cells. These varied on two dimensions: the coinsurance rate the patient paid and the maximum amount of money per year that the patient could spend out of pocket. The coinsurance rates were 0, 25, 50, and 95 percent. The latter two groups were assigned out-of-pocket maximums of 5, 10, or 15 percent of family income per year, but that could never exceed $1,000. Those in the 0 percent coinsurance group had free care. All plans covered a comprehensive list of services including preventive care and prescription drugs. The few things not covered included nonpreventive orthodontia, cosmetic surgery, and outpatient psychotherapy visits in excess of 52 per person within a year (Manning et al. 1987).

One experimental group was called the "individual deductible" plan. In essence, it provided free inpatient care, but there was a $150 deductible (per person) charge for outpatient services. Researchers used this experimental group to examine whether hospital inpatient and physician outpatient services were substitutes or complements. To appreciate this, compare this group to those who received free care. If the two types of services are substitutes, then those in the individual deductible group would be expected to use more inpatient care than those with free care: Inpatient care was free to both groups, but since the individual deductible group had to pay for outpatient physician care, they would use less of that and substitute more hospital inpatient care. If, on the other hand, they used less inpatient care than the free care group, the services are complements: A rise in the price of outpatient physician care leads to less hospital use, consistent with a negative cross-price elasticity of demand.

Findings from the Experiment

Table 4.1 shows the effects of different coinsurance rates on utilization and annual expenditures for different types of services. The last column shows that the annual expenditures of people who had to pay 95 percent of charges were 28 percent less than those who paid nothing. From a policy standpoint, the finding that those facing a 25 percent coinsurance rate had expenditures that were 18 percent less than those with free care may be more relevant.

Numerous results from the study, summarized by Rice and Morrison (1994) are reprinted here with permission from Sage Publications.

Utilization and Costs

The study found that, in general, cost sharing affected the quantity of medical care demanded. Elasticities were approximately –0.2. With one exception

TABLE 4.1: Findings from the RAND Health Insurance Experiment

	Face-to-Face Visits	Outpatient Expenses (1984 $)	Admissions	Inpatient Dollars (1984 $)	Prob. Any Medical (%)	Prob. Any Inpatient (%)	Total Expenses (1984 $)	Adjusted Total Expenses (1984 $)
Free	4.55	340	.128	409	86.8	10.3	749	750
25%	3.33	260	.105	373	78.8	8.4	634	617
50%	3.03	224	.092	450	77.2	7.2	674	573
95%	2.73	203	.099	315	67.7	7.9	518	540

SOURCE: Adapted with permission from Manning, W. G., J. P. Newhouse, N. Duan, E. B. Keeler, A. Leibowitz, and M. S. Marquis. 1987, "Health Insurance and the Demand for Medical Care: Evidence from a Randomized Experiment." *American Economic Review* 77: 259.

(noted below), similar effects were found for both inpatient and outpatient care. More specifically, the HIE (Manning et al. 1987, except where otherwise indicated) found that:

- Coinsurance rates had a major effect on use and costs. Individuals with free care (i.e., a 0 percent coinsurance rate) incurred annual 1984 medical expenditures of $777 per capita, which were 23 percent higher than for those with a 25 percent coinsurance rate, and 46 percent higher than for those with a 95 percent rate.
- In contrast, there were no differences in utilization by groups with different out-of-pocket maximums. For this reason, almost all analyses were conducted by coinsurance category, grouping together the different out-of-pocket maximums.
- Deductibles, in and of themselves, reduced service usage. It was hypothesized that once people in the cost-sharing groups exceeded their annual maximums, they would seek care at the same rate as those with free care.
- Cost sharing reduced the number of medical care episodes for which treatment was sought. People with higher coinsurance rates were less likely to seek any inpatient or outpatient care. However, once care was sought, the amount received and its cost did not vary by the coinsurance. Thus, once an insured person enters the medical care system for an illness, coinsurance does not appear to affect the amount of care received or the prices charged (Keeler and Rolph 1983).
- People who received free inpatient care but had to pay for outpatient care did not substitute the former for the latter. If anything, the opposite was true. Those assigned to the individual deductible plan used less inpatient

care than those for whom inpatient and outpatient care were free, although this difference was not quite statistically significant. In economics terms, the cross-price elasticity of demand was negative, indicating that inpatient and outpatient care may be complements rather than substitutes. The most likely explanation is that people who have to share in the cost of outpatient services are less likely to enter the formal medical care system in the first place, and therefore less likely to be hospitalized.

- The effect of coinsurance was the same for children and adults with respect to outpatient care, but not with respect to inpatient care: There were no statistically significant relationships between coinsurance rates and the likelihood that a child would be hospitalized. In other words, cost sharing did not deter pediatric inpatient stays.
- Coinsurance reduced service usage and expenditures for all income groups. But it was difficult to discern the differential effect of alternative coinsurance rates by income level, because lower-income people had, by design, a lower out-of-pocket maximum.
- Coinsurance reduced service usage about equally for those who were healthy and those who were sick.
- Individuals subject to higher coinsurance rates reduced their demand for care in situations in which medical intervention was most likely to be effective as much as they did in situations in which medical care would likely provide the fewest benefits (Lohr et al. 1986), a finding further discussed later in the chapter.
- Coinsurance was a greater deterrent to low-income persons seeking care that was judged by researchers to be highly effective. For children of middle- and upper-income families, those assigned to coinsurance plans used 85 percent as much highly effective care as did similar individuals assigned to free care plans. However, among children from low-income families, those in coinsurance plans used only 56 percent as much highly effective care as did low-income children with free care. A related finding was that upper-income adults subject to coinsurance used 71 percent as much effective care as their counterparts with free care, while the corresponding figure for low-income adults was only 59 percent (Lohr et al. 1986).

Because those who faced cost sharing used fewer services than those with free care, it was possible to examine the effect of more generous health insurance policies on various measures of patient health. The HIE found that more medical care improved health status in few instances—the most notable exceptions being diastolic blood pressure and corrected vision. In interpreting these results, it must be kept in mind that the HIE only examined people with health insurance. Very different results emerge when examining the effect of owning *any* insurance on health status. Furthermore, it is possible that,

Health Status

by examining the effect of cost sharing on health status for only three to five years, the study could not detect changes that would manifest themselves only over a long period.

Specific findings of the HIE (Brook et al. 1983, except where otherwise indicated) that relate to health status included the following:

- Compared to those subject to coinsurance, adults who received free care did not fare better with respect to certain self-assessed health measures, including physical functioning, role function, social contacts, mental health, or health perceptions. Similarly, free care did not reduce cholesterol levels or weight.

- There were three areas in which those with free care experienced better outcomes: diastolic blood pressure, corrected vision, and risk of dying (for those who were at elevated risk). Having free care reduced diastolic blood pressure among the hypertensive or nearly hypertensive sample members by an average of 1.4 mm Hg; it improved corrected vision among those with uncorrected far vision problems from 20/25 to 20/24 (presumably because they were more likely to be diagnosed and to obtain eyeglasses); and it reduced the risk of dying among those at elevated risk by 10 percent (mainly due to the reduction in blood pressure).

- The reduction in blood pressure was achieved largely through additional physician contacts, during which problems were diagnosed and treatment was initiated. In addition, those with free care were more likely to reduce smoking and keep to a low-salt diet, and tended to follow medication regimens more closely (Keeler et al. 1985).

- As was the case with adults, there was little evidence that having free care improved children's health (Valdez et al. 1985). Among children of poor families who were at highest risk, however, those with free care were less likely to have anemia that those in the cost-sharing plans (8 percent versus 22 percent) (Valdez 1986).

- Low-income persons at elevated risk benefited most from free care. The reduction in diastolic blood pressure among low-income persons judged to be at elevated risk for hypertension was 3.3 mm Hg, versus only 0.4 mm Hg for people with higher incomes. Access to free care resulted in a statistically significant reduction in the risk of dying among low-income persons, although no risk reduction was detected among the group of higher-income persons who were also at the highest risk of dying.

- Low-income people in poor health with free care had the largest reduction in serious symptoms (Shapiro, Ware, and Sherbourne 1986).

- Similarly, cost sharing had a greater effect in deterring low-income individuals from receiving a general medical examination. Low-income adults in the cost-sharing groups received 46 percent fewer examinations than their counterparts with free care compared to a reduction of only 29 percent for other groups. For children of cost-sharing, low-income families, the comparison figures were 32 percent and 21 percent fewer examinations, respectively (Lohr et al. 1986).

There is one ostensible contradiction in these findings. If cost sharing reduces the use of highly effective care, why does it not also result in worsened health status? Lohr and colleagues (1986) list several possibilities: The effectiveness categories might not be valid; reductions in the use of highly effective care might manifest themselves only over a longer time period (i.e., after the study was completed); and those in the free care plans might have suffered from receiving too much unnecessary care.

The RAND HIE has been highly influential in health policy circles, due in large measure to its use of a true experimental design, which minimizes most potential research study biases. Experimental designs, however, do have their shortcomings, the primary one being the lack of generalizability to other settings.

Critique of the Experiment

Two major classifications encompass the *validity* of research studies: internal validity and external validity. Internal validity refers to how accurately study results represent what actually occurred in the specific setting being examined. For example, suppose a researcher studied 50 HMOs and found that they resulted in a 15 percent reduction in expenditures compared to fee-for-service medicine. The extent to which this study is internally valid is measured by how accurate this result is compared to the true (yet unknown) reduction in expenditures among that sample of HMOs. For a moment, let us say that the findings of this study appear to be reasonably accurate. But suppose the HMOs chosen were not representative of all HMOs, because they were all located on the West Coast of the United States. External validity refers to how well the results from a particular study can be generalized to other settings and/or populations.

With one possible exception, the health services research community generally agrees that the RAND Health Insurance Experiment had strong internal validity.[13] External validity is more of a concern. Issues include the exclusion of the elderly and the inclusion of only six sites in four states. Another concern is whether the study, which was conducted from 1974 to 1982, is still timely. During the 1980s and 1990s, hospital days per capita in the United States fell by 55 percent (Centers for Disease Control and Prevention 2001). If the study were conducted today, the results concerning the price responsiveness of hospital care might be much lower. Even if people had free hospital care, they might not want it or might be prevented from obtaining it.

An even greater threat to the external validity of the RAND study's utilization and cost findings exists. Consider the experimental design in the

RAND experiment. A random sample of individuals in six areas of the United States was chosen. Each site had an average of only about 1,000 study participants, many of whom were assigned to insurance plans that were equally generous as or more generous than those they had previously owned. Participants who were required to pay for care did indeed use fewer services. However, because only a small fraction of the population in each site participated—at most, 2 percent (Newhouse 1993a)—there was almost no effect on individual physicians' practices. Most doctors had, at most, only a handful of patients assigned to the high-coinsurance cells, so reductions in their service usage would not have markedly affected physician practice revenues. If everyone in an area had faced changing copayments—as might have occurred under various national health insurance proposals—the results might have been different. Suppose the plan called for coinsurance rates higher than the standard 20 percent level. Physicians might respond to the initial fall in business by inducing patient demand for services. This response could take the form of providing more follow-up services, more complex services, or even more surgery. The experiment examined only patient responses, not physician responses, to cost sharing.

The converse may also be true. Suppose a national health insurance plan removes all coinsurance. Subsequent demand may not rise as much as the RAND study would lead us to believe, for two reasons: (1) Physicians may have less financial need than before to induce demand, and (2) governmental and private payers are likely to introduce other measures (e.g., tighter utilization review, expenditure targets, global budgeting) to quell the initial increase in patient demand.

The RAND study's inability to deal with provider (and policymakers' regulatory) response has raised criticism since the inception of the experiment. In a discussion of these issues in 1974 (53–54), when the experiment began, James Hester and Irving Leveson wrote,

> The utilization of health services is the result of a complex balancing between demand for health care and the supply system that provides it. While the changing needs of one individual or small group will not affect this overall balance, the large-scale shifts in quantity and source of medical care that would result from a major national change in the financing of health care certainly would. Large changes in aggregate demand can be expected to produce substantial changes whose exact form is strongly influenced by specific administrative and financial regulations. . . . These changes will, in turn, feed back into the overall use patterns and costs, and influence again the users of the system.

In response, Joseph Newhouse (1974) noted that the study was not "designed to replicate what would happen if various health insurance proposals were enacted into law," and furthermore, that it "deliberately selected sites that vary considerably with respect to the amount of stress on the delivery system" (236–37). That is, the six sites varied with respect to provider-to-population ratios.

A number of economists, mostly from outside the United States, have provided similar criticisms of the generalizability of the RAND findings.[14] Testing this issue directly is difficult.[15] Thus, the RAND study results are more safely used to indicate the effect of cost sharing on patients' demand for services (independent of any resulting provider response) than to indicate ways in which overall utilization of services will change in response to large-scale policy initiatives concerning changes in patient cost sharing.

A full quarter century after the last subject left the experiment, John Nyman (2007) wrote an article that questioned its results and interpretation. He asserts that individuals assigned to the experimental groups with high cost sharing were less likely to agree to stay in the experiment if they anticipated, or later faced, high health expenditures. Nyman points out that fewer than 0.5 percent of those assigned to free care left the experiment early, compared to nearly 7 percent of those who faced cost sharing. This would mean that the experiment (1) underestimated the impact of cost sharing because some of the highest users were not included and, perhaps more importantly, (2) underestimated the impact of more medical care on improving health status. Such an interpretation calls into question one of the main study results: that cost sharing does little to harm health status.

The HIE's chief researchers were quick to respond (Newhouse et al. 2008), providing several reasons in defense of the experiment's findings, including the following:

- It would not be in a person's or family's financial interest to leave the experiment if they became sick.
- Other benign factors better explain the higher disenrollment of those in the cost-sharing groups.
- The HIE researchers had already analyzed attrition rates and found no patterns of concern.
- For the experiment's results to have been as biased as Nyman suggests, those dropping out of the experiment would have to have had extraordinarily high hospitalization rates upon leaving the study.
- The experiment's findings are consistent with other, nonexperimental research findings in the literature.

As this debate was occurring at the time the current chapter was being written, there is, as yet, no further discussion in the literature.

Newhouse and colleagues (2008) are right to point out that subsequent, nonexperimental research on the effect of patient cost sharing on the quantity of services demanded shows results consistent with those of the HIE. Most of the recent research has focused on prescription drugs, finding similar

More Recent Empirical Research on Demand

elasticities of demand. Of particular importance is the typical finding that when people have to pay more out of pocket for medications, their adherence falls (Chernew et al. 2008; Thiebaud, Patel, and Nichol 2008).

Perhaps the largest study with a major focus on demand after the HIE was the Medical Outcomes Study. It was carried out over four years, from 1986 to 1990, and followed those with chronic illness, including seniors, for 12 to 18 months. This differs from the HIE, which included a cross-section of the population under the age of 65. One key finding was that cost sharing reduced use of services for minor and serious symptoms (Wong et al. 2001). Not surprisingly, higher cost-sharing requirements reduced service use more than low cost-sharing requirements, but both reduced usage compared to free care. The odds of those with minor symptoms and low cost sharing using services were 20 percent lower compared with those with minor symptoms and free care. The odds for high cost sharing (compared to free care) were 61 percent lower.

There have been several reviews of the health services demand literature since the HIE (Rice and Morrison 1994). Ringel and colleagues (2002) find that most estimates center on an elasticity estimate of -0.17. Though this is technically inelastic (because the absolute value of that number is less than 1.0), it is reasonable to conclude that, considering the effect of cost sharing in the HIE shown in Table 4.1, service usage is reasonably responsive to price. That is, what economists consider inelastic often seems to be price responsive, at least in the healthcare area.

Moral Hazard, Part II: Mark Pauly's Model of Welfare Loss from "Excessive" Health Insurance

Some health economists have long contended that insured people in the United States and other developed countries are "overinsured," which results in a societal *welfare loss*. That is, people have more insurance than is optimal for them or for society at large. This might seem odd to the noneconomist, given the number of uninsured people in the United States. Moreover, we have already shown that a risk-averse person would do better by purchasing fairly priced health insurance.

The Welfare-Loss Argument

The microeconomics concept of *consumer surplus* is essential to understanding the debate about welfare loss from health insurance. In Chapter 2, we introduced the assumption that consumers try to maximize their utility through the bundle of goods they purchase. They therefore seek only those goods whose marginal utilities exceeded the market price. Consumers are often in the fortunate position where the market price of a good they seek is less than the maximum amount they would be willing to pay. The difference between how much consumers are willing to pay for a good or service and what it actually costs the consumer to purchase is called *consumer surplus*. This concept, first used in the mid-1800s by Jules Dupuit, a French engineer, to determine the value of railroad bridges, was popularized in the English-speaking world by Alfred Marshall (Ng 1979; Parkin 2007).

The calculation of consumer surplus is illustrated in Figure 4.3. Suppose the market price of a nurse practitioner (NP) visit is $30, at which price Paul is willing to purchase four per year (point B on demand curve D_1). Note, however, that he was willing to pay much more for the first three visits: $40 for the third visit, $50 for the second, and $60 for the first. Thus, in purchasing four NP visits, Paul has earned a surplus. He was willing to pay $180 for the four visits but only had to pay $120 (4 × $30), so he has earned a consumer surplus of $60. This is illustrated by triangle ABC in Figure 4.1.

The concept of consumer surplus comes into play not so much at the individual level as in the aggregate. If we add together all surpluses received by all consumers, we obtain the total consumer surplus, which is the difference between the value consumers receive from a good and how much they have to pay for it. Economists use this tool to determine whether society should embark on a publicly financed investment or project, and in applications such as calculating the welfare loss from excess health insurance.

Despite the fact that moral hazard in medical care is rational economic behavior, many economists are nevertheless troubled by its existence. This is because when people are fully insured, they may demand services that only

FIGURE 4.3: Derivation of Consumer Surplus

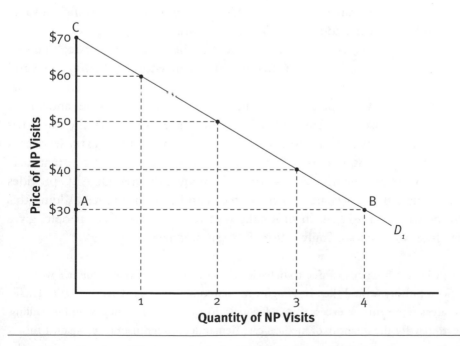

provide a small amount of benefit. But these services are likely to cost just as much as any other services. The benefits people derive from the purchase of these marginal services might be swamped by their cost.

In his famous article, Mark Pauly (1968) showed that a country might be better off without compulsory, government-sponsored health insurance. This was in response to an equally famous article by Kenneth Arrow (1963b), who contended that government might be justified in providing such insurance out of tax dollars if a private market did not exist.

Pauly's argument is as follows: Suppose a person is uninsured and has a 50 percent chance of staying well during a given year, a 25 percent chance of being mildly sick, and a 25 percent chance of being very sick. Further suppose that his medical expenditures will be zero if he is well, $50 if he is mildly sick, and $200 if he is very sick. These expenditure levels are indicated by the vertical axis and vertical demand curves D'_2 and D'_3 in Figure 4.4. Consequently, the expected value of his annual medical costs will be $62.50 [(0.5 × $0) + (0.25 × $50) + (0.25 × $200)]. Now suppose he has health insurance that pays 100 percent of costs. Assume that he continues to use no services if he is not sick, but spends $150 (instead of $50) if he is mildly sick, and $300 (instead of $200) if he is very sick. These expenditure levels are shown by the vertical axis and diagonal demand curves D_2 and D_3 in Figure 4.4. In this instance, the expected value of his annual costs will be $112.50 [(0.5 × $0) + (0.25 × $150) + (0.25 × 300)].

Pauly's point is that the person might be better off with no insurance and paying $62.50 a year out-of-pocket than with government-sponsored insurance and paying $112.50 in taxes. The person may have used more services with the insurance, but the services used might not be of sufficient value to him to justify the additional $50 in expenditures.

We can also use Figure 4.4 to calculate the welfare loss of health insurance for this particular person. Recall that in conventional theory, a demand curve shows the marginal utility associated with alternative quantities purchased. A mildly sick person who is provided insurance coverage, and whose expenditures rise from $50 to $150, accrues benefits equal to the lower triangle AGB. However, the cost to society of producing these extra services is indicated by the square AGBC (for convenience, we assume a constant marginal cost of producing services, MC). Consequently, triangle ABC provides an estimate of the welfare loss associated with health insurance. Adding this to the triangle DEF, which shows the welfare loss for very sick people, gives the total welfare loss. Pauly (1968, 534) summarizes,

> [T]he inefficiency loss due to behavior under insurance, if that insurance were compulsory, would then be roughly measured by triangles *ABC* and *DEF*. These areas represent the excess that individuals do pay over what they would be willing to pay for the quantity of medical care demanded under insurance. Against this loss must be offset the utility gain from having these uncertain expenses insured,

FIGURE 4.4: Pauly's Analysis of Welfare Loss

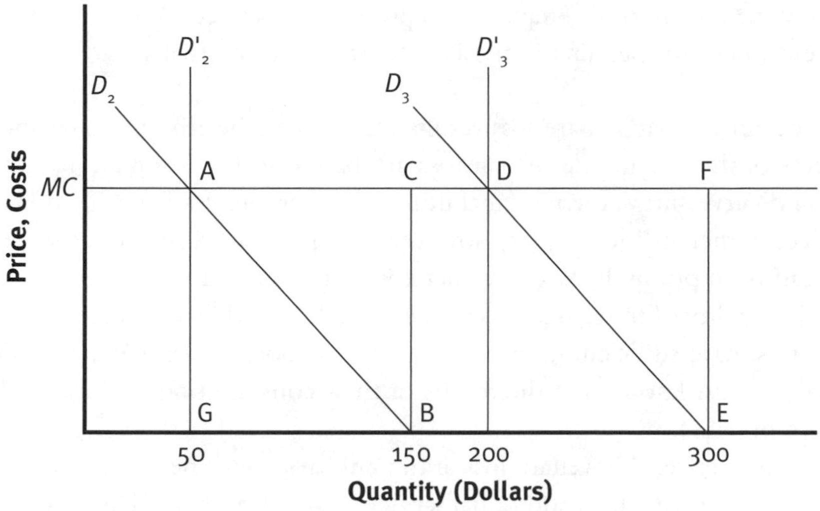

SOURCE: Reprinted with permission from Pauly, M. 1968. "The Economics of Moral Hazard: Comment." *American Economic Review* 58: 531–37.

but the net change in utility from a compulsory purchase of this "insurance" could well be negative.

The moral hazard that results from the possession of health insurance has made many economists conclude that a societal welfare loss is associated with the ownership of too much health insurance. This is an important conclusion; it implies that a society is not best off if its members have more health insurance than is deemed to be optimal. In a survey of U.S. health economists conducted in 2005, 65 percent agreed with the statement, "Third-party payment results in patients using services whose costs exceed their benefits, and this excess of costs over benefits amounts to at least 5 percent of total health care expenditures" (Morrisey and Cawley 2008).

A number of researchers have computed the magnitude of this welfare loss for the United States as a whole.[16] One well-known set of estimates was calculated based on the results of the RAND Health Insurance Experiment. Manning and colleagues (1987) used these results to estimate a total welfare loss of $37 billion to $60 billion, which represented between 19 percent and 30 percent of total national health expenditures.

A more recent set of welfare-loss estimates—also based on the RAND Health Insurance Experiment findings—come from a study by Feldman and Dowd (1991). This study provides a number of refinements over the previous one; in particular, it takes into account the fact that risk-averse individuals derive utility from being insured. It nevertheless concludes that the welfare loss associated with excess health insurance far outweighs the utility conveyed by owning insurance. Taking into account these conflicting components, the net welfare loss varied from $33 billion to $109 billion in 1984 dollars, depending on the assumptions employed, representing between 9 percent and 28 percent of health spending in the United States during that year.[17]

Critique of the Welfare-Loss Argument

The argument that welfare loss results from excess health insurance and estimates of the magnitude of that loss are based on the assumption that the demand curve shows the marginal utility a person derives from an additional service. Earlier in the chapter, however, we questioned that interpretation. Several assumptions have to be met for a demand curve to represent the marginal utility of purchases: Consumers must act rationally (Assumption 4), they must have sufficient information to make good choices (Assumption 2), and they must know what the results of their consumption decisions will be (Assumption 3).

In essence, the welfare-loss argument says consumers must be able to determine how much an additional service is worth to them. They then compare this number to the price of the service to determine if it is worth their while to purchase it. People who have insurance will have to pay less; consequently, they will be more likely to purchase a service that conveys little utility. The difference between the cost of the service and the utility received equals the welfare loss from the purchase of that service.

We need to consider, then, whether consumers can accurately estimate the marginal utility they receive from additional services. A method of testing this ability exists, but the method has some problems.

Welfare loss occurs because consumers with health insurance have an incentive to purchase additional services (compared with what they would purchase without insurance) that provide little benefit to them. We can determine whether that occurs by observing the kinds of services that consumers forgo when they are provided with less comprehensive insurance coverage. Our point is to carefully examine whether these services really seem to be of use to them. It is possible that these are important services. If this is true, it would cast doubt on whether there is a welfare loss when well-insured people actually do buy them.

The nature of this test is clarified in Figure 4.5, which is taken from an earlier work of one of the authors (Rice 1992). The horizontal line indicates the marginal cost (MC) of producing a service, which can be viewed as the cost to society—that is, the resources expended in providing a service. In a competitive market, this will equal its price (P). The curved line, which is a demand curve, shows the marginal utility of each additional service. At a zero price—that is, with comprehensive insurance—the consumer will demand Q_0 services; the last such service provides little utility.

Now suppose two types of services are available—those that are highly effective (HE) and those that have low effectiveness (LE). Further suppose

FIGURE 4.5: Change in Demand for Services of Differing Effectiveness

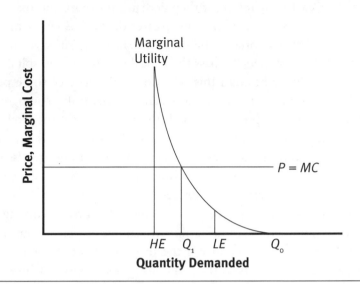

SOURCE: Reprinted from *Journal of Health Economics,* Thomas Rice, "An Alternative Framework for Evaluating Welfare Losses in the Healthcare Market," ©1992, with permission, from Elsevier Limited.

that the person no longer has health insurance, and his demand for care has declined from Q_0 to Q_1. Figure 4.5 demonstrates that the person would forgo the low-effectiveness service, *LE*, because its benefits are now outweighed by its costs. But he would still purchase service *HE* because its benefits exceed its costs, even in the absence of insurance coverage. If people actually behaved as the figure predicts, then we could confidently say the demand curve for medical care shows the marginal utility consumers obtain from additional services. This, in turn, would provide support for the welfare-loss estimates we discussed earlier.

A problem has been raised with this test. John Nyman (1999a, 811–12, italics added) notes that

> economic theory predicts that, if there were two procedures that were alike on every dimension except effectiveness (*and the effectiveness of the two procedures was known and greater effectiveness was valued by consumers*), the quantity demanded of the more effective procedure would exceed the quantity demanded of the less effective procedure, at any given price. The empirical evidence supporting this prediction is found in the many patients who bypass their local community hospital to travel to the Mayo Clinic (or any other similarly highly regarded medical center) to receive their coronary bypass or other procedure. . . . Given that the quantity demanded of high effectiveness procedures exceeds that of low effectiveness procedures other things equal, economic theory would predict that as the price rises, both quantities would decline, consistent with the Lohr et al. findings.

The key assumption in the above quotation is that when consumers are faced with choices between alternative medical procedures, they know the effectiveness of each. Therefore, if they demand more of one than another, they know that the procedure with the greater demand is either more effective or cheaper than the other. The only evidence Nyman gives to support this belief is that consumers "bypass their local community hospital to travel to the Mayo Clinic." Although this is undoubtedly true of some people, it provides little evidence that consumers can systematically compare the effectiveness of alternative procedures with their cost. It is more likely that, as empirical evidence (some of which we discussed earlier in this chapter) suggests, consumers were never aware that certain procedures are less effective than others, and never made utility-maximizing comparisons between the effectiveness and prices of alternative procedures.

The problem with implementing this test, of course, is coming up with a way to determine the marginal utility consumers receive from a service. The proxy used here is a measure of the medical effectiveness of a service, as judged by medical experts. Although consumers and experts may differ in what they think is important, common sense tells us consumers would prefer the most effective services.

As part of the RAND Health Insurance Experiment, Lohr and colleagues (1986) grouped services into categories based on their expected medical effectiveness:

Group 1. Highly effective treatment by medical care system
Group 2. Quite effective treatment by medical care system
Group 3. Less effective treatment by medical care system
Group 4. Medical care rarely effective or self-care effective

The category into which a particular service falls is shown in Table 4.2, which is taken from the study. Lohr and colleagues (1986, S32) found that

> cost sharing was generally just as likely to lower use when care is thought to be highly effective as when it is thought to be only rarely effective, [nor] was there any obvious trend suggesting that cost sharing would deter care seeking more as one moved "down" the effectiveness ranking.

They concluded that

> cost sharing did not lead to rates of care seeking that were more "appropriate" from a clinical perspective. That is, cost sharing did not seem to have a selective effect in prompting people to forego care only or mainly in circumstances when such care probably would be of relatively little value. (Lohr et al.1986, S36)

Another component of the RAND study reached a similar conclusion regarding the effect of coinsurance on appropriate versus inappropriate hospitalization (Siu et al. 1986).

TABLE 4.2: Medical Effectiveness Groupings in the Lohr and Colleagues Study

Group 1: Highly Effective Treatment by Medical Care System

Medical care highly effective: acute conditions
  Eyes—conjunctivitis
  Otitis media, acute
  Acute sinusitis
  Strep throat
  Acute lower respiratory infections (acute bronchitis)
  Pneumonia
  Vaginitis and cervicitis
  Nonfungal skin infections
  Trauma—fractures
  Trauma—lacerations, contusions, abrasions

Medical care highly effective: acute or chronic conditions
  Sexually transmitted disease or pelvic inflammatory disease
  Malignant neoplasm, including skin
  Gout
  Anemias
  Enuresis
  Seizure disorders
  Eyes—strabismus, glaucoma, cataracts
  Otitis media, not otherwise specified
  Chronic sinusitis
  Peptic and nonpeptic ulcer disease
  Hernia
  Urinary tract infection
  Skin—dermatophytoses

Medical care highly effective: chronic conditions
  Thyroid disease
  Diabetes
  Otitis media, chronic
  Hypertension and abnormal blood pressure
  Cardiac arrythmias
  Congestive heart failure
  Chronic bronchitis, chronic obstructive pulmonary disease
  Rheumatic disease (rheumatoid arthritis)

Group 2: Quite Effective Treatment by Medical Care System

Diarrhea and gastroenteritis (infectious)
Benign and unspecified neoplasm
Thrombophlebitis
Hemorrhoids
Hay fever (chronic rhinitis)
Acute middle respiratory infections (tracheitis, laryngitis)
Asthma
Chronic enteritis, colitis
Perirectal conditions
Menstrual and menopausal disorders
Acne
Adverse effects of medicinal agents
Other abnormal findings

Group 3: Less Effective Treatment by Medical Care System

Hypercholesterolemia, hyperlipidemia
Mental retardation
Peripheral neuropathy, neuritis, and sciatica
Ears—deafness
Vertiginous syndromes
Other heart disease
Edema
Cerebrovascular disease
Varicose veins of lower extremities
Prostatic hypertrophy, prostatitis
Other cervical disease
Lymphadenopathy
Vehicular accidents
Other injuries and adverse effects

TABLE 4.2: *Continued*

Group 4: Medical Care Rarely Effective or Self-Care Effective	
Medical care rarely effective	Headaches
Viral exanthems	Cough
Hypoglycemia	Acute URI
Obesity	Throat pain
Chest pain	Irritable colon
Shortness of breath	Abdominal pain
Hypertrophy of tonsils or adenoids	Nausea or vomiting
Chronic cystic breast disease	Constipation
(nonmalignant)	Other rashes and skin conditions
Debility and fatigue (malaise)	Degenerative joint disease
Over-the-counter or self-care effective	Low back pain diseases and syndromes
Influenza (viral)	Bursitis or synovitis and fibrositis or
Fever	myalgia
	Acute sprains and strains
	Muscle problems

SOURCE: Data used with permission from Lohr, K. N., R. H. Brook, C. J. Kamberg, G. Goldberg, A. Leibowitz, J. Keesey, D. Reboussin, and J. P. Newhouse. 1986. "Effect of Cost Sharing on Use of Medically Effective and Less Effective Care." *Medical Care* 24 (Supplement): S31–S38.

A recent study by Hibbard, Greene, and Tusler (2008) reached a similar conclusion to those of Lohr and colleagues (1986) and Siu and colleagues (1986). The authors studied employees in a large firm, some of whom joined a high-deductible consumer-directed health plan (these are discussed in more detail later in the chapter). They used a list developed by the state of Oregon to classify acute and chronic physician office visits as high-priority or low-priority. If the traditional economic theory held, those who joined the high-deductible plan should have used fewer low-priority services. That was not the case, however; their service usage declined by about the same amount for all types of services.

Much research has been conducted since the HIE, albeit rarely with a true experimental design. Nearly all studies have found that when patients have to pay out of pocket, they use fewer services. The concern continues to be, however—as Lohr and colleagues (1986) showed—that people are forgoing services that will improve their health, and furthermore, that those with lower incomes are more likely to forgo such services.

Trivedi, Rakowski, and Ayanian (2008, 375) looked at the use of mammograms by about half a million Medicare beneficiaries ages 65–69, a group the HIE excluded. Examining Medicare managed care plans, they found a large increase between 2001 and 2004 in the proportion of such health plans that required modest copayments of $10 or more or coinsurance of 10 percent or more. They found that

[b]iennial screening rates were 8.3 percentage points lower in cost-sharing plans than in plans with full coverage. . . . The effect of cost sharing was magnified among women residing in areas of lower income or educational levels. Screening rates decreased by 5.5 percentage points in plans that instituted cost sharing and increased by 3.4 percentage points in matched control plans that retained full coverage.

Other research on Medicare beneficiaries has shown concern regarding cost sharing and the use of prescription drugs. Rice and Matsuoka (2004) reviewed five studies where it was possible to directly assess the impact of cost sharing on mortality, and 15 others where it could be inferred indirectly by examining the appropriate use of medications. In two of the five studies, they found that cost sharing led to higher incidence of death; in the other three there were no effects. Of the 15 studies, 12 showed evidence that cost-sharing led to less usage of appropriate medications, and three showed no effects.

This phenomenon is not confined to older adults. A study of more than half a million employees of 30 employers found that increased copayments led to substantial reductions in the use of prescription drugs for those with acute care illnesses, with reduced impacts for those with chronic illnesses (Goldman et al. 2004). The doubling of copayments reduces use of nonsteroidal anti-inflammatory drugs (NSAIDs) by 45 percent and antihistamines by 44 percent, for example. "Still," the authors conclude, "significant increases in co-payments raise concern about adverse health consequences because of the large price effects, especially among diabetic patients" (2344). Among diabetics, doubling copayments reduced use of medications by 23 percent. A recent study of one large employer showed that enrollment in a high-deductible consumer-directed insurance plan led to a large decrease in filling prescriptions among those who had high blood pressure or high cholesterol (Greene et al. 2008).

What does this mean for the theory of welfare loss from excess health insurance? The Lohr and colleagues (1986) study shows that consumers who face cost sharing reduce demand across the board, both for highly effective care and less effective care. More recent studies show reductions in the use of preventive services and drugs that can provide significant benefits to patients. But the welfare-loss argument rests on the supposition that the services foregone as a result of cost sharing will *only* be those that provide less utility; the RAND Health Insurance Experiment shows this is not the case, and the newer studies imply the same. Only services that provide the lower level of benefits (such as service *LE* in Figure 4.5) should be included in the welfare-loss calculation. More generally, welfare-loss calculations are hard to defend when consumers cannot accurately value the benefits and costs of the medical services they consume (Rice 1992, 89).

The view that patient demand curves show how much consumers buy at different prices, but not necessarily the utility they derive from such services, runs against the grain of conventional economic theory. It is not unique among economists, however. Randall Ellis and Thomas McGuire (1993, 142) wrote,

> [W]e are skeptical that the observed demand can be interpreted as reflecting "socially efficient" consumption, [so] we interpret the demand curve in a more limited way, as an empirical relationship between the degree of cost sharing and quantity of use demanded by the patient.

As we noted earlier, the argument against the welfare-loss calculations depends in part on a close correspondence between consumer preferences and experts' opinions of the medical effectiveness of alternative services. It seems likely that consumers would not want to use services that experts find to be of little value. However, we must consider the validity of Lohr and colleagues' categories, shown in Table 4.2. Feldman and Dowd (1993) note one example of a potential problem: Medical care is considered highly effective for the treatment of strep throat, but rarely effective for throat pain (although self-care is effective). Others have noted that it seems odd to include chest pain in the category where medical care is rarely effective. These concerns are important, but until a study exists that takes them into consideration, Lohr and colleagues' findings from the RAND study, in conjunction with the theory developed in Figure 4.5, must at least give us pause before we accept the conventional welfare-loss methodology and estimates.

There is a second argument against the association of welfare loss with excessive health insurance, developed and reported by John Nyman (1999b, 2002, 2007) in a book and a series of articles. Unlike the critique we just discussed, which assumes consumers face information problems, Nyman's applies even if consumers are well-informed.

The traditional economic model, from which welfare loss can be derived, assumes a single benefit of insurance to the purchaser: Risk-averse people can raise their utility by purchasing fairly priced insurance (as shown in Section 4.3). Nyman posits another, potentially even greater benefit of insurance: It allows people to afford expensive procedures that otherwise would be too costly to obtain. The conventional analysis implies that if insurance leads to more usage as a result of lower out-of-pocket price, there must be a welfare loss (e.g., triangles ABC and DEF in Figure 4.6). But Nyman says that if the cause of the higher usage is not the lower price but the ability to afford a service that was previously unaffordable, there is a gain, not a loss, in welfare.

He illustrates this with an example. Suppose a mastectomy costs $20,000 and breast reconstructive surgery costs another $20,000, for a total cost of $40,000. Now suppose an uninsured woman has breast cancer and can afford the surgery but not the reconstruction. In contrast, assume the woman has insurance and can afford both. Is there a welfare loss associated with the latter? Under the conventional theory there would be, since the woman demanded it when the (after-insurance) price fell. But Nyman (2007) argues that it is not the reduction in price but the increase in effective income that generates the demand for reconstructive surgery. Insurance has effectively raised the woman's income by making a $40,000 service affordable, and she chooses to spend this newfound wealth on reconstruction. He provides a hypothetical test: If, instead of paying her healthcare provider directly, the insurance company wrote her a $20,000 check, and she chose to use the money for the reconstruction rather than any other purpose, then purchasing the service is evidence of a gain rather than a loss in welfare.

In 2006, the United States spent $2.1 trillion on healthcare, with per capita expenditures exceeding $7,000 (Catlin et al. 2008). This constituted 16 percent of the national income. The last time comparable figures were available, for 2004, the U.S. proportion was 32 percent higher than the next highest, Switzerland, and 44 percent higher than third-ranked Germany (Anderson, Frogner, and Reinhardt 2007).

Policy Implications of the Critique

Where Is the Waste in Medical Care?

It is hard to fathom just how much money $2.1 trillion is. It may help to imagine 2.1 trillion one dollar bills lined up end to end. They would stretch from the earth to the sun, and back again.[18]

Economists are quick to point out that the figures $2.1 trillion and 16 percent do not provide any direct evidence that we are spending too much for medical care in the United States. Maybe, they contend, people really get more out of this high level of medical spending than they would from spending their money in alternative ways.[19] Indeed, some economists have claimed that the spending that results from new medical technologies passes a cost-benefit analysis with flying colors.

Since the early work of John Wennberg and colleagues,[20] experts have agreed that many of the services provided are not medically necessary. Although little consensus has been reached on the magnitude of unnecessary services used, the rate for some procedures is estimated to be as high as 30 percent (Leape 1989; Schuster, McGlynn, and Brook 1998). As a result, one of the leading health services research efforts now being conducted is determining what services are and are not medically effective. This research is manifesting itself in two major forms: by disseminating and using practice guidelines for various medical conditions, and by "profiling" individual physicians' service provision rates. Managed care plans can then use the profiles to assess physicians' medical decision making.

Where, then, is the waste in medical care? Under the traditional theory, the source is clear: Patients with comprehensive insurance coverage demand too many services. The alternative presented here is that most of the waste is in the provision of services that do little or nothing to improve the patients' health.[21]

These alternative theories are not totally contradictory—some services could be deemed wasteful under both approaches (e.g., a person with complete insurance demands a service that brings him little utility and that experts believe will have little or no effect on his health). Nevertheless, the policy implications of the two approaches differ. The conventional theory suggests policies that make the user of services more sensitive to price. In contrast, if the problem is the provision of services that are not useful, policies should target service providers.

The idea of pursuing supply-side rather than demand-side policies will be explored in greater detail in Chapter 10. The key point here is that most public policies aimed at controlling costs in the United States—and in the rest of the world—are aimed at the supply side rather than the demand side. This contradicts conventional economic theory, which suggests consumers should decide what services they receive, because only they can measure the utility a given service will bring.

The supply-side policies that are most common now—putting physicians at risk through capitation or other forms of incentive reimbursement, such as "pay for performance," utilization review, and technology controls and global budgets in many countries—are designed to influence the types of services provided without consulting the patient. Thus, the policies are based, in part, on the belief that someone other than the consumer is the best judge of what medical services should be delivered.

Some analysts—economists as well as practitioners of other disciplines—believe managed care strategies based on capitating health plans offer the best hope for controlling U.S. health costs. These strategies are aimed at changing what services are provided rather than changing consumer demand. In the HMO approach to cost containment, copayments have historically been *lower* than patient payments in fee-for-service medicine. If these strategies are designed to reduce waste, it seems clear that policymakers believe waste is generated through the provision of unnecessary services, far more so than through excess demand by patients. And if this is the case in the United States, it must be even more so in other developed countries, where copayments tend to be lower, and where almost all cost-control activities are focused on providers. Chapter 10 and the appendix discuss the policies and experiences of some of these countries.

Should Patient Cost Sharing Be Encouraged, or Should We Use Other Policies?

The thrust of the welfare-loss literature is that more patient cost sharing will benefit society. We can modify Figure 4.4 to show how institution of a patient coinsurance rate would reduce the welfare loss of complete health insurance coverage. In Figure 4.4, the triangles ABC and DEF showed the original welfare loss from full insurance. With the institution of coinsurance, CI, it would be cut to the sum of triangles AHI and DJK in Figure 4.6.

Analysis of this sort can be dangerous, as Robert Evans (1984, 49) notes: "The welfare burden is minimized when there is no insurance at all."

FIGURE 4.6: The Impact of Coinsurance on Welfare Loss

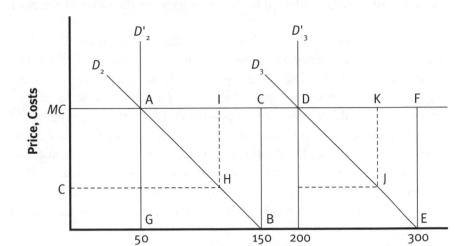

Conventional analysis will always show that higher patient cost-sharing requirements will result in a more efficient health system (Reinhardt 1992). By this rationale, the U.S. system is more efficient than the Canadian system or any of a number of European systems, not because of a comparison of outcomes to costs, but simply because the United States imposes patient copayments, which in turn reduces utilization. Although this conclusion might seem surprising, it follows directly from the viewpoint that the demand curve provides our best estimate of the benefits derived from the use of additional services.

Non-U.S. health economists have been more willing to accept that a healthcare system can be efficient even if patient cost sharing is low. Canadian economist Robert Evans and colleagues (1983) argue that the case for patient cost sharing is difficult to make if four questions can be answered in the affirmative:

- Is the service really health related?
- Does the service work?
- Is the service medically necessary?
- Is there no better alternative?

If a service passes all of these tests, "the standard argument against user charges, that they tax the sick, seems wholly justified" (Evans et al. 1983).

Two broad arguments can be made against employing patient cost sharing as a cost-control technique. First, of course, is the issue of equity.

Cost sharing is more burdensome on people with lower incomes. In this regard, one of the key findings of the RAND study was that the people whose health was most adversely affected by cost sharing were the sick and the poor (Newhouse 1993b).

The other issue concerns efficiency. Specifically, are there alternative ways to encourage efficiency and contain health costs besides cost sharing? Ellis and McGuire (1993, 135) have argued the benefits of what they deem a "neglected" area of reform, supply-side cost sharing, "which seeks to alter the incentives of healthcare workers to provide certain services." (One could make a compelling argument that this has not been neglected by analysts in other countries, however.) Supply-side policies, Ellis and McGuire argue, can achieve the same desired quantity as demand-side levers. Furthermore, they claim that supply-side cost sharing is clearly superior to traditional demand-side policies in one key respect: It does not result in a financial burden on patients.

Their main example is from the prospective payment system Medicare and some other payers use to reimburse hospitals in the United States. Because hospitals receive a fixed payment (based on diagnosis) irrespective of how long the patient stays, the hospital shares in the cost of additional usage. Just as a patient has an incentive to use less when he or she has to pay part of the price, in the case of supply-side cost sharing, the provider has a financial incentive to reduce service usage.

Nevertheless, economists tend to focus most of their attention on the role of the price the consumer faces. One possible reason, noted by Milton Friedman (1962), is that the focus on price is part of an overall division of labor between economics and the other social sciences. If each of the social sciences were equally influential in determining health policy, this would not present a problem. But economics seems to be paramount, so it is incumbent on health economists to consider other health policy levers as well.

Although one could imagine many possible policy levers—and indeed, we discuss several supply-side levers in Chapter 10—the focus here will be on a single, nonprice, demand-side lever: influencing behavior. Curiously, economists who are concerned about the purported welfare loss due to excess health insurance often do not focus on more tangible losses, such as the cost of "bad" behaviors (smoking, alcohol consumption, drug abuse, etc.). This is not to say health economists do not study such issues—they do—rather that these costs are not seen as welfare losses for society. This is particularly curious given the estimated sizes of these losses. In the United States alone, an estimated $181 billion was lost for drug abuse in 2002 (Executive Office of the President 2004), and $157 billion was lost in 1999 for smoking (*Morbidity and Mortality Weekly Report* 2002). These figures far exceed all estimates of the welfare losses from health insurance.

Sociologists and psychologists are concerned with the factors that influence behavior and the ways in which it can be altered. The field of health education focuses on how behaviors can be changed. David Mechanic (1979, 11) has stated,

> Reducing needs involves the prevention of illness or diminishing patients' psychological dependence on the medical encounter for social support or other secondary advantages. Reducing desire for services requires changing people's views of the value of different types of medical care, making them more aware of the real costs of service in relation to the benefits received, and legitimizing alternatives for dealing with many problems.

Changing behavior is not easy, however. Mechanic (1979, 12) writes, "it is prudent to recognize the difficulty of the task, the forces working against change, and the depths of ignorance concerning the origins of these behaviors and the ways in which they can best be modified."

The point is not that economists need to conduct this research. Rather, (1) health economists who are proposing policy need to recognize policy levers like these, and (2) relying largely on conventional tools such as demand elasticities to recommend policy is inappropriate once some of the special characteristics of the health market are recognized.

Another generally accepted tool in the health economist's toolbox is the belief that the magnitude of patient coinsurance rates should be directly related to the elasticity of demand. More specifically, services for which consumers show a high demand elasticity should have higher cost-sharing requirements than services for which consumers are less price sensitive. As we shall see, the basis for this argument is similar to the one economists use to argue a welfare loss associated with excessive amounts of health insurance.

Should People Pay More for Price-Elastic Services?

Ellis and McGuire (1993, 137) summarize the issue as follows:

> [T]he optimal insurance literature has been based on the assumption that the demand curve correctly reflects the marginal benefits of services. As a result, it has held that the greater the demand response to what consumers/patients must pay for health care, the higher should be demand-side cost-sharing.

Why is this the case? Suppose one views the demand curve as indicating the marginal benefits a consumer derives from a service. In Figure 4.7, point P_1 shows the price of medical care in the absence of health insurance, and point P_2 shows the price when insurance pays 80 percent of medical costs. Thus, at point C, which represents the quantity of medical care purchased with insurance, the marginal benefit derived from the last service is only one-fifth as great as at point A, where the person is uninsured—since the price paid is equal to the marginal benefit of the last service provided.

Under the conventional theory, this results in a societal welfare loss equal to the difference between the cost of producing the last service, Q_2—

FIGURE 4.7: Relationship Between Demand Elasticity and Welfare Loss

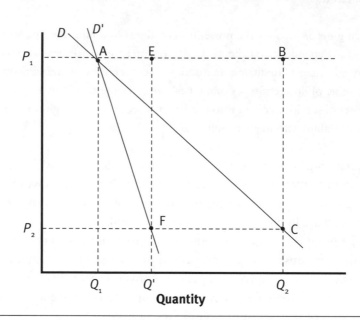

indicated by point B—and the benefits, shown at point C. But that welfare loss is only associated with the last service. Welfare loss also occurs for all other services purchased between Q_1 and Q_2. The total welfare loss is therefore equal to the triangle ABC. [22]

Now suppose the demand curve is steeper, or less elastic (curve D'). When the person obtains insurance, thereby lowering the price of care, his consumption increases only to Q'. In this case, the welfare loss will be smaller, equaling the triangle AEF. One can predict that if the demand curve is more gently sloped (that is, more price elastic), health insurance will result in a larger welfare-loss triangle.

If the possession of insurance leads to a large increase in utilization, then welfare loss will be larger because more services will be purchased where the marginal costs exceed the marginal benefits. Higher patient coinsurance rates for such services would reduce usage, thereby improving social welfare. In contrast, if utilization rates are not sensitive to the possession of insurance, then there is little welfare loss, and less need to charge high coinsurance rates.

Conventional theory calls for higher coinsurance rates when services are more responsive to out-of-pocket price. We therefore need to consider what services are most price elastic, since those should have the highest patient cost-sharing requirements.

The major source of data to answer this question is the RAND Health Insurance Experiment. Its results in this regard are somewhat ambiguous because the calculated elasticities vary depending on the level of coinsurance. In the study, patients were assessed 0 percent, 25 percent, or 95 percent of the total charge.[23] Therefore, one can examine price responsiveness to alternative coinsurance rates only between these intervals.

Table 4.3 shows these elasticities. In general, they do not vary much by type of service. One exception is well-care services, which, while showing a comparable elasticity to other outpatient services (acute and chronic) in the 0 to 25 percent range, had a much larger one in the 25 to 95 percent range (Phelps 1997). Dental services also showed a relatively high elasticity in the 25 percent to 95 percent range. The well-care services considered in the study include preventive care and other services.

The implications of the standard economic model are clear: If preventive services are the most price responsive, they should have the highest patient coinsurance rates, which will discourage usage. This is true even if some of these services are particularly effective in improving health and/or well-being.

Of course, alternative criteria could be used to determine the patient copayment levels that are in the best interest of society. A public health model would make preventive services free of any copayments—the opposite of what the economic model would recommend.

Five justifications for basing copayment rates on factors other than price elasticities are possible.

1. If consumers do not have sufficient information, they are likely to underestimate the value of such things as preventive services.
2. Even if the appropriate information is available, consumers may not use it correctly. As we noted earlier, it is difficult for consumers to make choices based on counterfactual information. Furthermore, cognitive dissonance may cause consumers to avoid seeking services that are valuable to them.
3. Medical experts may understand the benefits of certain services better than individuals do—and these experts routinely recommend more services than people are obtaining.
4. Consumers might be shortsighted in their views, particularly when they are young.
5. Preventive care is something society wants to encourage: If it makes you healthy we want you to have it, but the free-rider effect (discussed in Chapter 5) will prevent us from subsidizing you. Subsidized low copayments could meet this demand.

In summary, certain policy implications follow the assumption that a demand curve for medical services represents the marginal benefits consumers receive from services. One such implication is that patients should be charged more for services for which demand is price sensitive. But if one does

TABLE 4.3: Arc Price Elasticities of Medical Spending in the RAND Health Insurance Experiment

Range	Acute	Chronic	Well	Total Outpatient	Hospital	Total Medical	Dental
0–25	−0.16	−0.20	−0.14	−0.17	−0.17	−0.17	−0.12
25–95	−0.32	−0.23	−0.43	−0.31	−0.14	−0.22	−0.39

SOURCE: Keeler, E. B., J. L. Buchanan, J. E. Rolph, et al. 1988. "The Demand for Episodes of Medical Treatment in the Health Insurance Experiment." R-3454-HHS. Santa Monica, CA: RAND, 1988. Copyright RAND 1988. Reprinted with permission.

not make this assumption, a different set of policy prescriptions is more appropriate. One example is reducing patient prices for preventive services even if such services are more price responsive than others—a conclusion directly in conflict with conventional theory.

Recently, some researchers have suggested tailoring cost sharing to the usefulness of the service, which is consistent with what we propose. Under their Value-Based Insurance Design (VBID) (Chernew, Rosen, and Fendrick 2007; Fendrick and Chernew 2006), "cost sharing is still put to use, but a clinically sensitive approach is explicitly adopted to mitigate the adverse health consequences of high out-of-pocket spending" (Chernew, Rosen, and Fendrick 2007, W196). They believe this approach "relaxes the questionable assumption that when faced with cost sharing, consumers will balance costs and clinical value optimally."

The researchers suggest two possibilities for operationalizing VBID: (1) reducing everyone's copayments for services shown to be very effective from a clinical standpoint and (2) tailoring the cost sharing requirements to the individual patient's needs and characteristics—obviously, a bigger challenge. Under the latter, insurers would identify which patients are likely to benefit from which services, and target those for lower cost sharing. Some early adopters have focused on diabetes, a condition for which there is general agreement on appropriate treatment and drug regimens.

4.5 New Health Insurance Products That Rely on Increased Patient Cost Sharing

As we discussed earlier, a key implication of the traditional economic model as applied to healthcare is that higher patient cost sharing—deductibles, coinsurance, copayments—is desirable for society. This is because it reduces the welfare loss associated with overutilization. Recall that the architects of the RAND Health Insurance Experiment claimed that by implementing cost-sharing requirements, the eight-year, $282 million (in 2008 dollars) experiment would have paid for itself in a week. Much of our discussion has centered on flaws in this argument.

Nevertheless, recent years have seen a movement toward health insurance products that do rely on greater patient cost sharing, specifically health savings accounts and consumer-directed health plans.

Health Savings Accounts

A good deal of policy interest in the United States is currently directed toward health savings accounts (HSAs), which rely heavily on patient cost-sharing. These are a reworking of a concept called medical savings accounts (MSAs). Under most MSA proposals, people (usually employees) are able to choose a health plan with a large annual deductible (often several thousand dollars), but that covers medical expenses above that amount in full. The (tax-favored) savings in premiums could be used to make payments toward the deductible, or alternatively, to spend (or save) as the consumer desires. MSAs have been used abroad as well. Advocates suggest that MSAs have the advantage of offering protection against catastrophic health costs while discouraging people from using services needlessly.

HSAs, which are based on the MSA concept, were introduced in the United States in the mid-2000s as part of a revision of the federal tax code.[24] In essence, they provide health insurance and a tax-favored vehicle for savings. A person can only open an HSA account if she chooses a health insurance policy with a high deductible, defined in 2008 as a minimum of $1,100 for individual coverage and $2,200 for family coverage. To protect people from buying insurance that provides coverage that is too thin, out-of-pocket costs cannot exceed $5,600 for an individual or $11,200 for a family (excluding premiums).

HSAs work as follows. An individual can contribute up to $2,900, and a family $5,800, to a tax-sheltered account. They can use this money toward qualifying medical expenses that they incur during the year, or they can save it for future medical expenses. The idea is that they will think twice before spending it, because spending would take away from how much they save. Moreover, because their health insurance policy has, by definition, a high deductible, they would consider paying for a particular service more carefully. In theory, they would spend less on medical care, and the welfare loss from excessive health insurance would be reduced.

We will focus on three issues that follow from the discussion of HSAs. The first is whether HSAs will indeed quell the demand for services. Although consumers with HSAs will likely forgo some minor services, the vast majority of medical spending goes toward big-ticket items. For example, in a particular year, 2 percent of the U.S. population is responsible for 38 percent of expenditures (Berk and Monheit 2001). Because any hospitalization or procedure is likely to meet the annual deductible, the financial incentive to curb medical spending will not be strong. For that reason, HSAs would not result in de-pressed demand for expensive medical technologies.

Second, the idea behind HSAs is that individuals can make informed choices about whether to seek treatment for a particular illness. As we showed earlier, however, consumers' ability to perform this task well is questionable.[25] Findings from the RAND Health Insurance study indicate that patients are as likely to forgo effective medical services in the presence of cost sharing as they are to forgo less effective care (Lohr et al. 1986; Siu et al. 1986).

Third, selection bias could cause various problems for a country em-barking on adoption of HSAs. Those who are less likely to need medical care seem most likely to purchase the accounts. This would cause two problems. First, patients who are sicker—and who therefore might need more incentive to consider costs when making medical care decisions—would tend to not en-roll in HSAs, and therefore would not be subject to any efficiency-enhancing incentives that derive from cost sharing. Second, the markets would be seg-mented, with healthier people in these less expensive plans and sicker people pooled together in non-HSA plans, making the non-HSA plans even more expensive. This could result in a premium death spiral for non-HSA plans, as we will discuss later.

Selection bias can be a major force, undermining health plans that are unlucky enough to attract sicker enrollees. Competitive-based reform propos-als place intense pressure on health plans to attract enrollees by keeping pre-miums at a competitive level. One way to do this is through instituting true efficiencies, but another is to try to obtain a *favorable selection* of patients. It is in the interest of health plans to avoid groups whose costs are likely to be high and individuals with chronic conditions (Light 1995).[26] In theory, risk adjust-ing premiums for the health status of enrollees could ameliorate adverse selec-tion, but few employers or government sponsors do so, and when they do, they generally use age and gender rather than the health status of enrollees.

In addition, because enrolling in better health plans is likely to be more expensive, the lowest-cost plans in an area might be the least desirable ones—for example, those having a limited provider network, offering little choice, paying for only the most basic services, making it difficult to obtain referrals, and so forth (Rice, Brown, and Wyn 1993). Indeed, to the extent that putting providers at considerable risk is effective in controlling costs, one would expect less expensive plans to employ more severe physician incentives to conserve resources.

One dramatic consequence of adverse selection is a premium *death spiral*. This occurs when one health plan is the recipient of sicker enrollees, which in turn results in higher costs, and, during the next open enrollment period, higher premiums. These higher premiums then dissuade all but the sickest enrollees to sign up; eventually, premiums can become so high that almost no one can afford them.

A dramatic example of a death spiral occurred in the University of California health benefits system. As Buchmueller (1998) reported, the university adopted a fixed contribution policy in 1994, whereas previously it had essentially paid the costs of all plans except a high-cost, fee-for-service option. The new policy ultimately saved the university money, as plans had an incentive to compete with each other on the basis of premiums, and employees had an incentive to switch to lower-cost plans. A spillover effect was that the only fee-for-service plan, Prudential High Option, experienced a premium death spiral resulting from an adverse selection of enrollees. In 1993, the year prior to the change, 10 percent of employees enrolled in this plan, paying $750 annually for single coverage. Just three years later, premiums had more than quadrupled to almost $3,300, and enrollment had fallen to 1 percent of employees. The death spiral continued unabated; in 2001, the annual premium had risen to almost $17,000 for single coverage, and over $40,000 for family coverage (University of California 2001). As a result, only a handful of members remained and new enrollment was barred.

The trade-off between cost savings and adverse selection is also illustrated in Cutler and Reber's (1998) study of Harvard University's health plans. A preferred provider organization (PPO) and several HMOs were offered, and until 1995, the PPO was heavily subsidized compared to the other plans. In 1995, Harvard adopted a fixed contribution policy. Because the PPO had an adverse selection of patients, out-of-pocket premium costs rose dramatically. A death spiral occurred as the people leaving the PPO each year were less costly than those who remained. By 1997, just three years after the fixed contribution policy was adopted, the PPO plan was driven from the market, and only HMO and point-of-service plans remained. Cutler and Reber note that even though Harvard saved some money from the policy, social welfare declined because people who wanted a PPO plan could no longer choose one.

Since HSAs are so new, there is little experience from which we can glean lessons. One study published soon after the introduction of HSAs found, perhaps surprisingly, that they did not increase patient cost sharing much, and would likely have little impact on service usage (Remler and Glied 2006). Another found that by making health insurance more affordable, HSAs could reduce the number of uninsured in the United States by about 3 million (Feldman et al. 2005), but since their introduction the number of uninsured has continued to rise.

Even with MSAs, their earlier iteration, experience is minimal. The best-developed model is that used in Singapore, but analysts disagree on its effect. One common viewpoint is that although Singapore has had some success controlling its health costs, this is not due to MSAs, but to supply-side controls such as the rationing of hospital beds and physicians and regulation of fees (Yip and Hsiao 1997; Barr 2001).

Consumer-Directed Health Plans

During the mid- to late 2000s, "consumer directed" or "consumer driven" health plans (CDHPs) have received a great deal of attention. It is noteworthy, however, that the attention seems to outweigh enrollment. Even in 2007, several years after these plans were introduced into the marketplace, only 2 percent of the U.S. population was enrolled in them. A greater proportion of the population—about 11 percent—were in high-deductible plans that did not possess the characteristics of consumer-directed plans (Fronstin and Collins 2008).

Unfortunately, the term "CDHP" encompasses various insurance products with disparate characteristics. The most common type is sometimes called a "health reimbursement arrangement" or HRA, and that will be our focus here.[27]

HRAs are not terribly different from HSAs, which we discussed earlier. Two of the main differences are that in an HRA, the employer rather than the employee owns the account, and that the employee does not retain any remaining balance if he or she leaves the firm (Buntin et al. 2006).

A typical HRA may be designed as follows. An employer purchases a high-deductible insurance plan for an employee. For example, the annual deductible might be $1,500 for individual coverage and $3,000 for family coverage. At the same time, the employer provides a spending account for the employee. It might be half the value of the deductible—in this case, $750 for an individual and $1,500 for a family. When an employee or family member uses a medical service, the cost comes out of the spending account. But when that is exhausted, all costs within the gap (sometimes called the "doughnut hole") between the amount of the spending account (here, $750 or $1,500) and the deductible (here, $1,500 or $3,000) must be paid out of pocket. This would give the employee an incentive to think twice before receiving another medical service. Once the deductible is met, the insurance policy would cover most if not all additional spending during the remainder of the year. Certain services, such as preventive care, may be carved out so that payment for them does not come out of the spending account, as a way of encouraging their usage. A key component of a good CDHP is sufficient information for enrollees to make intelligent decisions about their care.

At the time of writing, CDHPs (including HRAs and HSAs) were responsible for only 5 percent of total enrollment in employer-provided plans (Claxton et al. 2007).

Several studies have been conducted on early CDHPs. Rosenthal, Hsuan, and Milstein (2005) examined 14 actual plans, seven of which could be characterized as HRAs. They provided a grade, from A to F, on several characteristics of HRAs related to cost containment and quality, and on two other types of CDHP models. While the HRAs did better than the others, grades were low. HRAs received As for two components involving higher consumer cost sharing and cost containment, but Fs for incentives to control spending after one has already met the annual deductible, equity for low-income enrollees, incentives encouraging quality care, and sufficient information for selecting cost-effective providers.

Feldman, Parente, and Christianson (2007) followed CDHP enrollees over a three-year period and compared them to employees at the same firm who chose another kind of health plan. Spending rose more for the CDHP enrollees than for those in other plans. This is probably because once someone in such a plan enters the hospital, he will have spent enough to meet his annual deductible, and therefore will have few remaining incentives to control his expenditures.

So-called selection effects remain a concern. Many have speculated that healthier enrollees will choose CDHPs because they do not fear the higher out-of-pocket costs. They also seem to be more popular among wealthier people. In one study, the average income of an employee choosing a CDHP was $93,000, compared to $52,000 or $70,000 for two other plan types (Feldman, Parente, and Christianson 2007). In another study, those with incomes higher than $80,000 were almost twice as likely as other employees to choose a CDHP option (Lo Sasso et al. 2004). Finally, a national survey of over 4,000 working-age adults conducted in 2007 found that a disproportionate number of CDHP enrollees had high incomes, with 31 percent in households earning more than $100,000, up from 22 percent two years earlier. They were also in better health, had fewer chronic conditions, and were less likely to smoke and more likely to exercise than those in conventional health insurance plans (Fronstin and Collins 2008).

Some researchers have raised serious concerns about the movement to CDHPs. A number of those concerns fit into the theme of this book:

- Exposing consumers to higher out-of-pocket prices will discourage them from using services that may be beneficial to their health. Earlier, we noted a study by Greene and colleagues (2008), who found that those enrolled in a high-deductible CDHP often stopped filling prescriptions for high blood pressure and high cholesterol medications.
- The information consumers need to make case-by-case decisions about what services to use is either not available or extremely difficult for all but the most expert to use.
- CDHPs have a greater appeal to those who are in better health and who do not have chronic conditions, which leads to the potential for serious adverse selection and increases in premiums for those who do not join such plans.
- Nearly every aspect of CDHPs has the potential to harm disadvantaged populations. These groups of people have lower incomes and therefore are less likely to be able to afford increased copayments. They are also less likely to be able to use what information is available, which is usually only

on the Internet (Bloch 2007). Bloch (2007, 1322) calls this the "reverse Robin Hood" effect, with "redistribut[ion of] money from the less advantaged to the prosperous."

- Studies to date have shown that CDHPs do not result in decreased expenditures. Rather, expenditures are often just as high or higher because there are no cost-containment mechanisms in place once the deductible has been met.

There are various ways to ameliorate these problems. For example, cost-sharing requirements could be linked to income or premium subsidies could be provided for those who earn less—but these are unlikely to be enacted in the wake of budgetary concerns.

In spite of these problems with CDHC, there appears to be a movement toward increased consumer cost sharing. Consumers are skeptical of tightly managed care arrangements, and the United States shows little movement toward a system that relies more on regulation and less on price competition. One of the few tools available is the price mechanism—charging people more (e.g., through higher deductibles or copayments). But if people do not understand the consequences of their choices, if information systems cannot provide ready help to many facing medical decisions, and if affordability concerns are ignored—then the problems just noted are likely to magnify as these trends continue into the future.

4.6 Chapter Summary

In this chapter, we questioned the effectiveness of reliance on markets in bringing about an economically efficient healthcare system. We challenged several assumptions, most of them related to consumers' ability to make good choices in the face of asymmetric information and, more recently, an overwhelming choice set. We applied this theory to the health insurance and health services markets and, along the way, questioned the belief that society suffers from a welfare loss as a result of excessive health insurance. We argued that much of the waste in medical care is due not to consumers demanding too much, but rather to the provision of wasteful services that do little good. Furthermore, we raised a variety of concerns about high patient cost-sharing requirements, which led to further questions about new insurance products, such as consumer-directed health plans, that rely on charging patients more.

Notes

1. This assumes that society is satisfied with the distribution of income, which will be discussed further in chapters 5 and 9.
2. Others have employed Dr. Pangloss in their critiques of contemporary economics. See, for example, Culyer (1982) and Evans (1983).

3. The primary caveat is that no important externalities exist, because in the presence of important yet uncorrected externalities, there will be market failure. Externalities are discussed in some detail in Chapter 5.

4. Recall that all points along the contract curve in Figure 2.24 are Pareto optimal, each corresponding to a different distribution of wealth.

5. Ten years later, the summer 1988 issue of the *Journal of Health Politics, Policy and Law* (volume 13, number 2) was devoted to a follow-up of these issues. The fall 1989 issue included a critique of some aspects of this follow-up (see Rice and Labelle 1989; Wedig, Mitchell, and Cromwell 1989).

6. We will take up this issue of asymmetric information between the provider and patient in Chapter 6, where we consider supply-side issues in health economics.

7. This quotation, from Dr. Harvey Mandell, is from Hoerger and Howard (1995). The Hoerger and Howard article contains a good review of the literature on consumers' search for physicians.

8. For a review of alternative ways of increasing consumer voice in the managed care market, see Rodwin (2001).

9. This is a critical point, one with which many economists would disagree. In fact, some practitioners have tried to show that many seemingly self-destructive human behaviors, such as drug addiction and even suicide, are the result of utility-maximizing decisions. There is a body of literature—known as rational addiction theory—that purports to show drug and alcohol addiction to be consistent with rationality. Becker and Murphy (1988, 675, emphasis added), for example, claim that "addictions, even strong ones, are usually rational in the sense of involving forward-looking maximization with *stable preferences*," and that even though unhappy people often become addicted, "they would be even more unhappy if they were prevented from consuming the addictive goods" (691). This viewpoint defies not only common sense, but the professional opinions of the vast majority of health professionals. Thus, this view of rationality is rejected here. Instead, we define rationality as indicating *reasonable* behavior.

10. This assumes that we control for the loading costs of insurance—administration, marketing, and profits. If the price of insurance goes up, not because the costs of care rise, but because of these loading costs, then we would not expect demand for insurance to rise.

11. Another reason we see first-dollar insurance coverage is that most people cannot tailor their own health insurance. Rather, their coverage is determined by the firm for which they work and sometimes by the insurance company. Some firms prefer first-dollar coverage for preventive services because they believe it will encourage healthy behaviors, and perhaps even lower costs, in the long run.

12. This has been called the "cookie jar effect." The idea is that if people save these inducements rather than treat them as normal income—putting them in a cookie jar—then the results of the experiments would be biased. Specifically,

the estimates of the impact of higher copayments would be biased downward. Such persons would be less put off by paying for care because they would have stored funds for such an event.

13. Not everyone agrees with this, however. In addition to the critique by John Nyman discussed below, criticisms have been leveled by Welch and colleagues (1987) and Hay and Olsen (1984). For responses to these criticisms by those who carried out the experiment, see Newhouse and colleagues (1987) and Duan and colleagues (1984).

14. See, for example, Evans (1984) and Mooney (1994). One U.S. economist who has made the same point is Alain Enthoven (1988, 17), who wrote,

> There are . . . problems in applying the results of the RAND experiment to national policy. RAND studied the behavior of about 7,700 people in six different cities. Thus, the proportion of the population affected by the experiment in any city was too small to have a noticeable effect on doctors' incomes, but the effects might be very different if everyone in a city were changed from a coverage with little co-insurance to one with a great deal. Initially, visits to the doctor would drop, but as the doctors found more time on their hands, all our experience suggests they would find other ways to make themselves useful: extra visits and consultations for hospitalized patients, more frequently advising patients who telephone that they should come in to be seen, and the like. What applies to a small sample might not apply to the whole community.

15. The only U.S. study that addresses this issue was a small natural experiment analyzed by Marianne Fahs (1992), on the experience of one multispecialty group practice located in Appalachia in 1977. Fahs compared utilization in the year before the institution of cost sharing with that during the two years following its institution, for two groups: mine workers who faced increasing cost-sharing requirements and steel workers who did not. The study found that physicians responded to the imposition of cost sharing on their mine worker patients by changing their practice behavior for their steelworker patients. Fahs concludes that "when the economic effects of cost-sharing on physician service use are analyzed for all patients within a physician practice, the findings are remarkably different from those of an analysis limited to those patients directly affected by cost-sharing" (Fahs 1992, 25–26).

16. The first such estimates were developed by Martin Feldstein (1973).

17. This calculation is based on figures provided in Levit and colleagues (1985).

18. A dollar bill is 6 inches, or ½ foot long; 2.1 trillion of them would therefore equal 1.05 trillion feet. As there are 5,280 feet in a mile, 1.05 trillion feet is 198.86 million miles. The average distance from the earth to the sun is 93 million miles. So the line of dollar bills would stretch from the earth to the sun and back again, with about 13 million miles to spare—enough to go to the moon and back another 27 times!

19. Survey data show that about two-thirds of all Americans believe the country spends too little on health (Blendon and Benson 2001).

20. Perhaps the best-known article is Wennberg and Gittlesohn (1982). For a thorough review of the early literature, see Paul-Shaheen, Clark, and Williams (1987). For some of the recent research, see Fisher and colleagues (2003a).

21. Other writers have advocated calculating welfare losses based on the provision of unnecessary services. See Phelps and Parente (1990), Phelps and Mooney (1992), Dranove (1995), and Phelps (1995).

22. As we noted earlier, one must weigh the welfare loss in the conventional theory against the welfare gain from the reduction in risk brought about by the insurance. For convenience, we disregard the latter element here, but this does not affect the substance of the argument.

23. Some patients were charged 50 percent coinsurance rates, but they were not used in the analysis of demand elasticities.

24. Detailed current information can be found at www.ustreas.gov/offices/public-affairs/hsa/.

25. There is also concern whether consumers will make rational choices about contributions to programs such as HSAs. In a study of university employees' contributions to tax-deductible flexible spending accounts, Schweitzer, Hershey, and Asch (1996) found that employees did not act rationally. Relatively few contributed to such accounts, even though it would have been in the best financial interest of most to have done so. And those who did contribute tended to give the same dollar contribution each year, even when changing financial circumstances would have been expected to result in different contribution amounts over time. The authors conclude that "[t]he pervasiveness of these patterns raises concerns that healthcare reform plans that rely on financial incentives at the consumer level—for example, proposed medical savings accounts—will be inefficient" (Schweitzer, Hershey, and Asch 1996, 583).

26. One way to deal with this problem would be to "risk adjust" payments to health plans—that is, to pay them more if they have sicker patients. Although health services researchers are devoting much attention to this problem, there are few instances in which employer-sponsored health plan contributions use risk adjustment, and in most of those cases, adjustments are done based just on demographic characteristics of enrollees, such as age and sex.

27. Gabel and colleagues (2004) mention two other types of CDHPs: personalized or design-your-own plans and customized-package plans. Rosenthal, Hsuan, and Milstein (2005) call the other types of CDHPs "tiered models," which they further subdivide into "customized-benefit-design" models and "point-of-care" models.

5

SPECIAL TOPICS IN DEMAND: EXTERNALITIES OF CONSUMPTION AND THE FORMATION OF PREFERENCES

While Chapter 4 covered and critiqued some of the main topics in consumer demand as applied to health—the demand for health, health insurance, and health services—it hardly exhausted the subject. This chapter raises other issues in the same area, specifically those that relate to three assumptions of the traditional model (from Table 3.1) that have received less attention from health economists:

Assumption 6. There are no negative externalities of consumption.
Assumption 7. There are no positive externalities of consumption.
Assumption 8. Consumer tastes are predetermined.

Section 5.1 addresses the first two of these assumptions, and Section 5.2, the last of them. Regarding the latter section, if preferences are not predetermined, how are they formed? This issue is central to some of the other social sciences but economists have not taken it up (much). The belief that preferences are formed within the context of the society in which a person is raised and lives brings up serious concerns about the policy prescriptions that fall out of the competitive marketplace. In Section 5.3 we provide an application of these issues, positing that consumers might find themselves with too much choice. As an example, we look at the number of Medicare prescription drug plans available to senior citizens in the United States.

5.1 Externalities of Consumption

The Role of Externalities in Market Performance

This subsection addresses the issues of externalities in general and consumption externalities in particular. Externalities exist when the actions of one person or firm affect the well-being of others. There are two broad types of externalities: production and consumption. Production externalities exist when one firm's production affects other firms or individuals. The classic example of a negative production externality is pollution. Firms can maximize their profits if they pollute, but this results in a cost to others in the form of poor air or water quality. Thus, allowing them to pollute as much as they want without paying any associated costs is not optimal for society at large.

There are positive externalities of production as well. The existence of a tree farm is an example. Trees absorb carbon dioxide and therefore reduce that particular form of air pollution.

The most famous essay on negative production externalities is Garrett Hardin's (1968) "The Tragedy of the Commons." He uses the example of a common pasture that herdsmen use to graze their cattle. The herdsmen increase the size of their herds until the number of cattle is such that the land will be overgrazed. For the group as a whole, it would be better to establish limits so that all will continue to benefit from the common pasture. But to each individual, it is better to acquire another head of cattle, since that one animal will provide revenue upon its sale but will only have a negligible impact on the viability of the grazing land. Of course, since everyone faces the same incentives, the ultimate impact is hardly negligible; rather, it is the destruction of the common good. In Hardin's (1968, 1244) intentionally dramatic prose,

> the rational herdsman concludes that the only sensible course for him to pursue is to add another animal to the herd. And another; and another . . . But this is the conclusion reached by each and every rational herdsman sharing a commons. Therein is the tragedy. Each man is locked into a system that compels him to increase his herd without limit—in a world that is limited. Ruin is the destination toward which all men rush, each pursuing his own best interest in a society that believes in the freedom of the commons. Freedom in a commons brings ruin to all.

Hardin (1968) used this example to discuss the threat of nuclear war, environmental pollution, overfishing the oceans, and his main concern, population growth. Regarding the last, he makes the sobering point that an "appeal to conscience" to "control the breeding of mankind" (1246) will lead to a curious result: Those who heed the call will have fewer children, and those who do not will have more. Hardin (1968) quotes Charles Darwin: "It may well be that it would take hundreds of generations for the progenitive instinct to develop in this way, but if it should do so, nature would have taken her revenge, and the variety *Homo contracipiens* would become extinct and would be replaced by the variety *Homo progenitivus*" (1246). In other words, those who practice family planning will, over time, disappear from the population.

One of Hardin's key points is that there is no *technical* solution to a problem of the commons. Rather, any solution must be political, and will abridge individual freedoms. The quintessential economic solution is the privatization of property. But that alone does not solve the problem, because what a property owner does upstream can have deleterious effects downstream—literally and figuratively. An unregulated private entity will continue to have an economic incentive, say, to pollute, since this will save a great deal of money, but the incremental degradation of the environment will be shared by all.

Economists often suggest that we should tax negative externalities and provide subsidies for positive ones, so that individuals and firms have an incentive to act in a way that is more consistent with society's goals. Although perhaps coercive, it does not rely on overt government regulation—a firm can still choose to pollute, but it will have to pay a tax to do so. One can try to formulate these taxes so that the firm's marginal benefit from polluting is equal to society's marginal costs (which is the sum of the firm's productive costs and the costs the rest of society bears from the pollution). In the coming years, we may see more of this—for example, through the establishment of carbon taxes and credits.[1]

The other class of externalities relates to consumption. One of the key assumptions with regard to the advantages of competition is that there are no externalities of consumption—or alternatively, that any such externalities are explicitly dealt with through public policy. A consumption externality exists when one person's consumption of a good or service has an effect on another person's utility. There are positive and negative externalities of consumption. With a positive externality, one person's consumption of a good raises another person's utility. With a negative externality, the consumption lowers another person's utility.

Certain consumption externalities have received much attention from health economists. Perhaps the classic example of a positive externality of consumption is immunizations. If we receive an immunization, we will not be the only beneficiaries, because if others cannot catch the disease from us, they are less likely to get it. But because in a competitive market an individual bears the full cost of the immunization, either directly or through an (unsubsidized) insurance premium, too few immunizations will be purchased. Recall that consumers purchase goods until the ratio of the marginal utility of each to its price is equal across all goods (Equation 2.4). A positive consumption externality implies that society's marginal utility is greater than that of the individual, so consumers, acting on their own, will not purchase a socially desirable quantity of such goods.

A parallel argument can be made about negative externalities such as smoking. If smoking lowers your utility, society's marginal utility from our smoking will be lower than our own. In making consumption decisions through equalizing the marginal utility and prices of all goods, people will smoke more than is in society's best interest.

The existence of important externalities like these means the operation of a competitive market, by itself, will not result in a socially optimal outcome. One way to improve matters is through government intervention. In the case of a positive externality like immunizations, government can subsidize their provision, even providing them free of charge. Most taxpayers would contribute, which seems desirable, since so many people are benefiting. Dealing with a negative consumption externality like smoking is somewhat more problematic. Although it is easy to tax smokers, it is much harder to ensure that this revenue from special taxes on the production and sale of cigarettes is disbursed to those who are most affected by smoking. As a result, governmental bodies in the United States have taken an additional route by prohibiting smoking in many public places. They also sometimes fund smoking-cessation programs, which partially mitigates the externality.

Concern About Status

Recall Equation 2.1, in which a consumer's utility (U) was assumed to depend on the various quantities of the n possible goods and services possessed, three of which are labeled X, Y, and Z:

$$U = f(X, Y, Z \ldots, n) \tag{5.1}$$

It was also assumed that having more of each good is better. No consideration is given to how one's bundle of goods and services compares to, affects, or is affected by the bundles of goods and services other people possess.

Let us suppose a person's utility function is more complicated; it depends not only on the quantity of goods X, Y, and Z a person has, but also on how this compares to how much other people have, on average (as indicated by the horizontal bars above the letters). We will denote this as follows:

$$U = f(X, Y, Z, \bar{X}/X, \bar{Y}/Y, \bar{Z}/Z) \tag{5.2}$$

This states that a person's utility is determined not only by what he or she has, but by how this compares to the average of the population. A more realistic formulation might use those people with whom a person has most contact, or those in the same social class, for comparison.

Alternatively, one could imagine a utility function in which *only* one's position relative to others matters,[2] as shown in Equation 5.3.

$$U = f(\bar{X}/X, \bar{Y}/Y, \bar{Z}/Z) \tag{5.3}$$

A few well-known economists have, over the years, noted the substantial implications for the competitive model if one believes that relative as well as absolute wealth matters. Lord (Lionel) Robbins (1984, xxii–xxiii) writes:

> If the remaining groups regard their position relatively, they may well argue that
> the spectacle of such improvement elsewhere is a detriment to their satisfaction.

This is not a niggling point: a relative improvement in the position of certain groups *pari passu* with an absolute improvement in the position of the rest of the community has often been a feature of economic history; and we know that has not been regarded by all as either ethically or politically desirable.

Francis Bator (1958, 378) states the issue in a more technical manner:

[M]arket efficiency is neither sufficient nor necessary for market institutions to be the "preferred" mode of social organization. . . . If, e.g., people are sensitive not only to their own jobs but to other people's as well, or more generally, if such things as relative status, power, and the like, matter, the injunction to maximize output, to hug the production-possibility frontier, can hardly be assumed "neutral," and points on the utility frontier may associate with points inside the production frontier.

We therefore need to ask which of the above equations is the best representation of actual behavior. Intuition tells us that Equation 5.1 is implausible, if not downright wrong. This equation implies that people are indifferent about their rank in society, have no concern about status, and do not worry about "keeping up with the Joneses." Rather, all they care about is what they themselves have, irrespective of whether this is more or less, better or worse, than others with whom they have contact.

If this is true, then:

- How can one account for much if not most advertising, which tries to convey how favorably one will be viewed by others if one owns a particular car, wears a particular type of jeans, or drinks a particular brand of beer?
- How can one account for people's concern about their coworkers' salaries?
- How can one account for the following example, similar to one suggested by Robert Frank (1985): Give each of two siblings one piece of candy, and both children will be happy. But give two pieces to one child and three to another, and the child who receives the smaller share will be less happy than if each received only one. As Uwe Reinhardt (1998) quips, "the trait has its onset in early childhood and lingers until about, say, age 100, even among economists" (28).

A. C. Pigou (1932, 90), one of the founders of modern economics, quotes and affirms John Stuart Mill's statement that "Men do not desire to be *rich*, but to be richer than other men." (In a lighter vein, Frank [1985, 5] notes that "H. L. Mencken once defined wealth as any income that is at least one hundred dollars more a year than the income of one's wife's sister's husband.") Lester Thurow (1980, 18) has stated that once incomes exceed the subsistence level, "individual perceptions of the adequacy of their economic performance depend almost solely on relative as opposed to absolute position."

It is perhaps not unnatural to think that, while other people may behave in this manner, we are above such petty concerns about rank and status. Such a viewpoint is hard to hold, however, after considering the following thought experiment provided by Robert Frank (1985, 116–17):

> In this experiment you are to imagine yourself in the following situation: As a high-income resident of the United States, you are suddenly confronted with an opportunity to be transported to a much richer planet. The trip will be free of charge, but with no option of return. You are a genuine standout here on Earth. You earn $100,000 per year and live in a tastefully decorated home in a quiet, fashionable neighborhood. Your children are enrolled in the best schools and are very popular among their classmates. You are happily married to a person you hold in high esteem, who regards you likewise. You are a person of integrity, a highly respected expert in your profession, and are in good health. You enjoy peace of mind and the admiration and affection of a large group of friends, who regard you as one of the most charming and caring people they know.
>
> On the new planet your income would be $1,000,000 per year. But instead of being near the top of the income scale as you are here, you would be at the bottom. The home you would be able to afford there is much larger and better appointed than the one you live in here. Yet it is located in a marginal neighborhood, one that people urge their children not to venture into. You would pursue the same occupation there as you do here. But the people on the new planet are so skilled that they regard your profession in the way we think of repetitive, assembly tasks here. The schools your children would go to there compare very favorably with the ones they go to here, but among schools on the new planet they are thought to be ill-equipped and poorly staffed. Although your children will amass more knowledge in those schools than they do in the ones here, they will struggle there on the academic borderline, instead of bringing home A's as they do here. Although your children are much sought after by their classmates here, you will discover on the new planet that most parents attempt to steer their children to more suitable playmates. You will recount the same anecdotes there as you do here, but your friends there will regard them as simple and boring, instead of clever and erudite as your friends here regard them. Although your spouse will love you equally there as here, you know that, once there, he or she cannot fail to notice how the achievements of others surpass your own.

Frank contends that you would be willing to give up $900,000 in income in order to retain your current status. It is hard to disagree.

The discussion thus far has been intuitive, so it is natural to ask whether there is any evidence supporting the superiority of Equation 5.2 or 5.3 over Equation 5.1. Two classic sets of studies are relevant here. James Duesenberry (1952, 31) developed the *relative income hypothesis*. Under this hypothesis, people's drive for self-esteem makes them wish to emulate the consumption habits of those who are on a higher rung of the socioeconomic ladder. Duesenberry states that "this drive operates through inferiority feelings aroused by unfavorable comparisons between living standards" and is heightened by frequent contact with people who have higher standards of living. The theory predicts that people with lower incomes will save a smaller proportion of their income because they will have more frequent contact with those in the economic class just above them, whose consumption patterns they will mimic. This prediction has been verified through empirical studies.

Further evidence is provided by Richard Easterlin's (1974, 1995, 2001, 2005) studies of human happiness conducted over the past 30 years. He has found that in a given country at a given time, wealthier people tend to be happier than poorer people. However, in a given country over time, happiness levels are surprisingly constant, even in the wake of rising real incomes. Furthermore, average levels of happiness are fairly constant across countries; people in poor countries and wealthy countries claim to be about equally happy. The only way such findings can be reconciled is if relative wealth matters more than absolute wealth. From this, Easterlin (1995, 35) concludes:

> Today, as in the past, within a country at a given time those with higher incomes are, on average, happier. However, raising the incomes of all does not increase the happiness of all. This is because the material norms on which judgments of well-being are based increase in the same proportion as the actual income of the society. These conclusions are suggested by data on reported happiness, material norms, and income collected in surveys in a number of countries over the past half century.

Table 5.1 provides 2004 data from the United States, where it is clear that those with higher incomes declare themselves happier. Figure 5.1 provides historical data from 1960 across several countries—some wealthy, some poor—showing no apparent correlation between the wealth of a country and the happiness of its people. Figure 5.2 shows that over a 16-year period, among the people of nine European countries, there is no upward trend in happiness within countries, even though real gross domestic product rose between 25 and 50 percent in each country (Easterlin 1995). Moreover, in a study of happiness levels in the United States over three decades, through 2004, the percentage of people stating that they are "very happy" was nearly identical with what it was in the early 1970s (Yang 2008).

Evidence on the Impact of Relative Deprivation on Happiness and Health

TABLE 5.1: Distribution of Self-Reported Global Happiness by Family Income, 2004

	Percentage Indicating Global Happiness at Family Income of			
Response	Under $20,000	$20,000–$49,999	$50,000–$89,999	$90,000 and over
Not too happy	17.2	13.0	7.7	5.3
Pretty happy	60.5	56.8	50.3	51.8
Very happy	22.2	30.2	41.9	42.9

SOURCE: From Kahneman, D., A. B. Krueger, D. Schkade, N. Schwarz, and A. Stone. 2006. "Would You Be Happier If You Were Richer? A Focusing Illusion." *Science* 132 (June 30): 1909. Reprinted with permission from AAAS.

NOTE: The question posed was "Taken all together, how would you say things are these days—would you say that you are very happy, pretty happy, or not too happy?" Sample size was 1,173 individuals.

FIGURE 5.1: Personal Happiness Rating and GNP per Capita, 1960

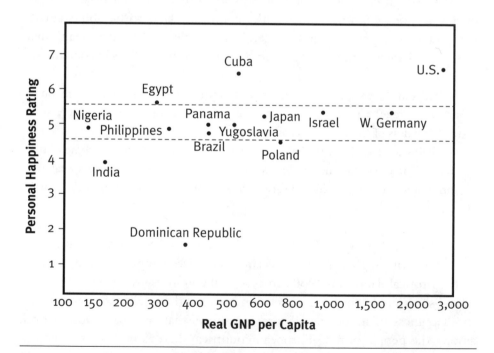

SOURCE: Reprinted with permission from Easternlin, R. 1974. In *Nations and Household in Economic Growth: Essays in Honor of Moses Abramovitz,* edited by P.A. David and M.W. Reder, p. 106. New York: Academic Press.

FIGURE 5.2: Percentage Very Satisfied with Their Lives in General, Nine European Countries, 1973–1989

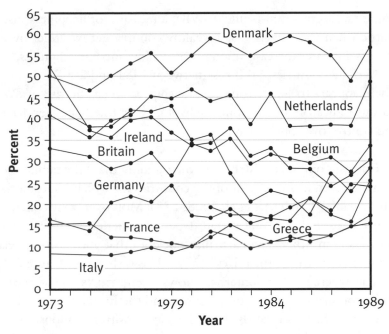

SOURCE: Reprinted with permission from Easterlin, R. A. 1995. "Will Rasing the Incomes of All Increase the Happiness of All?" *Journal of Economic Behavior* 27(1): 13. Copyright © 1995 Published by Elsevier Science.

NOTE: Inglehart et al. 1992. The question asked is, "Generally speaking, how satisfied are you with your life as a whole? Would you say that you are very satisfied, fairly satisfied, not very satisfied, or not at all satisfied?" Ordinary least squares regressions (not shown) yielded time trends that were not significant for five countries, significant and positive for two, and significant and negative for two.

Perhaps the most dramatic illustration of the fact that rising wealth over time within a country does not lead to more happiness is exemplified by post-war Japan. As summarized by Easterlin (1995; 2005, 39–40),

> Between 1958 and 1987 real per capita income in Japan multiplied a staggering five-fold, propelling Japan to a living level equal to about two-thirds that of the United States. . . . Consumer durables such as electric washing machines, electric refrigerators, and television sets, found in few homes at the start of the period, became well-nigh universal, and car ownership soared from 1 to about 60 percent of households. . . . Despite this unprecedented three decade advance in level of living, there was no improvement in mean subjective well being. . . .

A recent study, however, casts some doubt on these assertions, indicating that happiness may be higher in wealthier nations, and that it may have risen *within* countries in recent years. Using longitudinal survey data from 52 countries and examining trends from 1981 to 2007, Inglehart and colleagues (2008) conclude that:

- While "subjective well-being" (SWB), a measure of happiness, rises only a little when the citizenry of a wealthy country get wealthier over time, there is a greater increase among those in low-income countries.
- In 45 of 52 countries, SWB rose between 1981 and 2007.
- There appears to be a strong relationship between the rise of SWB and various indicators of freedom, such as greater tolerance, gender equity, and control over one's own life.

This last point is consistent with their finding that "the public's sense of freedom increased in 79 percent of the countries for which a substantial time series is available" (Inglehart et al. 2008, 273). Moreover, they conclude that "[t]he evidence indicates that certain types of societies are more conducive to happiness than others—in particular, societies that allow people relatively free choice in how to live their lives" (279). This is shown in Figure 5.3, from their article, where the horizontal axis shows changes in "sense of free choice" in various countries over the study period, and the horizontal axis shows the corresponding changes in SWB. There is a clear positive relationship between the two. The authors posit that, within countries, as sense of free choice (a barometer of social freedom) increases, it causes an increase in SWB.

As the Inglehart study was published soon before this book went to press, it is too early to know whether the findings will be replicated by others, and their conclusions adopted.[3]

Although these studies do not explicitly refute the concept of the indifference curve, the research helps provide an understanding of why people might behave in a way that is so contradictory to the predictions of traditional economic theory. Easterlin (1974) reports the results of a study by Hadley Cantril (1965) based on 1960s surveys of individuals living in the United States and India, concerning what makes them happy. Following are several quotations from the surveys that indicate that the things that make people happy vary dramatically with their circumstances:

India. I want a son and a piece of land since I am now working on land owned by other people. I would like to construct a house of my own and have a cow for milk and ghee. I would also like to buy some better clothing for my wife. If I could do this then I would be happy. [35-year-old man, illiterate, agricultural laborer, income about $10 a month]

India. I wish for an increase in my wages because with my meager salary I cannot afford to buy decent food for my family. If the food and clothing problems

FIGURE 5.3: Changes in Subjective Well-Being and Sense of Free Choice

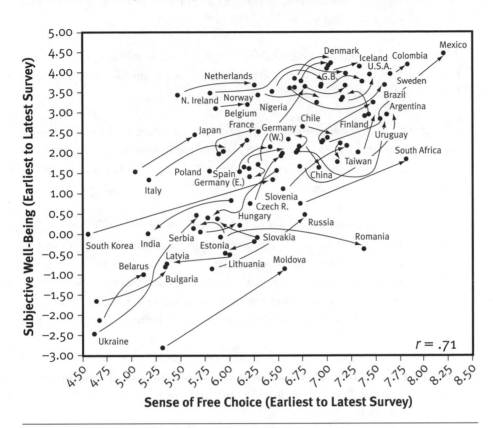

SOURCE: Inglehart, R., R. Foa, C. Peterson, and C. Welzel. 2008. "Development, Freedom, and Rising Happiness: A Global Perspective." *Perspectives on Psychological Science* 3 (4): 264–85. Reproduced with permission of Blackwell Publishing Ltd.

were solved, then I would feel at home and be satisfied. Also if my wife were able to work the two of us could then feed the family and I am sure would have a happy life and our worries would be over. [35-year-old sweeper, monthly income around $13]

India. I should like to have tap water and a water supply in my house. It would be able to have electricity. My husband's wages must be increased if our children are to get an education and our daughter is to be married. [45-year-old house-wife, family income about $80 a month]

India. I hope in the future I will not get any disease. Now I am coughing. I also hope I can purchase a bicycle. I hope my children will study well and that I can provide them with an education. I also would sometime like to own a fan and maybe a radio. [45-year-old skilled worker earning $30 a month]

United States. If I could earn more money I would be able to buy our own home and have more luxury around us, like better furniture, a new car, and more vacations. [27-year-old skilled worker]

United States. I would like a reasonable enough income to maintain a house, have a new car, have a boat, and send my four children to private schools. [34-year-old laboratory technician]

United States. I would like a new car. I wish all my bills were paid and I had more money for myself. I would like to play more golf and to hunt more than I do. I would like to have more time to do the things I want to and to entertain my friends. [24-year-old bus driver]

United States. Materially speaking, I would like to provide my family with an income to allow them to live well—to have the proper recreation, to go camping, to have music and dancing lessons for the children, and to have family trips. I wish we could belong to a country club and do more entertaining. We just bought a new home and expect to be perfectly satisfied with it for a number of years. [28-year-old lawyer] (Cantril 1965, as quoted in Easterlin 1974, 114–15)

These quotations, which are poignant in their own right, provide a glimpse into why people in two cultures can be equally happy with different quantities of goods: People's utility depends less on what they have than on what they have relative to the social norm.

Suppose one accepts the notion that people care about how they compare with others, as well as what they themselves have irrespective of others (i.e., Equation 5.2). It could still be argued that, even if concern about relative position does exist, it is irrational or a character flaw that the analyst or policymaker should ignore. But this argument fails for two reasons. First, traditional economic theory does not evaluate where preferences come from or whether they are good or bad. Instead, it views preferences as what have to be satisfied for an individual, and ultimately a society, to be in a best-off position. Although we disputed this notion in Chapter 4, economic theory does not view any individually held preferences pejoratively.[4]

Second, it is not at all obvious that concern about one's status is an irrational or even undesirable character trait. Tibor Scitovsky (1976, 115) makes a strong argument to the contrary:

The desire to "live up to the Joneses" is often criticized and its rationality called into question. This is absurd and unfortunate. Status seeking, the wish to belong, the asserting and cementing of one's membership in the group is a deep-seated and very natural drive whose origin and universality go beyond man and are explained by that most basic of drives, the desire to survive.

Similarly, Uwe Reinhardt (1998, 28) writes,

Envy probably is among the most basic of all human traits. It is the very engine of economic growth. Normative economic analysis that abstracts from this common human trait, because it is deemed unsavory, might be useful on other planets. It misses the core of the human experience on planet Earth.

In this regard, what others have can also be viewed as necessary information for formulating a person's individual desires. It shows what can be had, and what is reasonable to expect.

Let us now return to the question of how this negative externality—concern about status and rank—affects the competitive model. Recall that competition leads to Pareto optimality, in which it is impossible to make someone better off without making someone else worse off. In the absence of the human characteristics discussed here, it is easy to see the appeal of relying on competition. Why not let people engage in trade until they are satisfied with their lot and no longer wish to engage in further trades? Why not enact policies that convey benefits to some people and no cost to others? Wouldn't encouraging such trade, and enacting such policies, be in everyone's best interest?

We have tried to show that the answer to the last question is, perhaps surprisingly, "not necessarily." This is because if people feel worse off when they find themselves falling relative to others, competition is not necessarily the best means of improving societal welfare. If, for example, by buying a fancy car, you make us unhappy because our cars no longer seem as appealing, then society's marginal utility from your purchase of the car will be lower than your personal marginal utility. By extension, if social competition leads to everyone purchasing fancier cars than they need, society will hardly be better off, and the resources used to produce the cars could instead be used in ways that most people would find more beneficial.[5]

Without some sort of intervention (or intensive psychological therapy to get us to stop caring about what others have), a competitive market will overproduce goods and services that convey status.

When an externality exists, economists try to come up with taxes or subsidies to correct it. In this case, Frank (1999) suggests one possibility: a progressive consumption tax. For example, above a certain level of spending (say, $50,000 a year), government could charge a 20 percent tax on the next $10,000 in spending, a 21 percent tax on the next $10,000—up to, say, a tax of 70 percent on annual spending above $550,000.[6] The idea is that if everyone has to pay much higher taxes as they spend more, they will have more of an incentive to seek out nonstatus goods, such as greater leisure time from not working as many hours or taking more vacation time. Whether such a plan is politically feasible, however, is doubtful.

Where does all this leave us? It is our hope that the reader now has some appreciation for the notion that an economic system that is based on competition and encourages production, but not necessarily the redistribution of wealth, does not always make society better off. One application of this, which has been analyzed extensively in the literature, concerns how the *distribution* of income in society—over and above individuals' own incomes—affects population health.

Does the Distribution of Income Affect the Health of the Population?

Economic theory focuses on absolute, not relative, relationships. An individual is assumed to care about only the bundle of goods he or she possesses, not what others have. A natural extension of this theory is the belief that absolutes are what matter when it comes to the population as a whole. A wealthier nation should be a happier nation if utility is determined by the value of the goods possessed. As we showed earlier, however, there is mixed evidence on this.

What about health? Nearly all research shows that more income improves most measures of health among the poor, but has a much smaller effect on those whose incomes were higher to begin with. This is true not only at the individual level, but in the aggregate. Wealthier countries exhibit better population health up to a certain income threshold, but beyond that point, little relationship is apparent (Daniels, Kennedy, and Kawachi 2000).

The issue is whether there is also a relationship between health and the *distribution* of income. At any given level of income, do countries (or states or cities) where wealth is spread more evenly among the population exhibit better health outcomes? If so, then narrowing the distribution of income would make the populace healthier.

Why might such a relationship exist? Three possible pathways are noted here (Kawachi and Kennedy 2001; Wilkinson 1999). The first relates to stress. In an inegalitarian society, those on the bottom of the income distribution are more likely to feel pressure, which can have negative physiological and psychological consequences. This stress can result from various factors, such as being unable to make ends meet, feeling anger at one's lot, or being "picked on," either directly or indirectly, by those in higher social classes.

The Whitehall studies of British civil servants (Marmot et al. 1997), the first of which began in the 1960s and the second in the 1980s, support the idea that social standing affects health. The first study found that over time, lowest-level civil servants, such as clerks, had twice the mortality as those in the highest level, such as administrators. The second study found differences of about 50 percent in coronary heart disease, much of which was the result of how much control workers felt they had over their work. But why does control matter? Michael Marmot and his coauthors (1997, 239) write:

> The putative pathophysiological mechanisms by which psychosocial factors cause [coronary heart disease] involve activation of the autonomic nervous system and the hypothalamic pituitary adrenal axis, which in turn leads to metabolic changes

that increase cardiovascular risk. Work conditions are not the only way to activate these neuroendocrine pathways: low control in other areas of life, a self-image of low efficiency, and hostility may be other social or psychological factors that activate these pathways.

Researchers have not confined their inquiry to *Homo sapiens.* Studies of other primates, such as wild baboons (Sapolsky, Alberts, and Altmann 1997) and captive monkeys (Shively and Clarkson 1994), show how low social standing among these species can also lead to a greater risk of coronary disease and other health risks, apparently as a reaction to continual stress. As interpreted by Robert Evans (1999, 17):

> If you are constantly under the pressure of fight or flight, slowly you will, in fact, find your health deteriorating in various ways. [One study] found that the sub-dominant animals were in a state of permanent arousal—partly because of constant threats from the dominant animals and partly because once that state was triggered, physiologically they were changed in ways that made it difficult for them to turn off that fight-or-flight switch. In other words, they were physiologically changed by the experience of their rank and position.

Although difficult to demonstrate directly, the analogous theory is that humans who find themselves on the lower rungs of employment and social structures will experience similar reactions.

The second pathway relates to the effect of income distribution on the resources available to those in lower classes. In a nearly egalitarian society, people are more likely to feel empathy toward others because most everyone is in a similar position. Of course, some people will be more disadvantaged than others, but when the bridge across classes is smaller, more societal resources are likely to be transferred to those who are more in need. In contrast, a society with a large gulf between classes is less conducive to such empathy, and may encourage overt hostility instead. In such a situation, the well-to-do may provide fewer resources to help others. Daly and colleagues (1998, 319) have hypothesized that "political units that tolerate a high degree of income inequality are less likely to support the human, physical, cultural, civic, and health resources needed to maximize the health of the population." This theory has garnered some empirical support (Kaplan et al. 1996). Related research indicates that social investment in disadvantaged children is particularly important to their development (Hertzman 2001); areas with greater income disparity tend to provide fewer such investments.

A third pathway, closely related to the second, concerns some of the potential deleterious effects of a more stratified society, including a lack of trust, less individual investment in personal capital, and more violence—each of which may affect health. These issues are discussed in Chapter 9, with the introduction of the concept of *social capital.*

Unfortunately, it is difficult to test whether income distribution affects health status through the mechanisms noted above. The main problem is specifying and collecting data on all the factors that are likely to affect health status. The distribution of income is related to other characteristics—social, environmental, even behavioral—that may also affect health outcomes. If these are not controlled for, empirical analyses can inappropriately attribute causal effects to the distribution of income. Moreover, the ability to properly distinguish between the effects of individual characteristics (i.e., a person's income) and aggregate traits (i.e., the distribution among all people in a particular area) on the income–health relationship is essential.

Another difficulty with conducting this research is that we would expect to find a correlation between health and income distribution—even if none of the causal factors mentioned above matter.[7] This may seem counterintuitive, but it is illustrated in Figure 5.4.[8] Suppose each point on the curve represents a particular person in an area. Further suppose two areas each have the same average income, but one exhibits a narrow distribution of income, ranging from A to B, whereas the other has a wide income distribution, ranging from Y to Z. Mathematically, the average health status is shown as the midpoint (M) of a line segment connecting these points. In the area with more equal incomes, average health status will be H_2, which is higher than the health status (H_1) where there is greater income inequality. This means that "[o]verall population mortality increases when inequality increases, even though every individual's risk of mortality depends only on their own income level and not on the income level of anyone else" (Gravelle 1998, 383). This would hardly support the viewpoint that relative income matters through the pathways outlined above. It does confirm, however, that societal redistributions of income from the wealthy to the poor should increase health status—for the simple reason that the marginal impact of more income on health is greater for poorer people (Subramanian and Kawachi 2004).

A substantial body of literature reports on whether income distribution affects health status, but unfortunately, there is little agreement among researchers, and the issue is far from settled. One of the earliest studies was conducted by Rodgers (1979). Using data from 56 countries, he found that, controlling for the level of income, measures of income distribution had a large effect on infant mortality and life expectancy. Compared to those in a stratified society, members of a relatively egalitarian society have life spans of five to ten years longer. Using data from the United States, Kennedy, Kawachi, and Prothrow-Stith (1996) found that the states with the widest distribution of income had higher total mortality and infant mortality rates. Other studies have also found evidence that narrower income distributions improve health.[9]

Significant literature, however, criticizes studies that have found a relationship between income inequality and health and provides some counter-

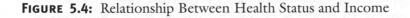

FIGURE 5.4: Relationship Between Health Status and Income

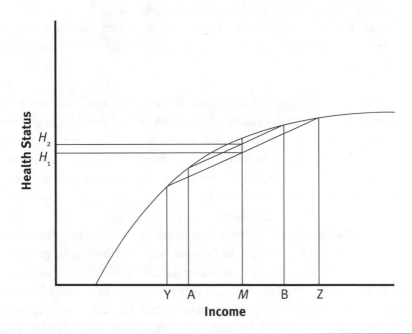

evidence. One of the main criticisms is that these studies do not adequately control for other factors related to income distribution and health status (and thus suffer from "omitted variables bias"). Judge (1995) finds no relationship between several alternative measures of income inequality and life expectancy among developed countries. Mellor and Milyo (2001) use data from several dozen countries at a particular time period and over time and find no evidence of the relationship, nor do they find evidence of it when looking at nine different measures of health status across the different states in the United States. Similarly, Deaton (2001) finds no evidence of a relationship between income inequalities and health, but he does posit that inequalities other than income might be important. Moreover, Lorgelly and Lindley (2008) find no association in the United Kingdom. In a review of the literature, Wagstaff and van Doorslaer (2000) conclude that little convincing evidence exists that income inequality affects health.[10] But a more recent review of about 50 studies (Macinko et al. 2003) finds more mixed results.

Some data sets are richer than others, however. If one wishes to distinguish between the roles of absolute and relative incomes in regard to health, a data set that includes both individual-level characteristics and area-level ones is essential. Subramanian and Kawachi (2004) review the results of over 20 such studies across a number of nations. The results are mixed, with a little more than half of the U.S. studies finding a relationship between income distribution and health, but almost none of the international studies finding such a relationship. This could be because there is less income inequality, and more social programs and solidarity, in other countries.

In the United States, the geographic entity where such findings exists tend to be the state, which, the authors believe, indicates that politics play a role:

> The state-level associations seem to suggest the importance of political mechanisms, such as the relation of economic disparities within each state to patterns of spending by state legislatures on social goods such as health care, education, and welfare. In other words, economic polarization leads to political polarization, as reflected by state variations in the generosity of benefits to the poor. (Subramanian and Kawachi 2004, 81–82)

Although there is certainly no consensus in the literature, most recent studies have not found a strong link between the distribution of income and health. More research with access to better data undoubtedly is forthcoming. This is critical because in many countries—particularly the United States—income inequality has been rising (Subramanian and Kawachi 2004; Brandolini and Smeeding 2007), a trend certainly correlated with and probably a result of the growing role of markets (Kuttner 1997).

There is, however, one firm conclusion reached by many of the authors: Even if the distribution of income does not matter, income itself certainly does—as do the many factors with which it is correlated, such as wealth, home/land ownership, education, occupation, and social class. Two sets of authors state this particularly well:

> Regardless of the relationship between income inequality and health . . . nearly every study has confirmed the importance of individual income on health outcomes—even within countries with universal insurance and relatively generous social welfare policies. This suggests that one benefit of research on income inequality is that it has highlighted the role of economic and social resources and their impact on health inequalities . . . (Macinko et al. 2003, 435)

> Although we found little evidence to support a direct effect of income inequality on health, this should not be interpreted to mean the factors that drive unequal income distribution at the system level are not important to individual and population health. Reducing income inequality by raising the incomes of more disadvantaged people will improve the health of poor individuals, help reduce health inequalities, and increase average population health. (Lynch et al. 2004, 83–84)

A natural (though not necessarily inevitable) consequence of greater reliance on markets is a reduction in the role of the welfare state (Coburn

2000). One reason is that greater use of markets goes hand in hand with lower tax rates; with lower tax revenues, less money is available to finance welfare-related programs. As these quotations imply, a pullback in welfare-related governmental policies is likely to worsen these health-related consequences.

Concern About Others

In this section we deal with a different type of consumption externality: concern about the well-being of others. If we care about other people's needs as well as our own—be they specific needs like food or medical care or somewhat more vague concerns about how happy the people are—then a positive externality of consumption exists. As we noted earlier, a competitive market, by itself, will not provide enough of the goods and services for which there is a positive externality.

In the previous section, we argued that people are concerned about their status relative to others. But this does not mean that they cannot be concerned about others' well-being at the same time. People might feel that others should have certain things, such as adequate food or medical care or even happiness, but they might also feel envy when others have things they do not. Most plausible, perhaps, would be that people want those who have less than they have to have more—although not as much as themselves, as suggested by the Mencken quotation—and, at the same time, want to have as much as those who have more.

Even though we are talking about concern for others, our focus here is on *economic efficiency*. We noted earlier that a competitive market is not designed to improve the distribution of resources among the population, so one might ask how its failure to deal with distributional issues can be raised as an efficiency problem.

The answer to this question is that there are two distinct reasons for redistributing income.[11] The one that might be most familiar to readers concerns issues of *social* or *distributive justice*—in essence, that redistribution is the "right thing to do." John Rawls's (1971) book, *A Theory of Justice*, provides a strong philosophical foundation for this belief. The economic tools we provided earlier illustrate the concept of social justice. Refer back to the Edgeworth Box in Figure 2.24. Suppose we are at economically efficient point C, where Jane has most of the wealth and Paul has little. If one views this situation as unfair, a possible justification for redistributing income from Jane to Paul would be to correct this inequity. Much of Chapter 9 will be devoted to examining these issues.

A second possible reason exists, however, for redistributing resources: to satisfy people's preferences. Suppose I care about poor people and want them to have more food and medical care. To increase my own utility, I would want to give some of my resources to the poor, stopping at the point where the marginal utility I gain from contributing the last dollar equals the marginal utility I gain from spending it on something else.

Why doesn't everyone just donate their optimal amount to charity, thereby maximizing their personal utility? The problem is that many, if not most, people will attempt to become free riders, which will result in less redistribution than is optimal. Assume again that people care about others and want the poor to have more food, housing, medical care, and so forth. If this is done through a competitive model, an unfortunate thing happens. The Joneses will recognize that the poor will do about as well if everyone except the Joneses provides donations. But if many or most people act in this way, too little money is redistributed. The outcome therefore remains inefficient; society would be better off if there were a way to redistribute the optimal amount of resources rather than the lesser amount that occurs under competition.

Some Theory on the Use of Taxes to Change Income Distribution

The standard answer to this problem in traditional economics is to rely on a competitive marketplace to allocate resources efficiently, and then to employ just the right amount of special taxes and subsidies to redistribute income. These are called *lump-sum* taxes and subsidies.

The idea is to come up with a way to tax, say, the wealthy, to subsidize—presumably—the poor, without changing (in any important way) the efficiency-enhancing incentives of a competitive market. If no such methods are feasible, market competition is problematic when there are consumption externalities: If we do not redistribute income, the market is inefficient because people want poorer people to be better off than they are. But if we do redistribute income, we damage the efficiency that the marketplace is designed to create.

The problem with the lump-sum solution is the virtual impossibility of establishing true lump-sum taxes and subsidies. We would need to come up with a way of transferring income that does not affect the incentives of the payer of the tax or the recipient of the subsidy.[12]

The taxes we use most commonly do not meet these requirements, because they would alter incentives. An income tax, for example, results in a reduction in net wages from the provision of additional labor. Standard theory assumes laborers will work until their *opportunity cost*—forgone leisure—equals the wage rate. If the imposition of an income tax causes a decrease in net wages, workers are likely to substitute more leisure for labor because the value of labor will be lower. This results in a lower overall production of goods and services. The other commonly employed tax is a sales tax. The problem with a sales tax is that it results in the consumer paying a higher price than the producer will receive. A condition of Pareto optimality is that consumers' marginal rates of substitution must be equal to the economy's marginal rate of transformation (as discussed in Chapter 2). This is no longer the case when there is a sales tax; allowing competition with sales taxes in place will not result in an economically efficient allocation of resources (Nath 1969).

It is equally difficult to come up with an incentive-neutral method for subsidies. A typical way of transferring money to the poor is through welfare payments, but this results in a work disincentive. Receiving a smaller welfare check when your income rises is no different from facing an income tax; as we just saw, a competitive market with income taxes is not economically efficient. (This is one of our arguments for the superiority of in-kind over in-cash transfers for the poor in Chapter 9.)

One sort of tax and subsidy might work in theory, but not in practice. This is a *poll tax*—a tax levied irrespective of income. But as J. de V. Graaff (1971, 78) writes,

[a poll tax] is not very helpful in securing desired redistributions unless we tax different men differently. But on what criteria should we discriminate between different men? Ethical ones? And what if a man cannot pay the tax? If we start taxing the poor less than the rich, we are simply reintroducing an income-tax. If we tax able men more than dunderheads, we open the door to all forms of falsification: we make stupidity seem profitable—and any able man can make himself seem stupid. Unless we really do have an omniscient observing economist to judge men's capabilities, or a slave-market where the prices they fetch reflect expert appraisals of their capacities, any taxing authority is bound to be guided by elementary visible criteria like age, marital status and—above all—ability to pay. We are back with an income tax.

The problem gets even more ticklish when we consider issues of fairness. Suppose we decide to tax people based not on their income, per se, but on their *ability* to generate income. This would mean that those who are less able to earn would be taxed less than those more able. As Paul Samuelson (1947, 247–48) notes,

Analytically, the problem resembles that of determining . . . a fair "handicap" for golfers of different ability. We wish to equalize opportunity for all contestants, but we do not want them to hold back from playing their best because of a fear of losing their favorable handicap. . . . Thus, we might decide that everyone should have at least a minimum income, that Society will make up the deficiency between what the less fortunate can earn and this minimum. Once this is realized by those who fall below the minimum, there is no longer an incentive for them to work at the margin, at least in pecuniary material terms. This is clearly bad social policy.

The aim of the foregoing discussion was to show the near impossibility of devising workable lump-sum taxes and subsidies—which are necessary if we are to retain economic efficiency in the wake of externalities of consumption. What, then, is the implication? Simply this: In making policy, it is impossible to separate issues of resource allocation from issues of resource distribution.

Dealing with Allocation and Distribution Concurrently

Several economists have pointed out the impossibility of separating allocative and distributional economic activities in a variety of contexts, but this anomaly has received little attention from the profession at large. The traditional economic method, in which competitive forces are allowed to prevail and distribution is only done afterward, is not necessarily appropriate—especially in the presence of consumption externalities.

A more reasonable approach to dealing with this problem, particularly in the healthcare system, is for society to grapple with allocative and distributive issues concurrently. Rather than saying, "we will take whatever the competitive market gives us, and then institute the necessary taxes and subsidies," a reasonable society might contend that "we will start with certain redistributive principles, and once they are established, allow the market to operate around these principles."

Uwe Reinhardt (1992, 315) provides a similar philosophy:

> [T]o begin an exploration of alternative proposals for the reform of our health system without first setting forth explicitly, and very clearly, the *social values* to which the reformed system is to adhere strikes at least this author as patently *inefficient*: it is a waste of time. Would it not be more *efficient* merely to explore the *relative efficiency* of alternative proposals that do conform to widely shared *social values*?

This method, and not the method the competitive model advocates, is how policy has traditionally been made in the United States and almost all developed countries. In the United States, public programs like Medicare and Medicaid were established *outside* of the competitive marketplace to ensure that our priority—access to medical care services for the elderly and the poor—was met. Of note, however, is that in recent years we have been moving away from this. Increasingly, Medicare is relying more on competition among private insurers, both through Part C (managed care plans) and Part D (prescription drug plans). This is not surprising, since the Republican administrations that controlled the presidency and the two houses of Congress from 2000 to 2006 believed in the superiority of markets over government. Such a movement is in line with the traditional economic prescription of redistributing resources and then letting market forces dictate the ultimate allocation.

Further Applications to Health Policy

The belief that we should start with principles of fairness and then proceed to considerations of efficiency is the foundation on which most other health systems have been built. In their comprehensive study of financing and equity in nine health systems in Europe and the United States, Adam Wagstaff and colleagues (1992, 363) found that:

> [t]here appears to be broad agreement . . . among policymakers in at least eight of the nine European countries [studied] that payments towards health care should be related to ability to pay rather than to use of medical facilities. Policymakers in all nine European countries also appear to be committed to the notion that all citizens should have access to health care. In many countries this is taken further, it being made clear that access to and receipt of health care should depend on need, rather than on ability to pay.

One of the best ways to deal with this concern is to enact policies that ensure that those in need have access to goods and services, even if they do not have the economic resources to purchase them in the marketplace. Programs like Medicare and Medicaid in the United States—which are not in keeping with some economists' recommendations for reliance on competition and then redistribution of resources through cash subsidies—offer good examples of how society grapples with such problems.

Evidence that U.S. health policy has eschewed the competitive prescription dates back many years. Beginning with the post–World War II period, the subsidization of the building and expansion of hospitals under the Hill-Burton Act (1948) and subsequent subsidization of physician training costs directly reflected a belief that poorer, rural areas of the United States should not be disadvantaged *relative to* wealthier, urban areas of the country. By basing the need for hospitals on the per capita availability of beds, the philosophy behind Hill-Burton was that no areas of the country should have greater access than others to hospital care.[13]

State mandates concerning the content of health insurance coverage provide more recent evidence. One implication of the competitive model is that insurance companies are allowed to provide whatever health insurance coverage they wish. Economists have argued that mandating health insurance coverage could have deleterious consequences, including raising insurance costs, lowering wages, and lowering health insurance coverage rates (Jensen and Morrisey 1999).

Public policy makers not have followed economists' advice, however. States, which have almost all regulatory authority over the sale of insurance, have enacted mandates concerning eligibility for and content of health insurance policies. One study found that by 1988, there were more than 730 mandates across the different states (Gabel and Jensen 1989). For example, 37 states required insurers to cover alcohol treatment, 28 required that mental health services be covered, and 18, maternity care. A more recent study found that the number of state mandates had grown to about 1,000 by 1997 (Council for Affordable Health Insurance 1997). In 1996, the most common mandates were for mammography screening (46 states), alcohol treatment (43 states), and services provided by psychologists and chiropractors (41 states each) (Jensen and Morrisey 1999). Special interest groups provide much of the support for these mandates; nevertheless, consumer groups, and particularly people who need certain services (or know someone who does), also tend to support them, indicating that the public does not want insurance coverage decisions left solely to the marketplace.

Examining the political fallout from the Oregon proposal for Medicaid reform, which required "rationing" of services, reveals similar evidence for this viewpoint. Early versions of the proposal met with opposition, mainly because program beneficiaries would not be able to receive coverage for the same services as the rest of the population. Rather, the services paid for would depend on how much money was available. Less cost-effective services would not be covered if program money was exhausted after paying for more cost-effective services. This prompted Bruce Vladeck (1990, 3), who later became director of the federal government's Health Care Financing Administration (currently the Centers for Medicare & Medicaid Services), to write,

> [T]his will be the first system in memory to explicitly plan that poor people with treatable illnesses will die if Medicaid runs out of money or does not budget correctly, and providers will be excused from liability for failing to treat them. The Oregonians argue that it is healthier for society to make such choices explicitly, but it is hardly healthy to establish rules of the game that require such choices.

In fact, federal officials cleared the proposal only after the methodology was revised substantially to ensure that disabled individuals would not face discrimination in coverage (Fox and Leichter 1993), and after the state made it clear that all essential services would be provided.[14] After the modified proposal had been implemented, a survey of Medicaid beneficiaries in the state found that one-third had needed a service that was not covered. In 38 percent of these cases, the service was not covered because funding was insufficient. About half of these people obtained the service with their own money. Among the other half, 60 percent said that their health had deteriorated as a result (Mitchell and Bentley 2000).

Indeed, the Oregon program has faced many subsequent hurdles, with Oberlander (2006) commenting on the "unraveling" of the program around 2003. The state had tried to expand eligibility to cover more people who were near-poor, but in charging substantial premiums and requiring cost sharing for a reduced set of benefits, it lost most of the people it wanted to insure. Oberlander writes, "Oregon failed to anticipate how price-sensitive . . . enrollees were and their troubles navigating the new system, a cautionary tale for states enamored with consumerism and the prospect of having Medicaid recipients put more 'skin in the game' through added cost sharing" (W100). In 2008, the state even held a lottery to allot 3,000 new spaces among over 90,000 applicants, with one newspaper calling it "a jarring reminder of just how broken the U.S. healthcare system really is" (Glascock 2008).

A final example of how U.S. health policy operates in conflict with the competitive model with respect to concern about others relates to coverage for new technologies. Imagine a new technology that can help save lives, but is very expensive. Is society better off if we allow only the rich to purchase it, as the Pareto principle would imply? It might seem that the answer is yes, because we do allow people to spend their own money for such procedures as long as the procedures are legal. But further reflection reveals that something quite different is going on.

Traditionally, new and potentially effective technologies are considered experimental until their safety and efficacy are established. Once they are proven safe and effective, insurers almost always cover them; failure to do so results first in strong pressure from policyholders and eventually in lawsuits that claim the insurer is withholding necessary medical care. Having these technologies covered by public and private insurance ensures that the majority of the insured population has access to them. Uwe Reinhardt (1992, 311) writes,

> Suppose [that a] new, high-tech medical intervention [is available] and that more of it could be produced without causing reductions in the output of any other commodity. Suppose next, however, that the associated rearrangement of the economy has been such that only well-to-do patients will have access to the new medical procedure. On these assumptions, can we be sure that [this] would enhance overall *social welfare*? Would we not have to assume the absence of *social envy* among the poor and of guilt among the well-to-do? Are these reasonable assumptions? Or should civilized policy analysts refuse to pay heed to base human motives such as envy, prevalent though it may be in any normal society?

If public policy were based on market competition, we would see a gap between the services available to the wealthy and those available to the rest of the insured population. We do not see such a gap; once a procedure is found to be safe and effective, everyone with private health insurance is potentially eligible to receive it.[15] And, if insurers are not quick to adopt new procedures, states can and do mandate their provision.[16]

This is not to say that policy has ensured equal access for all Americans. In fact, the uninsured population tends to use fewer services and to benefit from fewer new medical technologies (Institute of Medicine 2001). Until now, however, most have been able to benefit from a safety net of public hospitals and community clinics, as well as "cross-subsidization" of uninsured patients by their insured counterparts.

5.2 Formation of Preferences

The Formation of Preferences in the Traditional Model

Of all of the assumptions in the traditional economic model, perhaps most often forgotten is the notion that consumers' tastes are already established when they enter the marketplace. This assumption is extraordinarily important. In this section we will attempt to show that when established taste is not taken into account, the competitive model loses some of its advantages.

Economics is almost universally viewed as a social science. Social sciences seek to understand how individuals and/or groups of people behave. But each social science views human behavior through its own lens. Sociology, for example, focuses on how behavior is affected by society's organization, social stratification, group dynamics, and the like (Mechanic 1979). Political science examines how individuals and groups attempt to obtain what they want through such means as "conflict, influence, and authoritative collective decision making in both public and private settings" (Marmor and Dunham 1983, 3). Social psychology attempts to understand "the influences that people have upon the beliefs or behavior of others" (Aronson 1972, 6).

One facet of these other social sciences is that, in general, they seek to determine how people and groups actually behave. In contrast, Thurow (1983, 216) contends, "while the reverse is true in the other social sciences that study real human behavior, prescription dominates description in economics." In this regard, in economics one commonly sees the word "ought" (e.g., people *ought* to maximize their utility, otherwise they are being irrational; to maximize social welfare, a society *ought* to depend on a competitive marketplace).

According to Gary Becker (1979, 9), three things distinguish economics from the other social sciences. First, economics assumes that people engage in "maximizing behavior"—that is, individuals strive to obtain the most utility possible, firms work for the greatest profits, and so on. Second, the milieu in which people operate is the market. And third, "preferences are assumed not to change substantially over time, nor to be very different between wealthy and poor persons, or even between persons in different societies and cultures." Similarly, George Stigler and Gary Becker (1977, 76) go even further than this, claiming that

> tastes neither change capriciously nor differ importantly between people. . . . [O]ne does not argue over tastes for the same reason that one does not argue over the Rocky Mountains—both are there, will be there next year, too, and are the same for all men.[17]

Not only are preferences assumed to be immutable, but they are also assumed to be determined outside of the economic or even social system in which the person exists. In economic theory, individual tastes and preferences "simply exist—fully developed and immutable" (Thurow 1983, 219). This is what Kenneth Boulding (1969, 2) has referred to as the "Immaculate Conception of the Indifference Curve," because "tastes are simply given, and . . . we cannot inquire into the process by which they are formed."

Milton Friedman (1962, 13, emphasis added) provides an explanation for this that is consistent with our discussion of how economics differs from the other social sciences:

> [E]conomic theory proceeds largely to take wants as fixed . . . primarily [as] a case of division of labor. The economist has little to say about the formation of wants; this is the province of the psychologist. *The economist's task is to trace the consequences of any given set of wants.*[18]

Critique of the Traditional Model

Henry Aaron (1994, 7) has pointed out the importance of recognizing that individual behavior influences, and is influenced by, the community.

> It is then essential to recognize how changes in individual beliefs and values alter the environment in which individual actions occur. The environment is important both because people's preferences are shaped by pressure from peers and neighbors and because community attitudes shape the actual payoffs to various kinds of individual behavior.

It is beyond the scope of this book to fully demonstrate that people's tastes and behaviors are mutable. The field of social psychology deals with this particular issue. Good overviews of the field, as well as evidence from some of the more noteworthy experiments, are provided in Aronson (1972) and Ross and Nisbett (1991).

Overwhelming evidence suggests that people's decisions—market related and otherwise—can indeed be influenced by their environment. Consider the case of advertising. The reader, who is likely well-versed in media tactics, will probably admit that most consumer advertising is not aimed at providing objective information to minimize consumers' search for the best value. Rather, advertising is designed to (1) *minimize* the search process itself, and more generally, (2) change consumer tastes, in part by exerting social pressure. It is hard to claim that the tastes people develop as the result of exposure to this sort of advertising are sacrosanct. In fact, people often make nonmaximizing decisions by acting on the message—the hallmark of a successful advertising campaign.

Although it does not deal with market behavior directly, one particular set of social psychology experiments is reviewed here because it shows graphically how people's beliefs and behaviors can be distorted by their environment.

These are Stanley Milgram's (1963) renowned studies of obedience in the face of authority.[19] These results have been used to explain, among other things, the behavior of Nazi officials during the Holocaust (Ross and Nisbett 1991).

In one version of the experiment (Milgram 1963), 40 male volunteers aged 20 to 50 are solicited to participate in a study of memory and learning at Yale University. An "experimenter" has two individuals—one a naive subject and the other an imposter—draw lots to determine who will be the "teacher" and who the "learner." By design, the naive subject always becomes the teacher, and he or she is instructed to give electrical shocks to the learner (who is stationed in a different room) when the latter provides incorrect answers on a memory test. Although the shocks are, of course, fake, participants have been told that they are real and that "although the shocks can be extremely painful, they cause no permanent tissue damage" (Milgram 1963, 373). The experimenter tells the teacher to administer a shock of 15 volts for the first wrong answer, and to increase this by 15 volts each time a subsequent wrong answer is given, to a maximum of 450 volts. The apparatus that supposedly gives the shocks is labeled to indicate their severity, going from "slight shock" to "danger: severe shock." At 300 volts, the victim starts banging on the walls, begging that the experiment be discontinued. After 315 volts, even these protests stop, at which point the victim no longer provides any answers. But the experimenter urges the subjects to continue, because no answer is to be construed as a wrong answer, until the maximum 450 volts is administered.

Not surprisingly, as the experiment proceeds, some subjects question the experimenter about whether they should go on, and/or whether the recipient of the shocks is all right. When this occurs, the instructor insists that they continue to participate, although no loud voice or threats are used.[20]

Much to the surprise of the researchers (and subsequently, to much of the civilized world), most people continued to administer shocks all the way to the maximum level. In this particular study, all 40 participants continued to shock the victim up to a level of 300 volts, and 35 continued even after the wall banging. A full 26 (65 percent) continued to the maximum 450 volts.

It is especially curious that subjects continued to administer the shocks, given that they were clearly not predisposed to such behavior. As Stanley Milgram (1963, 375) reports,

> Many subjects showed signs of nervousness in the experimental situation, and especially upon administering the more powerful shocks. In a large number of cases the degree of tension reached extremes that are rarely seen in sociopsychological laboratory studies. Subjects were observed to sweat, tremble, stutter, bite their lips, groan, and dig their fingernails into their flesh. . . . One sign of tension was the regular occurrence of nervous laughing fits. . . . The laughter seemed entirely out of place, even bizarre. . . . In the post-experimental interviews subjects took

pains to point out that they were not sadistic types, and that the laughter did not mean they enjoyed shocking the victim.

Why people can be influenced to behave in a way that so contradicts their personal values has been debated for years and has still not been satisfactorily explained (Ross 1988). Milgram himself offered 13 reasons in his 1963 article. Some of the reasons clearly reflect the peculiar nature of the situation.[21] The point being made here is that people's tastes (here, to inflict harm on others) are not predetermined or fixed, but rather are subject to innumerable cognitive and social forces.

Why, then, does economics consider tastes predetermined and fixed rather than subject to the forces of change? The primary tenet of modern economics is the sanctity of consumer choice. Most economists believe that the consumer is the best judge of what will maximize his or her utility. Consequently, to maximize overall social welfare, we should set up an economic system that best allows consumer choices to be satisfied. Where these choices come from, as Friedman (1962) said, is beside the point.

But if what you want depends on what you had in the past or on the influence of peers or advertisers, then it is not clear that a competitive marketplace is the best way to make people better off (Pollack 1978). True, if certain conditions are met, a competitive market will result in allocative efficiency; however, a major assumption attached to this is that the things people demand are really the things that will make them best off. We pursue this issue more broadly in Chapter 4. Here we focus on the specific issue of whether satisfying consumers' tastes, as indicated by their demand for particular goods and services, will necessarily maximize their utility.

The following paragraphs provide three examples in which people's market behaviors are not predetermined but rather are a result of their past or present environments. In each case, it is not clear that fulfillment of their personal choices would make them best off.

The first and perhaps least important example concerns addiction. Suppose that, while growing up, you are in a peer group that smokes cigarettes and you become addicted. Once you leave that peer group, you will still have a "taste" for cigarettes and are more likely to demand them than someone who is not addicted. Can we really say, in such an instance, that satisfying this taste through the marketplace is efficient from a societal standpoint in the same way satisfying the demand for bread or literature would be? Might not you be better off if cigarettes were taxed so prohibitively (or even banned) that you stopped smoking?[22]

A second and much more general application is habit formed by past consumption patterns.[23] Suppose you live in a community that has not discovered the joys of music. A resident of such a place will therefore not have developed a taste for music. But, as Alfred Marshall (1920) once noted, "the more good music a man hears, the stronger is his taste for it likely to become" (94). The aforementioned resident might be better off with music than without, but he or she has not been sufficiently educated to know this.[24, 25]

This is a problem for competitive markets. If people demand goods based on their prior experience—as they certainly must—and furthermore, if their prior experience is colored by the economic environment in which they live, they will demand things that are characteristic of that environment. This implies a strong advantage for whatever is the status quo; familiarity breeds preference (as opposed to breeding contempt), so what exists now will continue to be demanded in the future.[26]

If tastes are determined in this way, a society might be better off pursuing some goods and services that are not demanded most strongly by the public. This is because people might not know what alternatives are available that might make them better off. But if consumer tastes are viewed as predetermined, as they are in the economic model, people get stuck with whatever they demand because they are assumed always to know best.

The third example concerns occupational choices. The traditional economic model assumes that people make occupational choices by weighing all alternatives, considering factors such as how much satisfaction they obtain from the work and the wages it offers. Whatever choice is made in a competitive labor market is assumed to be utility maximizing. But this might not be the case if tastes are a product of one's environment.

Suppose, for example, that a person grows up in a factory town and later decides to work in the factory. This might not necessarily be utility maximizing; it is possibly a poor choice, made because of the person's limited horizons. As another example, imagine that one person works to perform house-cleaning services for another. This may not reflect the personal preferences of the worker as much as lack of good alternatives (Buchanan 1977). In this regard, John Roemer (1994, 120) states that "people learn to live with what they are accustomed to or what is available to them. . . . Thus the slave may have adapted to like slavery; welfare judgments based on individual preferences are clearly impugned in such situations." The status quo would be favored by competitive markets, even though people might be better off if society intervened in these choices.

In the following subsection, we provide one health application of the view of preferences as something that, rather than being endemic to a person and immutable to misinformation, can in fact be influenced by firms in the marketplace.

Government-Sponsored Health Education and Intervention

The traditional economic model assumes that consumer tastes are predetermined. People come into the marketplace knowing what they want, and what they want is intrinsic to them; it is not shaped by past consumption or external forces. If, however, individuals' consumption patterns are influenced by the advertising and marketing of items that contribute to poor health (e.g., tobacco), it may be necessary to enact policies that discourage the "choice" to use those products, or even to prohibit their sale.

How does advertising fit into all of this? There are really two types of advertising: that designed to provide purely objective information (e.g., prices, availability) and that aimed at shaping consumer tastes. (There is probably much more of the latter than the former.) Advertisers may pass along information to the consumer that, if he acts upon it, will not necessarily be in the consumer's best interest.

One policy implication of this concerns health education. Because economics concerns itself primarily with money-type variables (e.g., price, insurance, income), its practitioners tend to be less conversant with other policy interventions, such as education designed to change people's harmful habits. If, however, preferences are the product of advertisers' activities, medical education may have a role in undoing some of these deleterious effects.

Government has long been involved in trying to convince the public not to smoke. Part of this effort has been regulatory. Tobacco companies in the United States, for example, cannot advertise their products on television. Government has also been directly involved in antismoking campaigns, through explicit advertisements as well as requirements that tobacco companies include various health disclosures on their packaging. One wonders if more of this involvement, extending into other consumer behaviors (e.g., drinking) is warranted. The need for these efforts is heightened if consumer tastes are malleable rather than predetermined.

Nutrition provides another example. The incidence of obesity is steadily rising in the United States and other developed countries (Flegal et al. 2002), with the majority of research concluding that it results in serious health consequences (Kopelman 2000) and increases healthcare costs, perhaps quite substantially. Kenneth Thorpe and colleagues (2004) conclude from U.S. population surveys in 1987 and 2001 that obesity was responsible for 27 percent of the increase in inflation-adjusted per capita health spending between 1987 and 2001.

The proliferation of unhealthful food options and their marketing raises the issue of whether people are making the right decisions for themselves. Government involvement has been most prevalent among children, with some school districts banning snack food and sugary drinks from their sites. Cities have even issued moratoria against the opening of more fast-food outlets (Hennessy-Fiske and Zahniser 2008).[27] There is also a fast-growing movement toward requiring restaurants to include nutritional information on their menus.

Economists believe that providing information is enough. But what if people don't heed the information? At the time of writing, a movement is taking place in the United States toward banning a particular ingredient, trans fats, from restaurant food. In July 2008, following the example of New

York, California passed a law banning more than small amounts (0.5 grams per serving) of trans fats from all restaurant food, effective in 2010. The reason, according to Governor Arnold Schwarzenegger, who signed the bill into law, was that "Consuming trans fat is linked to coronary heart disease" (McGreevy 2008). Some researchers have determined that eliminating trans fats from the food supply could reduce heart-related deaths by 6 to 19 percent per year. For this to occur, however, they would also have to be banned from food sold in grocery stores.

Clearly in some cases government goes beyond just educating. The trans fat ban is extreme in the sense that it eliminates consumer choice. In some instances it may be inadvisable to proscribe choice, and a better option might be to guide it by giving consumers a "nudge." This term, which is the title of a book by Thaler and Sunstein (2008), champions an idea they had previously developed, called "libertarian paternalism." The idea is not to limit choice so much as to push people toward wise choices. One health example they provide relates to organ donation. When people have to fill out a form to indicate they are willing to donate their organs if their brain ceases to function, relatively few do so. But if government changes the law and instead says that people must fill one out *not* to donate, the supply of organs for donations can rise substantially. They cite a study that found

> [t]he effect on consent rates is enormous. . . . consider the difference in consent rates between two similar countries, Austria and Germany. In Germany, which uses an opt-in system, only 12 percent of citizens gave their consent, whereas in Austria [which employs opt-out], nearly everyone (99 percent) did. (Thaler and Sunstein 2008, 178–79)

5.3 Can There Be Too Much Choice?[28]

Economists believe that more choice is better. This makes sense, as long as people understand the information available to them, can resist being swayed by misleading claims, and have the wherewithal to sift through all of the available choices. If not, there may be *too much choice*, and government may wish to help consumers navigate through it, or alternatively, to limit choices.

The idea that cognitive limitations may hinder people's ability to make the best choice from among many goes back to the writings of Herbert Simon (1955). Simon developed the notion of *bounded rationality* to describe the computational limitations (e.g., memory) individuals face—limitations that render the assumptions of rational choice theory unrealistic. Indeed, Simon questioned the idea that individuals are able to sift through all of the information available to them with the aim of maximizing their expected utility. Note that this was well before the so-called "information age" and complaints of "information overload."[29]

More recently, psychologist Barry Schwartz (2004) has written extensively on this issue. In his book, *The Paradox of Choice: Why More Is Less*, he combines his own experiences with an extensive review of the literature in making the point that we would often be better off with fewer product options. This could be true for several reasons: People may fail to even make a choice if there are too many options, or if they do, it might be the wrong one; the process of decision making could, in and of itself, lead to a great deal of disutility; and after making a choice a person might regret her decision.

Schwartz begins recounting his own harrowing search for a pair of blue jeans as well as a stop at his local grocery store, where he finds 285 varieties of cookies, 61 sunscreens and tanning oil, 40 toothpastes, 75 instant gravies, and 275 cereals. He cites the work of Iyengar and Lepper (2000), who compared the behavior of individuals who faced a limited number of choices versus others who faced more extensive choices in a series of psychological experiments.

The first, sometimes called the "jam experiment," involved a tasting stand set up in a fancy grocery store in Palo Alto, California. On different days, customers were presented with a table that either had six or 24 different flavors of jam produced by a single company. The researchers recorded what percentage of customers stopped by the table on the alternative days, and whether they ultimately purchased jam with a discount card offered to them. They found that more people stopped by to taste when there were 24 flavors, but far fewer actually made a purchase: only 3 percent, versus 30 percent when there were just six choices. The authors conclude that with so many choices, consumers were not confident that they would make the right choice, and thus did not make a purchase.

Their second experiment involved chocolate. College students were presented with either 6 or 30 different flavors of Godiva chocolate and were asked questions about their tasting experience. Afterward, participants were asked whether they preferred being compensated for their time in cash or in chocolate. Those who were given a choice of six flavors were far more likely to choose compensation in the form of chocolate (48 percent) than those given 30 choices (12 percent). Finally, the researchers set up an experiment involving extra-credit essays for a college class. Students were given a choice of either 6 or 30 specific topics about which they could write. The researchers found that those given the smaller array of choices were more likely to write an essay, and to write a better one.

The too-much-choice literature has also examined whether people make good investment choices for their retirement. Historically, people have not done so. Common errors include investing too little (given the tax-favored nature of such investments); investing too conservatively; paying too much in "loading costs" when cheaper, no-load funds are available that historically have performed just as well; not adjusting portfolio composition over time; investing too much in the stock of the company for which one works; and using overly simple formulas to allocate the distribution of one's contributions to different investments.

There is some evidence that people would invest more successfully if less choice were available. Sethi-Iyengar, Huberman, and Jiang (2004) used data from over 750,000 employees in retirement plans administered by a leading broker of 401(k) plans, a major vehicle for retirement savings in the United States. Controlling for a number of factors, they found that as the number of investment choices increased, the amount employees invested fell. Overall, as another ten fund choices were added, participation fell by 1.5 to 2 percentage points.

In the health sector, a strong argument can be made that there is too much choice for Medicare beneficiaries in the United States with respect to coverage for pharmaceuticals. Beginning in 2006, Medicare began covering prescription drugs for program beneficiaries, mainly seniors. There are two ways of getting the coverage, which is provided only through private insurers that contract with Medicare: One can enroll in a stand-alone drug plan, or in a managed care plan. In 2008, the typical state had 53 stand-alone drug plan choices; when one counts managed care plans, the number was often over 100 (Kaiser Family Foundation 2008b).

Is there too much choice? Senior citizens in the United States seem to think so. Nearly 70 percent say they would prefer a handful of drug plans rather than dozens (Kaiser Family Foundation and Harvard School of Public Health 2006). The fact that so few people switch to another plan during the annual open enrollment period supports the belief that there is too much choice. Switching rates hover around 10 percent (Neuman et al. 2007), but an estimated 43 percent could save money—on average, several hundred dollars a year—if they did switch (Domino et al. 2008).

An experiment conducted by one of the current authors (Hanoch et al. 2008) tested how two factors—number of choices and age—affected the quality of decisions people make about hypothetical prescription drug plans. The experiment took place in Claremont, California, about 30 miles east of Los Angeles. Participants (half of whom were older than age 65) were randomly given 3, 10, or 20 drug plans from which to choose. After giving them data similar to what they would encounter on the Medicare website, participants were asked a number of factual and subjective questions about the material they'd received. Older participants did worse than their younger counterparts on the factual questions, and those with more choices also fared worse. One curious finding was that seniors, on average, were more confident that they had done well on factual questions even though they did worse than younger people—a strong indication that just thinking you can handle a lot of choice does not mean that you can.

To deal with these sorts of problems, economists usually recommend providing more information—although, in Chapter 4, we saw that this often did not do much, if any, good. The problem is even greater for seniors who have to make choices about Medicare drug plans, since many do not use the Internet.

One policy option that one of the current authors has suggested by is to have Medicare limit the number of drug plans that can be marketed to seniors (Rice, Cummings, and Kao 2008). Under this proposal, Medicare would sort through all companies that wish to sell to seniors and choose a handful (the authors suggest ten) of the best values, some of which would have relatively high benefits and costs, and others, lower benefits and costs. Drug insurers would still compete to be among the ten chosen plans; moreover, those ten plans would still compete for enrollees. With only ten plans from which to choose, however, the choice facing the senior would be less daunting.

5.4 Chapter Summary

This chapter focused on several special topics in demand by questioning three key assumptions of the traditional model. If one examines key externalities that pervade healthcare and questions how consumer tastes come into being, different policy implications arise compared with those that fall out of a traditional market model. It becomes clear, for example, that government intervention can play a critical role in ensuring that societal desires and values are met for helping those without coverage, providing information to consumers that counteracts what is available in the marketplace, and, we argue, even limit the amount of choice to a more manageable level.

Notes

1. There is more to this issue, but as it does not affect the other material in the chapter, it is noted only here. An influential concept of modern economics called the Coase Theorem, after economist Ronald Coase, relates to this issue of production externalities. In his article "The Problem of Social Cost" (1960) Coase takes on the *previous* solutions for negative production externalities like pollution, which were to (a) tax the polluting firm by an amount determined by government, (b) hold the firm legally liable for the damage it causes those nearby, or (c) prohibit such firms from locating in residential areas. He argued that in the absence of large transactional costs, the optimal solution for society could be reached without government interference by allowing the affected parties to negotiate a settlement. This solution would have the lowest cost to society. More remarkably, however, was that the assignment of property rights did not matter: The same economically cost-minimizing solution to the pollution problem would be reached whether the polluter had to pay the victim or the victim had to pay the polluter. Such a neat outcome, however, is not necessarily feasible when there are large transactional costs—for example, when thousands of people are affected by the pollution and a negotiated settlement cannot be worked out.

2. Yet another possibility is that one's absolute wealth matters up to a subsistence level, after which only relative wealth matters.

3. A Google Scholar search conducted February 20, 2009, found only one reference (a book chapter) to the paper. In contrast, other pieces by Inglehart and colleagues published earlier in the decade had over 100 citations, implying that the 2008 study is likely to be vetted thoroughly over the next few years.

4. This tenet of modern theory also has its detractors. Joan Robinson (1962, 49), for example, notes that under this theory, "Preference is just what the individual under discussion prefers; there is no value judgment involved. Yet, as the argument goes on, it is clear that it is a Good Thing for the individual to have what he prefers. This, it may be held, is not a question of satisfaction, but freedom—we want him to have what he prefers so as to avoid having to restrain his behaviour. But drug-fiends should be cured; children should go to school. How do we decide what preferences should be respected and what retrained unless we judge the preferences themselves? It is quite impossible for us to do that violence to our own natures to refrain from value judgments." This echoes the sentiments of Pigou (1932, 17), who wrote, "Of different acts of consumption that yield equal satisfaction, one may exercise a debasing, and another an elevating influence."

5. Frank (1999) suggests several things in which we could invest, where there are few if any negative consumption externalities (because none of these is a status good): more vacation time, more leisure time (from less work) to spend with family and friends, and shorter commute times from more investment in transportation.

6. Frank argues that this could be carried out without explicitly keeping track of expenses, by adding a single line to the federal income tax form. Essentially, taxable consumption would simply be income earned minus income saved. Thus, the system would have the added advantage of encouraging more savings.

7. For a fuller discussion of conceptual problems in distinguishing between alternative hypotheses, see Wagstaff and van Doorslaer (2000).

8. This graph is similar to one provided by Kawachi (2000) and Subramanian and Kawachi (2004). The argument is based on a critique of the literature by Gravelle (1998), as well as that provided by Subramanian and Kawachi (2004).

9. For a collection of such studies, as well as the views of dissenters, see Kawachi, Kennedy, and Wilkinson (1999).

10. This was also a finding in a review of the literature by Lynch and colleagues (2004, 5), where they conclude that the "strongest evidence . . . is among states in the United States, but even that is somewhat mixed."

11. A good discussion of the distinction can be found in Wagstaff and van Doorslaer (1993).

12. For further discussion of problems in enacting such taxes and subsidies, see Graaff (1971, 77–82) and Samuelson (1947, 247–49).

13. In fact, because of greater driving distances in rural areas, subsidies were aimed at giving them higher bed-to-population ratios than urban areas. The construction and expansion of hospitals was subsidized up to a level of 5.5 beds per 1,000 people in areas where there are fewer than six persons per square mile, versus only 4.5 beds per 1,000 in areas exceeding 12 persons per square mile.

14. Politics undoubtedly entered the decision as well. The first Bush administration had blocked approval of the plan, but soon after taking office, the Clinton administration approved it. See Pollack and colleagues (1994).

15. Some HMOs have tried to ration the use of medical technologies, with varying degrees of success. This is one of the primary reasons for the so-called consumer backlash against managed care, a consequence of which has been a movement away from heavy-handed cost-control techniques (Gabel et al. 2001).

16. Currently, states cannot mandate provision of services under employer-sponsored health plans that fall under the jurisdiction of the Employee Retirement Income and Security Act. This has effectively reduced the strength of state mandates, since they normally only apply to nongroup coverage.

17. Stigler and Becker (1977) also imply that there is no need for social sciences other than economics. Recall that demand is a function of prices, incomes, and tastes. If tastes do not differ among people or change over time, all consumer behavior can be determined simply by understanding changes in price and income. Indeed, they argue that "the economist continues to search for differences in prices or incomes to explain any differences or changes in behavior" (76).

18. Becker (1979, 9) provides a second explanation for this assumption: "The assumption of stable preferences provides a stable foundation for generating predictions about responses to various changes, and prevents the analyst from succumbing to the temptation of simply postulating the required shift in preferences to 'explain' all apparent contradictions to his predictions."

19. According to Lee Ross (1988, 101), "Perhaps more than any other empirical contribution to the history of social science, [Milgram's] have become part of our society's shared intellectual legacy—that small body of historical incidents, biblical parables, and classic literature that serious thinkers feel free to draw on when they debate about human nature or contemplate human history." It is very unlikely, however, that today's human subjects committees would approve such a study, not only because it relies on deception, but also because subjects might be harmed.

20. When questioned, the experimenter would say "please continue." If the subject balked, he would then say, in order, "the experiment requires that you continue," "it is absolutely essential that you continue," and "you have no other choice, you *must* go on" (Milgram 1963, 374).

21. The experiment was sponsored by a noted university; it was purportedly for a worthy purpose—to study how to enhance learning; the "victim" supposedly

volunteered and was randomly chosen to be the recipient of the shocks; the experimenter did not bend in his conviction that the subject continue administering the shocks; the subject was told that no permanent physical damage would result from the shocks (Milgram 1963).

22. Note that this argument does not hinge on the negative externalities associated with smoking. Prohibitive taxes could also be enacted so that your smoking results in fewer negative side effects on others.

23. For a good discussion of these issues, see Hahnel and Albert (1990).

24. Stated in economic terms, the tangency between their indifference curve and budget constraint is not utility maximizing.

25. The idea of having the economic system not only reflect given preferences but also nurture "more refined" preferences has been a theme of some radical economists. Herbert Gintis (1970, 12), for example, has said that a person can use his existing preferences to demand what he has demanded before, or alternatively, to "*improve* his preference structure so as to be capable of increased satisfaction based on available material goods." Gintis believes that the commodities contained in people's utility functions should not be viewed as ends in themselves, but rather, as instruments for obtaining higher welfare.

26. For a review of health studies that show a preference for the status quo, see Salkeld, Ryan, and Short (2000).

27. For an argument against this policy, see Hicks (2008).

28. Some of the ideas in this section were originally expressed in Rice and Hanoch (2008).

29. In 2008, the nonprofit Information Overload Research Group was formed. According to its website, it is "a group of industry practitioners, academic researchers, and consultants dedicated to reducing information overload, a problem which diminishes the productivity and quality of life of knowledge workers worldwide." E-mail is considered one of the main culprits. See www.iorgforum.org/.

SUPPLY

Besides demand, the other key element in understanding microeconomics is supply. Supply is defined as the amount of goods and services firms wish to sell at alternative prices. In a competitive market, the point at which demand and supply are equal indicates the price at which goods and services will be exchanged and the amount that will be exchanged.

In the economic theory of competitive markets, supply plays a relatively passive role. Suppliers react to changes in demand, but they are unable to induce demand or set prices. Another characteristic of competitive markets is that the supplier's motivation to produce is purely profit oriented.

In healthcare markets, however, suppliers are not just passive producers of whatever is demanded nor are they takers of whatever market price exists. Rather, as in the case of the physician who acts as the patient's agent, suppliers can play a major role in determining what services the consumer chooses to purchase. In some healthcare markets, such as hospital services, suppliers may have some control over prices.

Healthcare suppliers may have motivations other than profits, such as responding to community needs and maintaining high-quality care. The common perception is that nonprofit hospitals have these types of motivations, and that they lead to greater expenses and less efficiency than that associated with for-profit hospitals. In healthcare markets that are predominantly for-profit, such as nursing homes, for-profit goals may conflict with consumer needs for quality care.

The supply of the healthcare workforce, where there are concerns over the adequacy and distribution of professionals such as physicians and nurses, constitutes another important difference between the healthcare market and typical competitive markets. In traditional economic theory, these shortages and maldistributions would be corrected by wage and salary increases and other employment incentives. This does not seem to happen in healthcare.

The following three chapters cover these healthcare supply issues. Chapter 6 examines the extent to which healthcare supply approximates a competitive market. It focuses on four issues: supplier-induced demand, monopoly/

oligopoly behavior, cost shifting, and increasing economies of scale. Chapter 7 looks at the role of the profit motive in healthcare, exploring behaviors and outcomes in several markets, including hospitals, nursing homes, and pharmaceuticals. Chapter 8 discusses the healthcare workforce, focusing on physicians and nurses.

HOW COMPETITIVE IS THE SUPPLY OF HEALTHCARE?

In the traditional economic model, demand is key, while supply tends to play a supporting role. If, for example, demand shifts outward, causing a short-run increase in prices, quantities, and profits, supply will increase to meet demand. In contrast, a change in supply—perhaps due to a reduction in the cost of inputs—does not influence people's demand curves, which are primarily a function of tastes (or, in healthcare, of health status).

If policymakers wish to alter a competitive market, traditional economic theory would suggest focusing on demand. The main tool for doing so is price. Taxes can be used to raise prices, thus suppressing the amount of a good that is demanded, and subsidies can do the opposite. Similarly, deductibles or copayments can be raised (or lowered) in public or private insurance plans, which, as we showed in Chapter 4, would decrease (or increase) the amount of services used. A second policy lever might be to better inform consumers so that they can make the choices that are in their best interest. Beyond that, the list of demand-side tools is rather thin.

If, however, suppliers are more than passive participants in market operation, the list of available policy tools expands. Among the most prominent are incentives designed to influence providers' behavior. Capitation, diagnosis-related groups (DRGs), and practice guidelines are a few examples. In this chapter we examine the extent to which the assumptions of the competitive model regarding supply are met in the health services sector. We then discuss the policy implications of this analysis.

In the following sections, we critique three assumptions of the competitive model, which were presented in Table 3.1:

Assumption 9: Supply and demand are independently determined.
Assumption 10: Firms do not have any market power.
Assumption 11: There are not increasing returns to scale.

6.1 Are Supply and Demand Independently Determined?

The relationship between supply and demand is one of the most thoroughly studied issues in health economics, but it is also one of the issues on which there is the least agreement. Most of the focus has been on whether suppliers—particularly physicians—act totally in their patients' interest, or whether they can convince their patients to act in a way that also benefits them (the suppliers).

Two economic concepts come into play in this controversy. First, physicians act as *agents* for patients in that they help patients make decisions regarding their health and healthcare. Second, physicians tend to have more medical information about patients' conditions and treatments than do patients, which leads to *information asymmetries*. Even though patients are becoming more informed and active in their own care, their knowledge cannot match that of their physician. There seems to be consensus among health economists on both the agency relationship and the existence of at least some information asymmetry (Freebairn 2001).

However, just because physicians have more information than their patients and can exercise this informational power in terms of demand for healthcare does not mean that they will abuse this relationship by providing healthcare that benefits *them*. Physicians can still be perfect agents for their patients by making decisions in the interest of the patients alone. Whether they remain perfect agents or whether they become imperfect agents who *induce demand* is a controversial issue among health economists. One reason physicians might not induce demand is the cost to them: loss of leisure time and psychic discomfort. It will only be in the interests of physicians to induce demand if the benefits outweigh the costs (Evans 1974).

One reason demand inducement has engendered so much interest among health economists is that its existence is at odds with the competitive model. Normally, an increase in supply would lower price, but that is not necessarily the case if physicians induce demand. Furthermore, physicians would be expected to supply fewer services if they are paid less per service, but again, this would not necessarily be true if demand inducement were occurring.[1]

As we noted, there is little agreement on the issue, although most health economists believe that physicians are able to induce demand. In a survey of 359 U.S. health economists, 55 percent of respondents believed that physicians generate *substantial* demand for their own services, while just 29 percent disagreed. (Sixteen percent said they didn't know.) (Morrisey and Cawley 2008.)

This section is not intended to definitively answer the questions that surround demand inducement. Rather, we try to show that in spite of the difficulty of testing for demand inducement, enough evidence is available to make one doubt the independence of demand and supply curves in the physicians' services market. Readers wishing to examine both sides of the issue may want to consult a published debate.[2]

This section is divided into five subsections, the first three of which are devoted to different methods of testing for demand inducement, the fourth to summary remarks, and the fifth to supply-side mechanisms, such as managed care, designed to reduce unnecessary utilization.

Testing Demand Inducement Through Physician-Population Ratios

One of the earliest methods for testing whether physicians induce demand was to determine how a particular market measure, such as utilization or price, changes in response to a change in the number of physicians. The idea behind the test is straightforward: If there is an increase in competition among physicians, and physicians *can* induce demand, they will do so to maintain their revenues. Some studies have found evidence of demand inducement and others have not.[3] Because of the inherent difficulties in conducting such studies, it is unlikely that they will ever reveal uncontestable evidence.

Some of the problems can be seen in Figure 6.1, which is taken from earlier articles by Reinhardt (1978)[4] and by Rice (1983). D_0 and S_0 are the initial demand and supply curves, and S_1 reflects an independent increase in the physician-population ratio. D_1 is the demand curve if physicians induce demand in response to the increase in competition that results from the augmentation of the physician-population ratio. Clearly, just looking at whether utilization increases in response to an increase in the number of physicians does not allow us to distinguish between the competitive and demand-inducement hypotheses—both predict a utilization increase (from Q_0 to Q_c with no inducement, and from Q_0 to Q_i with inducement). But the problem goes even further. Suppose that equilibrium price and quantity move from point A to point C. Although this is consistent with the inducement model, note that it would also be consistent with a no-inducement scenario if the initial demand curve were D' rather than D_0, as shown by the dotted line. Since it is difficult to obtain data that determine the exact shape of a demand curve, it seems unlikely that examining changes in utilization can help us determine whether physicians induce demand in response to changes in the number of physicians in an area.

Another option is to look at what happens to price. But in Figure 6.1, both models predict a decline in price. If physicians do not induce demand, market price will decline from P_0 to P_c, and if they do induce demand, it will decline from P_0 to P_i. This may seem a bit artificial, however, because one can imagine D_1 drawn in such a way that price would actually rise above P_0. Thus, it appears that one way to determine whether physicians induce demand is to see whether price *rises* in response to an increase in the number of physicians. If it does, then it would seem that physicians are inducing demand—although a decline in price, as just demonstrated, would not provide evidence one way or the other.

Unfortunately, this method also presents problems, primary among which is a statistical issue known as *omitted variables bias*. Suppose we find that areas with more physicians have higher prices. This would be consistent

FIGURE 6.1: Effect of an Increase in the Number of Physicians in a Geographic Area

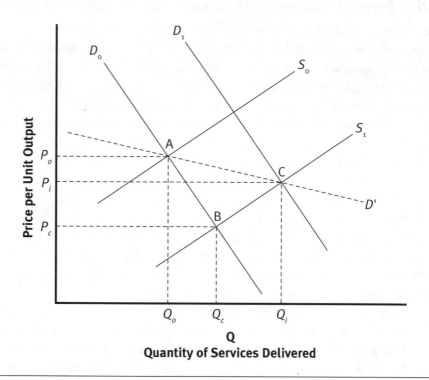

SOURCE: Reprinted from Reinhardt (1978).

with the demand-inducement hypothesis, but only if we control for factors that would make one area of the country more expensive than others. It might be that physicians gravitate to attractive urban and suburban settings with various cultural amenities, good schools, and the like—areas that tend to have higher price levels. If data are not available on all of these characteristics, we might incorrectly attribute higher physician prices to demand inducement. To correct for issues related to physician choice of location, a recent Australian study of physician fee response to changes in physician-population ratio included location variables related to the attractiveness of the location to physicians. This study found that general practice and specialist fees did not fall with a supply increase in the area (Richardson, Peacock, and Mortimer 2006).

Joseph Newhouse (1978) pointed out a final problem: Prices could be higher in areas with more physicians because their services are worth more. This would be the case if the physicians in these areas spend more time with patients and/or patients spend less time waiting. So we could see higher prices in areas with more physicians even if the market is competitive, because the product in those areas is of higher quality and is therefore more expensive.

Testing Demand Inducement Through Physician Payment Rates

Perhaps a somewhat more promising method of testing for demand inducement is to determine how physicians respond to changes in the payments they receive. One might expect that, without demand inducement, physicians would provide fewer services when they face a decline in payment—they would simply slide down the supply curve. But with demand inducement, they might behave differently—say, by increasing the provision of services in the wake of payment reductions to recoup lost income. Note that this sort of behavior is *not* consistent with the upward-sloping supply curve that is typical of competitive markets.

Most, but certainly not all, of the evidence these methods have produced supports the existence of demand inducement.[5] In one of the earliest sets of studies, researchers from the Urban Institute found that California physicians increased the quantity and intensity of services they provided to Medicare beneficiaries in response to a freeze in program payment rates during the early 1970s (Holahan and Scanlon 1979; Hadley, Holahan, and Scanlon 1979). In another set of studies, one of this book's authors found that physicians in urban areas of Colorado, who faced declines in their Medicare payment rates compared to their nonurban colleagues during the late 1970s, increased the intensity of medical and surgical services and the amount of surgery provided and number of laboratory tests ordered (Rice 1983, 1984). Other researchers have found that physicians responded to Medicare payment rate freezes during the mid-1980s by increasing the quantity and/or intensity of surgery, radiology, and special diagnostic tests (Mitchell, Wedig, and Cromwell 1989). A study of provider–client interaction in the Maine Addiction Treatment System in the early 1990s found evidence of provider control of quantity of services and demand inducement through persuasion (Lien, Albert Ma, and McGuire 2004).

Research regarding the Canadian experience through the early 1980s showed that the provinces that were least generous in raising physician payment rates over time experienced the greatest increase in the volume and intensity of services provided (Barer, Evans, and Labelle 1988). Unlike most other studies, this one could not be criticized for ignoring changes in patient out-of-pocket costs, because during this period Canadians received services without any copayments. In contrast, one confounding factor in most U.S. studies is that reduced physician payment rates often result in lower patient copayments because the copayment is a percentage of the charges. Thus, if the physician provides more services after the payment reduction, it is possible that part of the reason is that patient demand increased as a result of lower copayments.

Some counterevidence has been published, however. A study using data from some of the Canadian provinces found little relationship over a dozen years between the utilization of specific procedures and their fees (Hurley, Labelle, and Rice 1990). Some studies of Medicare payment rate reductions for "overvalued procedures" (mainly surgery and testing) in the late 1980s found little evidence that physicians increased the quantity of services provided (Escarce 1993a, 1993b). Other studies of the same payment reductions did find evidence of volume increases in the wake of Medicare payment reductions, however (Physician Payment Review Commission 1993).

Hurley and Labelle (1995) point out a problem with all of this literature. Results derived by examining response to physician payment rate changes may be consistent both with a demand inducement and with a competitive model of physician behavior, if physicians have a *backward-bending supply curve* (Hurley and Labelle 1995).

Figure 6.2 illustrates this concept. Recall that a normal supply curve, such as those shown in Chapter 2, has a positive slope throughout. Indeed, a large portion of the curve shown in Figure 6.2 has this typical slope, but at the top right, it bends backward.

With a normally shaped supply curve, if payment rates decrease—that is, if they move down the curve to the left, say, from B to A—we would expect the volume of services supplied to decrease. Suppose, however, that the services supplied actually increase when payment falls. That would seem to counter the traditional theory. In fact, some researchers (e.g., Rice 1983) concluded that increased provision of services in the wake of payment reductions is indeed evidence of demand inducement.

What Hurley and Labelle (1995) show is that such a conclusion is not necessarily accurate if there is a backward-bending portion of the supply curve. At that part of the curve, if payment falls, quantity actually rises (say, from D to C)—not because of demand inducement, but because of the shape of the curve.

Why would physicians have a backward-bending labor supply curve? One possibility is that physicians are not just interested in maximizing income. Physicians receive far better compensation than those in nearly any other occupation, so perhaps they are also interested in having more leisure time to enjoy their incomes as compensation gets to higher levels. At low levels of fees—for example, when moving from point A to B in Figure 6.2—higher payment rates will induce more work. At some level, such as point D, unit payment rates are so high that the physician may decide to enjoy more leisure. Thus, following the backward-bending portion of the curve from left to right to point C, a reduction in payment rates would lead to an *increase* in the quantity supplied. Note that this is the same result we would see under demand inducement—but in this case there is no inducement whatsoever. As Hurley and Labelle (1995, 424) note, "one cannot empirically distinguish

FIGURE 6.2: Backward-Bending Supply Curve

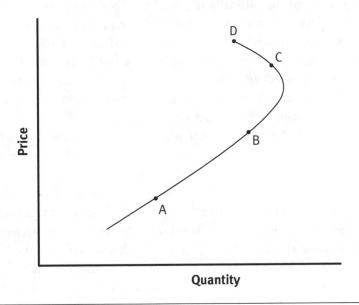

the inducement and no-inducement models based on predicted utilization effects."

More recently, some U.S.-based studies have explicitly taken into account the fact that physicians treat patients in more than one market—for example, Medicare and private insurance patients. In a theoretical piece upon which several subsequent empirical investigations have been based, McGuire and Pauly (1991) show that how physicians respond to fee changes depends on the relative importance of the *substitution effect* and the *income effect*. The substitution effect predicts that if one insurer reduces fees, physicians will treat fewer of its patients, substituting more lucrative patients from the other insurers. The income effect, in contrast, predicts that physicians will also spend more of their time treating the patients whose insurer reduced fees to compensate for the loss of income. The latter effect is consistent with the notion of demand inducement.

Like the literature discussed previously, studies testing this model have also been ambiguous. Yip (1998) examined the provision of coronary artery bypass grafting surgeries by physicians in two states. This study's findings tend to support demand inducement, in that the physicians who were most affected by cuts in Medicare fees were the ones who increased the volume of services—even Medicare services—the most. The results of other studies (Tai-Seale, Rice, and Stearns 1998; Mitchell, Hadley, and Gaskin 2000) varied according to specialty and type of service.

Other Research on Demand Inducement

Partly as a result of the difficulty of using the above strategies for analyzing demand inducement, some analysts have employed other means.[6] One novel approach has been to see whether physicians and their families use more or fewer medical services than other people. The theory is this: If physicians' families avail themselves of more services than other families, it could be argued that doctors aren't *inducing* their patients to purchase extra services, since they use as many or more themselves.

Two studies have found that physicians and their families use *more* services than others, contradicting the notion of demand inducement (Bunker and Brown 1974[7]; Hay and Leahy 1982). One problem with studies such as these, however, is the difficulty of controlling for the fact that physicians, other medical providers, and their families often get care at much lower prices. In addition, it is hard to account for other differences between physicians' families and those that do not have a healthcare connection.[8]

Another approach is to ask physicians how much money they would like to make or how many patients they would like to have, and compare this to their actual income or volume of services. It is then possible to determine whether this differential is correlated with their practice behavior. One such study found that the further physicians were below their targeted income, the more they charged their patients—evidence of demand inducement (Rizzo and Blumenthal 1996).[9] A Norwegian study compared physicians' preferred patient lists with their actual patient lists and found that physicians with a patient "shortage" (fewer patients than desired) performed more services—also evidence of demand inducement (Iversen 2004).

Finally, Labelle, Stoddart and Rice (1994) have argued that we should not only examine whether and to what extent physicians and other suppliers induce demand, but also (1) what the outcomes of the demand inducement are and (2) whether fully informed patients would have wanted to receive the services. Policies aimed at reducing demand inducement would be considered in this context. For example, there would likely be general agreement on the need to reduce services that do not contribute positively to health status, and those that fully informed patients would not have consumed. If, however, an induced service positively contributes to health and would normally be demanded by a fully informed patient, policymakers would need to engage in a cost-benefit analysis to determine if the benefits of the service exceed its cost. In those cases where it did, policymakers would not want to discourage physician-induced demand.

Summary Remarks on Demand Inducement

There will likely always be doubts about how much demand physicians induce among their patients. Part of this is a result of the inherent ambiguity in the tools available, as the above discussion implies. We simply do not have sufficient information to answer the question definitively. Gavin Mooney (1994) has stated that to understand whether patients are being induced to use more services than they really want, we need to know how many they would demand if they were as well-informed as the physician, but no such studies have ever been conducted. Uwe Reinhardt (1989, 339) makes a similar point:

> [H]ighly sophisticated econometric methods ultimately cannot define what proportion of observed utilization [is] simply *accepted* by sick patients (or their anxious relatives) and what proportion the latter would have *demanded* of their own free will, had they been as well-informed as their physicians.

Another reason may explain why agreement is unlikely ever to be reached. The issue of demand inducement seems to raise the hackles of followers of conventional economic theory. Reinhardt (1985, 187–88) makes this point:

> [O]ne suspects that vested interest in neoclassical economic theory has added at least some fuel to the flames. Mastery of the neoclassical framework requires a heavy personal investment on the part of the analyst. Among the payoffs to that investment is entree into a fraternity whose power has derived in good part from the unity of thought forged by this shared analytic paradigm. One need not be an utter cynic to believe that, quite apart from our profession's yearning for truth, the defense of that unifying framework can take on a life of its own.

Finally, and perhaps most important, the question of whether physicians can induce demand directly addresses the competitiveness of the marketplace for healthcare—the main focus of this book. The existence of demand inducement would mean that the healthcare market is radically different from most other markets, which calls for a different set of public policies. Indeed, much of Chapter 10 focuses on the supply-side policies that various developed countries have adopted to deal, in part, with the strong role of suppliers in this market.

Perhaps a good summary of the state of the art is provided by Jeremiah Hurley and Roberta Labelle (1995, 420), who conclude,

> It appears that, in response to economic considerations . . . physicians *can* induce demand for their services, they *sometimes do* induce demand, but that such responses are neither automatic nor unconstrained. Further, physicians do not always respond in ways that can be predicted.

Supply-Side Mechanisms for Reducing Unnecessary Utilization

The probable existence of physician-induced demand calls into question the effectiveness of the usual demand-side policies for managing unnecessary utilization. Patient copays, deductibles, and medical savings accounts that encourage patients to examine the value of medical services and limit their spending to services they value most may not work well when physicians influence their decisions. Fortunately, there are supply-side alternatives for reducing unnecessary utilization. Supply-side mechanisms focus on reimbursement systems, practice guidelines, utilization review, selective contracting, and other practices that discourage unnecessary healthcare utilization. We briefly discuss these mechanisms in the following subsections, ending with a discussion about managed care's role in their use.

Reimbursement Incentives

The supply-side policy tools that appear most likely to succeed in addressing unnecessary utilization are those that directly reduce incentives for physicians to prescribe unnecessary healthcare services. Both private and public payers have implemented supply-side policies aimed at reducing unnecessary healthcare utilization. Chief among these are reimbursement systems that move away from the cost-based, fee-for-service reimbursement of traditional health insurance, in which physicians or other providers are paid additional money for each additional patient they see and each additional service they perform, to prospective fixed payment systems, in which additional patients or services do not add to the providers' income (Hillman 1987).

An annual salary is an example of a reimbursement system in which neither additional patients nor additional services add to a physician's income. Being paid a capitated amount—a set amount per patient over a discrete time period that covers certain care in the negotiated contract with the physician—is a reimbursement mechanism that does not increase a physician's income for additional services per patient. If physicians provide fewer services, profits will be higher, since the capitation rate is unrelated to the number of services provided. Of course, if caregivers provide too few services, quality will be adversely affected, providers may face lawsuits, and patients will likely become dissatisfied and move elsewhere. In addition to salaries and capitation, payers may withhold physician fees for excessive utilization and pay bonuses for keeping utilization down (Hillman 1987).

To ensure that hospitals also have incentives to reduce unnecessary care, payers may reimburse them through DRGs. Initiated by the federal government for Medicare services in 1983, the DRG system pays hospitals a predetermined amount based on each patient's diagnosis.[10] Hospitals that have higher patient care expenses will generally not receive more in payment than those that have lower expenses. This motivates hospitals to reduce unnecessary treatments and to send patients home as soon as possible.

Per diem payments are another common hospital reimbursement. Hospitals receive payments for each day that patients are in the hospital, up to maximum lengths of stay. Per diem payments do not motivate hospitals to reduce lengths of stay (other than not going over the maximum), but they do provide incentives to keep daily expenses as low as possible.

These reimbursement systems may be less effective than intended because payers do not have tight control over the medical procedure coding process or the volume of cases. For example, providers can "game the system" by unbundling services (pricing services separately), upcoding (pricing using codes that bring more revenue), churning (increasing the number of visits), or risk selection (picking healthier patients) (Rice and Kominski 2007; Robinson 1993). Increasing the monitoring of these gaming behaviors, however, is not necessarily the best solution, because it adds to costs.

Pay for performance (P4P), also called pay for value, or value-based purchasing (VBP), is the newest reimbursement system being adopted by payers. It reimburses healthcare providers differentially based on whether they meet quality and efficiency targets. Quality and efficiency measures can be structural, process-oriented, or outcomes-oriented and tend not to be standardized beyond the individual payment system. The quality and efficiency targets may be threshold- or rank-based (Rosenthal et al. 2004).[11] Threshold targets are those in which payment is awarded when quality and efficiency values meet or exceed a set point. Rank-based targets are those in which quality and efficiency scores from a group of providers are ranked from high to low. Providers that fall into the higher percentiles are rewarded. In contrast to threshold and rank-based targets, graduated targets reward successively higher levels of quality and efficiency.

Pay for Performance

Most P4P programs involve physicians, but payers have also begun applying this system to hospitals. Originally, the focus was on quality, but efficiency criteria are being added to the targets (Adler 2006). Since many of the quality goals also reduce unnecessary care—the "waste" in the system—P4P can be seen as a way to reduce demand for services that do little to improve health. Nevertheless, the introduction of efficiency targets into performance evaluation is highly controversial (Rosenthal and Frank 2006).

P4P is estimated to have spread to nearly half of all HMOs by late 2006, involving more than 80 percent of HMO enrollees (Rosenthal et al. 2006). One large P4P project is being conducted by the Integrated Health Care Association (IHA) of California, which includes seven health plans and over 35,000 physicians (Adler 2006). This program rewards clinical quality, patient experience, and investment in and use of information technology (IT), and will add efficiency measures in the future (Adler 2006; O'Kane 2006). Bridges to Excellence (BTE) is another effort by a coalition of large employers (General Electric, UPS, Procter & Gamble, Verizon, and others) that reimburses for performance in diabetes, cardiovascular, and stroke care (O'Kane 2006).

The Centers for Medicare & Medicaid Services (CMS) joined the P4P trend by conducting a three-year (2004 to 2007) P4P demonstration project with Premier Inc., involving 280 not-for-profit hospitals nationwide (O'Kane

2006). CMS awards hospitals bonuses for high-quality care and gives penalties for poor-quality care for patients with heart attacks, heart failure, pneumonia, coronary artery bypass graft, and hip and knee replacements (Rosenthal et al. 2004).

Practice Guidelines

Practice guidelines hold some potential for improving the appropriateness of care. Guidelines recommend the best way to diagnose and treat patients presenting with certain symptoms or thought to have particular illnesses. Some guidelines use algorithms to guide clinical decision making, and some provide information about the costs of alternative treatments (McCarberg 2004). Guidelines aim to ensure that necessary and appropriate care is given and to eliminate inappropriate or unnecessary care. This does not mean that guidelines always result in reduced healthcare utilization and costs. The recommendations in some guidelines, such as those for certain cancers or psychiatric conditions, may result in a greater utilization of healthcare and costs.

Currently, the main evidence-based, standardized guidelines are available from the National Guidelines Clearinghouse, an initiative of the U.S. Agency for Healthcare Research and Quality (AHRQ 2008). The Clearinghouse was originally created by AHRQ in cooperation with the American Medical Association and the American Association of Health Plans. It collects many of the guidelines that various groups, including physician societies, have developed (McCarberg 2004; Boyd et al. 2005).

Utilization Management, Selective Contracting, and Other Mechanisms

Utilization management techniques are also used to reduce physician demand (Rice and Kominski 2007; Robinson 1993). To reduce the use of specialist care, some health plans require referrals from primary care providers. To reduce hospitalization and the use of other expensive modalities, precertification can be required prior to hospitalization and other major tests or treatments. To reduce hospital length of stay, a case manager reviews the patient's progress and plans discharge. The use of healthcare is even reviewed retrospectively, and payment for the care can be denied if the payer concludes that it was not warranted. Disease management for patients with complex or expensive diseases is an additional utilization management strategy that aims to reduce hospitalizations and other expensive care related to certain illnesses.

Another practice is for payers to selectively contract with providers who have acceptable resource utilization patterns. With this strategy, the payer will avoid contracts with physicians who, in the eyes of the payer, have too many outpatient visits, hospital admissions, or costly tests and treatments, or whose hospital lengths of stay are too long (Fisher 2006).

Outside of the United States, broader supply-side measures, such as guidelines on which conditions should be treated and reimbursed, technology controls, and global budgeting, are used to reduce unnecessary demand. Some of these are discussed in Chapter 10.

The mechanisms for reducing unnecessary utilization described in the previous paragraphs are typical of those used by managed care organizations (MCOs). MCOs flourished in the 1980s and 1990s amid hopes that they would lower escalating healthcare costs. Prior to the growth of managed care, traditional "indemnity" insurance plans merely paid the claims of patients who had received healthcare (that is, they indemnified the claims). The traditional insurance system paid providers retrospectively, and provided little or no preventive care such as annual check-ups and screenings. Other than patient copayments and deductibles, there were few incentives for consumers or providers to minimize unnecessary utilization.

MCOs were seen as the solution to high healthcare costs because they combine the functions of insurance with the management of care. MCOs maintain the copayment and deductible requirements of traditional insurance, but add healthcare management mechanisms to those incentives. Management tools include the selection of provider networks, requirements for consumers to stay within networks, requirements for consumers to see primary care providers before going to specialists ("gatekeeper" requirements), prospective reimbursement to providers (contracted amounts agreed upon prior to the delivery of care), utilization management, and quality management. Some MCOs use strong physician reimbursement incentives, such as capitation, incentives, and withholds. They may also pay hospitals on a DRG basis. Weaker reimbursement incentives for physicians include discounted fees, with the discounts negotiated through contracts. Hospitals may be paid on a per diem or discounted charges basis.

Since the 1980s, MCOs have evolved from being predominately HMOs which strictly manage care (by requiring that consumers stay in network and go through a gatekeeper, and by paying physicians on a capitated basis), to preferred provider organizations (PPOs), that allow out-of-network care, do not require a gatekeeper, and typically pay physicians and hospitals discounted fees for service and discounted charges, respectively. Several other types of MCOs have developed with characteristics that fall between those of HMOs and those of PPOs. One example is point of service plans, in which consumers can choose whether they will stay within network and/or see a gatekeeper with each episode of care. Even HMOs may now include plans that are both closed access (with gatekeepers and in-network requirements) and open access (with the ability to bypass the gatekeeper and go out of network for increased copayments).

Transformation of managed care over the past decades has led to the development of organizations that offer several different types of managed care plans. For example, Cigna offers a PPO, a POS, an HMO, and other plans, such as health savings accounts.

Given the shift in U.S. healthcare services from indemnity-based insurance with retrospective fee-for service provider payments to the management

The Role of Managed Care in Reducing Unnecessary Utilization

of healthcare under various types of prospective payment, we would expect that healthcare utilization and costs have been constrained. The next section discusses the empirical evidence.

How Successful Are Supply-Side Mechanisms at Reducing Unnecessary Utilization?

Some evidence exists regarding the success of supply-side efforts in reducing unnecessary utilization. Reimbursement mechanisms such as salary, capitation, and other types of risk sharing are associated with shorter or fewer physician visits in most studies (Debrock and Arnould 1992; Hillman, Pauly, and Kerstein 1989; Miller and Bovbjerg 2002), but not in all (Luft 1999; Miller and Luft 1994). Some studies show that such reimbursement incentives result in fewer hospitalizations (Debrock and Arnould 1992; Hillman, Pauly, and Kerstein 1989; Jordan 2001; Stearns, Wolfe, and Kindig 1992). Studies uniformly indicate that utilization review reduces admissions (Smith 1997; Wheeler and Wickizer 1990; Wickizer 1992; Wickizer, Wheeler, and Feldstein 1989) and hospital lengths of stay (Khandker and Manning 1992; Wickizer, Wheeler, and Feldstein 1989) and lowers the intensity of use of services (Robinson 1996) and hospital costs (Robinson 1991; Wheeler and Wickizer 1990; Wickizer, Wheeler, and Feldstein 1989), although the reductions in use are often modest.

Due to the newness of P4P programs, there are still few data about their outcomes. A noncontrolled evaluation of the IHA P4P program mentioned earlier showed quality improvement among 87 percent of physician groups. Physicians participating in the BTE diabetes program mentioned earlier were more likely to use the best practices guidelines and to deliver care at lower cost (due to patients having fewer emergency room visits and fewer hospitalizations) than those not in the program.

Two reviews of the literature on evaluations of paying for quality, one through 2003 and the other through 2005, show mixed results. The review of literature up to 2003 finds little evidence for quality improvements under P4P (Rosenthal and Frank 2006). The review of literature up to 2005 finds some evidence for quality improvement in 13 out of 17 studies (Petersen et al. 2006). The first review overlapped with the second in five studies, but it also included non–healthcare related studies, while the second review included several additional healthcare-related studies.

Due to the lack of strong evidence that P4P works as intended, policy analysts are cautioning against a rush to adopt this reimbursement mechanism, and are raising some possible problems associated with it. In a 2006 article, Elliot Fisher lists several important concerns: First, he asks, is the goal to improve the quality of care, or is it "efficiency," implying a potential danger of denial of care and underutilization? Second, are the measures adequate? Do they adjust for patient severity, allow for patients' preferences, take into account the effect of multiple providers on outcomes, and reflect an integrated healthcare system? Third, is the program feasible? Small physician practices will either have to collect the data by hand or spend a large amount of money on IT systems.

Fourth, will rewards be enough to compensate for the higher costs, and if so, will they reduce payments to others by too much? Finally, could there be unintended consequences, such as providers avoiding sicker patients?

Other unintended consequences are possible. Since P4P targets are only for certain patient problems, P4P could result in performing to the target (as in "teaching to the test" in education) (Clarke, Raphael, and Disch 2008). Providers could spend so much time reporting and monitoring that time spent delivering care could decline (Rosenthal and Frank 2006). Finally, rewarding the better performers and punishing the worst performers could cause a spiral to the bottom for those who start out on the low end.

Regarding practice guidelines, an Italian study finds that their use results in lower costs, shorter hospital stays, and lower consumption of hospital resources for stroke patients (Quaglini et al. 2004). Two U.S. studies find that the use of practice guidelines reduces drug prescribing, resulting in positive patient outcomes (Goode et al. 2000; Dubois and Dean 2006), whereas one study indicates that guidelines have no strong effect on prescribing behavior (Martens et al. 2006). In contrast with studies that indicate a reduction in utilization with practice guidelines, their use in the care of the elderly with multiple comorbidities has been found to result in the prescribing of too many medications with possible interactions and high costs (Boyd et al. 2005). In the treatment of mental disorders, current physician practices are often below practice guideline recommendations. For example, only 29 percent of patients with depression receive care that meets practice guideline recommendations (Fortney et al. 2001).

Since MCOs simultaneously employ many of the mechanisms discussed earlier, one way to assess the overall success of these mechanisms is to examine healthcare utilization under managed care. One study finds that from 1985 to 1993, hospitals in areas with high rates of HMO penetration and growth had slower growth in costs (Gaskin and Hadley 1997). Another found that patients in managed care plans had shorter hospital stays, lower charges, and less use of mechanical ventilation in intensive care units than those in traditional indemnity insurance plans (Rapoport et al. 1992). Hospital length of stay was shorter for patients in an independent practice association (IPA) HMO, compared with traditional insurance patients (Bradbury, Golec, and Stearns 1991). In an IPA, the HMO contracts with a physician group over fees and establishes referral and hospital admission guidelines that may include financial rewards for keeping hospital admissions down. Young and colleagues (2002) found that operating margins for HMO contracts in Florida hospitals fell from 1990 to 1997.

Physicians and consumers dislike many of these supply-side practices, and there has been a "backlash" on both fronts. First, given a choice, consumers have voted with their feet and have moved into the least restrictive healthcare plans—PPOs (Ginsburg 2005). Second, some states enacted protective

"Backlash" and Concerns About Access

legislation, such as any-willing-provider and freedom-of-choice laws, in the 1990s (Ginsburg 2005). These laws limit managed care's ability to selectively contract with physicians and to keep consumers in physician networks. In order to maintain market share and meet regulatory requirements, HMOs and other restrictive managed care organizations became less restrictive (Hall 2005; Robinson 2001). Some of the restrictions, such as patients having to stay within the provider network or having to go to their primary physician prior to seeing a specialist, have been relaxed or abandoned. One key result of this backlash against heavy-handed managed care was a rise in healthcare costs (Lesser, Ginsburg, and Devers 2003).

One issue consumers and providers have had with managed care is whether practices such as reimbursement incentives and utilization management truly weed out only unnecessary care (Luft 1999). Although there are many legitimate horror stories of denied care and poor quality, research on the quality of care under managed care does not strongly corroborate the negative impressions. In a 2000 review, it was found that some studies indicate a positive relationship between managed care and quality, some indicate a negative relationship, and some show no difference between managed care and indemnity insurance (Robinson 2000). Another study from 2000 reports increased readmissions in hospitals with shorter lengths of stay (Lessler and Wickizer 2000). In a review of studies through 2001, Miller and Luft (2002) conclude that HMOs provide comparable quality of care to indemnity plans. There is, however, a good deal of variation in performance. Compared to indemnity plans, HMOs tend to provide worse quality of care for the frail elderly, the chronically ill, and cancer patients. HMOs in California had generally better quality of care than HMOs elsewhere. There were no major differences in quality between group and IPA-model HMOs.

The mixed results on managed care and quality to date may be due in part to the difficulty in controlling for the different types of patients seen by managed care compared with indemnity insurance plans. Some managed care companies "cherry pick" the less sick patients, which could bias quality results in their favor (Cutler, McClellan, and Newhouse 2000). Although most studies control for patient characteristics to some extent, they may not fully capture the difference in patient population between managed care and indemnity insurance. Another consideration is that, as we discussed, over time managed care has had to drop many of the more restrictive practices, so the differences between managed care and indemnity insurance are decreasing.

It may also be the case that managed care practices have not had a negative effect on quality because physicians and other professionals try to take good care of their patients even when there is pressure to do things that might result in negative outcomes. In other words, healthcare professionals remain advocates for patients and may even overextend themselves to maintain quality of care for their patients. A final consideration is that perhaps it is not the "management" of healthcare per se that sets the stage for quality issues, but the type of organization that pursues this management, and to what end. Perhaps it is the "corporate" or for-profit nature of many of the managed care organizations that creates the potential for reduced quality. We will discuss this issue again in Chapter 7.

6.2 Do Firms Have Market Power?

Market Power and Its Impact

The issue of whether firms have market power has received significant attention from economists. As we defined it in Chapter 2, a firm has market power if it can set prices above its marginal costs and can raise prices without losing its entire market. A firm that has market power can charge more than a firm in a competitive market. It may also be able to charge different prices to different market segments. Under the conventional assumption that suppliers cannot influence demand, higher prices would mean that the amount of output sold would be lower than in a competitive market. However, in healthcare the reduction in quantity demanded may be tempered by supplier-induced demand.

A market consisting of firms that have some degree of market power is considered to be *imperfectly competitive*. There are different types of imperfectly competitive markets depending on the number of firms in the market. In *monopolistically competitive* markets, a number of firms compete with each other to some degree. However, each seller is offering a slightly different product, and as a result, firms are able to influence prices. To illustrate, each brand of laundry detergent is a little different, so if Tide or Cheer raises its prices, it would not lose all its customers—just some of them.

An imperfectly competitive market that includes only a small number of firms is an *oligopoly*. Whether there is collusion or competition between these firms depends on whether or not they cooperate.[12] If the firms collude, prices can be set higher. Collusion is difficult to maintain, however, because there is always the temptation for one of the firms to lower prices slightly in order to take business away from the others. At that point, all firms must lower their price if they are to maintain their market share. The firms end up competing over price. Although price competition is disadvantageous to the firms, it is beneficial to consumers, because it will result in lower prices. Collusion in oligopolistic markets usually is not formal or overt. It is done through the informal "leadership" of one firm setting a price that all other firms follow (see note 12). Formal collusion, in which agreements are drawn up among the parties, is illegal in most countries.

An example of oligopoly in healthcare markets is hospitals. Since the market for hospitals is the local geographic region, in areas where only a few hospitals operate, an oligopoly may exist. As we will discuss in the following sections, this market power may lead to higher prices for hospital care.

Whether or to what extent prices are higher in more concentrated hospital markets depends on whether insurance companies on the demand side can counter the supply-side power. In Cleveland, Ohio, for example, after the closure of several for-profit and inner-city hospitals, two hospital systems had garnered two-thirds of the market. As a result, health plans were less able to keep their hospital payments down (Christianson et al. 2000). Another example of an oligopoly is the health insurance market, in which a few companies divide up the state or local market for health insurance. For example, in 2000, a single health plan controlled 70 percent of the market in Lansing, Michigan (Devers et al. 2001).

The most concentrated of all markets is the monopoly, in which only one firm sells a particular product or service. This entity can set prices higher than those in competitive markets, and it does not need to collude or strategize to find an equilibrium price. Insurance companies and hospitals have monopoly power in some areas.

Market power can also occur on the demand side of the market. Usually, this involves demand for inputs such as materials, services, or labor. When demanders have power over the price of the good, service, or labor they are buying, they are called *monopsonists* or *oligopsonists*. One example in healthcare is the insurance industry, in which large, multistate insurance companies have bargaining power over what they pay providers. Another example is hospitals, which are one of the major employers of healthcare workers. Nurses and other healthcare professionals and workers have only one or a few potential employers in the area where they live. Even when wages, benefits, and working conditions are not good, they may have no other alternatives for employment. Whether hospitals exert monopsonistic power is discussed in Chapter 8. Chapter 10 discusses how governments in other countries often use their monopsonistic power to control health expenditures.

Market power can be achieved by various means. Existing entities can merge and enter into joint production. Sometimes mergers or takeovers result in the closure of one of the entities, which then enlarges the market share of the remaining facility. Less formal alliances, such as shared or cooperative services, contract management, or formal agreement, can increase market power (Freund and Mitchell 1985). Hospitals, for example, join together in systems with varying degrees of integration.

In some cases, economies of scale from the centralization of production and distribution cause a monopoly to develop in that industry. No obvious examples of these "natural monopolies" exist in healthcare, but in markets such as utilities, they are common. Finally, market power can result when facilities experiencing poor financial performance close, leaving remaining facilities with greater market share.

When organizations collaborate or join together along the same product line, the integration is called *horizontal*. Multi-institutional hospital systems are horizontal integrations. But when the collaboration or joint activity occurs along different, frequently dependent, product lines, the integration is described as *vertical*. The establishment of physician-hospital collaboration and mergers of hospitals and outpatient services or nursing homes are examples of vertical integration. The Kaiser Healthcare System consists of vertically integrated insurance functions, physicians, and hospitals.

Horizontal integration can result in production efficiencies through economies of scale (decreases in average cost of product due to the high volume produced) and market concentration through reduced numbers of sellers in the market (Gaynor and Haas-Wilson 1999). Whereas increased efficiency reduces production costs and could result in lower prices, increased market concentration allows for price increases. Another problem associated with horizontal integration is the potential for lower production quantities. If, through horizontal integration, a firm can raise prices, the quantity of services demanded by consumers will fall. The degree to which demand will be reduced will depend on whether consumers have insurance coverage, how much they will have to pay out of pocket, and whether supplier-induced demand exists.

Vertical integration may result in greater efficiencies through economies of scope (decreases in average costs due to production of multiple products, especially as a result of joint administrative and advertising costs) (Gaynor and Haas-Wilson 1999). However, at times vertically integrated organizations can engage in *tying arrangements* with their customers. These arrangements force the customer of one firm's product line to use the product of another line the same firm produces or has an investment in. These arrangements are considered anticompetitive (Pender and Meier 2005). Some examples of tying agreements in healthcare are when physicians "self-refer" (send patients to labs or radiology facilities that they own) and when hospitals discharge patients to their own home care agencies without giving them of the option of using another agency.

Because oligopolistic, monopolistic, and other anticompetitive behaviors can result in higher prices and less quantity demanded and produced, in the United States these behaviors can be challenged and prosecuted by the Department of Justice (DOJ) or the Federal Trade Commission (FTC), two agencies that monitor and regulate market competition. For mergers or collusive actions to be challenged, the offense must have resulted (or have the potential to result) in a major concentration of the market and/or the ability of the firm(s) to set high prices or otherwise control the market ("unreasonable" restraint of trade), and the market power must have been attained through "improper" means (not through a natural monopoly or independent actions) (Freund and Mitchell 1985; Hyman and Kovacic 2004; Nguyen and Derrick 1994).

In the past, healthcare organizations were exempt from most antitrust regulations. As a result, they competed not so much over price, but rather by distinguishing their services from competitors (e.g., on the basis of quality, services, or amenities). This medical arms race from competition resulted in higher, rather than lower, prices (Baker 1988; Devers, Brewster, and Casalino 2003). In this situation, regulators did not see market power in healthcare as a problem.[13] However, as competition over price has increased in healthcare markets, a great number of firms have come under antitrust scrutiny. The DOJ and FTC have challenged more conduct, and more cases have resulted in decisions against the healthcare organizations (Pender and Meier 2005). A 2005 FTC report of antitrust actions since the early 1990s lists two cases of "monopolization" and six cases of "agreements not to compete" by drug companies; 79 cases of "agreements on price" by physician groups, hospital systems, physician-hospital organizations, nursing homes, pharmacy associations, drug companies, and others; three cases of illegal tying; 21 hospital mergers that have been challenged; and many other antitrust activities (Pender and Meier 2005).[14]

Trends in Market Power in the United States

Through alliances, system-building, mergers, and closures, market power in U.S. healthcare markets has increased dramatically since the 1980s. From 1980 to 2005, the hospital industry saw a 15 percent decrease in hospitals under 200 beds, and a 4 percent increase in hospitals with 200 beds or more, with a 7 percent increase in hospitals with 500 beds or more.[15] The first half of the 1990s was the period of greatest merger and acquisition activity, which increased ninefold in that period (Williams, Vogt, and Town 2006). Since 1995, the number of stand-alone hospitals has declined, while the number of hospitals with a local partner has increased (Cuellar and Gertler 2005). Not only do several large national chains now exist,[16] but in 2000, 43 percent of nongovernment hospitals were in local systems (Cuellar and Gertler 2005). Nationally, from 1990 to 2003 the Herfindahl-Hirschmann Index (HHI), an indicator of market concentration, increased around 40 percent for hospitals, indicating a significant increase in market concentration (authors' calculations based on data from Williams, Vogt, and Town 2006).

Although the insurance industry seems to receive less attention, it has perhaps undergone the greatest consolidation of all. Between 1992 and 2006, 95 insurance and managed care companies consolidated into seven (American Academy of Family Physicians 2007). In 2002, just three insurers controlled 40 percent or more of the market in every U.S. state (Robinson 2004). The top three insurers in New Hampshire and Rhode Island captured 100 percent of the market in those states (Robinson 2004). In 280 local markets (around 90 percent of all U.S. local markets) in 2005, 30 percent of HMO and PPO patients were covered by one company. Only two insurers covered one-third of all enrollees nationally (American Academy of Family Physicians 2007).

In nursing home markets, while the existence of chain membership does not directly indicate local nursing home concentration, the ten largest national nursing home chains in 2002 owned 15 percent of all facilities and beds in the United States (Gulley and Santerre 2007). The largest chain—Beverly Enterprises—is composed of 452 facilities with a total of nearly 50,000 beds, while the smallest—National Healthcare Corporation—has 82 facilities and 10,000 beds. Nursing home closures and ownership changes have been common (Castle 2005).

Physicians, too, have joined together. Most practiced independently in the 1970s, but by 1995 only one-fourth of all physicians were still in solo practices (Gaynor and Haas-Wilson 1999). Many physicians have joined group practices or independent practice associations that allow independent physicians to contract with managed care as a group. As we mentioned earlier, physicians have also integrated vertically with hospitals.

Some degree of market power exists in most healthcare markets. Economists are concerned about the existence and growth of market power in the healthcare industry because it can affect prices and the quantity and quality of services. In the following subsections we discuss why market power may be problematic and how it affects healthcare markets.

Why Market Power May Be a Problem

Figure 6.3 (which is identical to Figure 2.22) shows how imperfectly and perfectly competitive firms compare with regard to pricing and output. Both types of firms maximize their profits by producing up to the point where the marginal revenue derived from providing an additional service equals the marginal cost of providing that service. But because imperfectly competitive firms can raise price without a complete loss of customers, they do not face the horizontal demand curve that would indicate a complete loss of demand with a change in price. Instead, their demand curve is downward sloping, reflecting a loss of some, but not all, quantity demanded with each price increase.

Because the quantity demanded at each price level drops as prices rise, marginal revenue, the change in additional revenue with an increase in price, also falls. Instead of being horizontal and identical with the demand curve, as in the competitive model, the marginal revenue curve for imperfectly competitive markets is downward sloping and positioned under the demand curve. Prices can be set at the highest level the market will bear, which is the point on the demand curve that corresponds to (i.e., is directly above) the profit-maximizing quantity of output, where marginal revenue equals marginal costs. In Figure 6.3, S_c and D_c are the supply and demand curves, respectively, in a competitive market, and MR_m is the monopolist's marginal revenue curve.[17] The output produced by competitive firms is indicated by point B, where the supply and demand curves, and the corresponding output levels P_c and Q_c, intersect. For the monopolist, however, the intersection of marginal revenue and supply is at point A. The monopolist produces less (Q_m) and charges more (P_m).

Even greater profits—and greater healthcare expenditures—are possible if, in addition to being able to influence the price of healthcare services,

FIGURE 6.3: Pricing and Output Decisions by Competitive Firms
and Monopolists

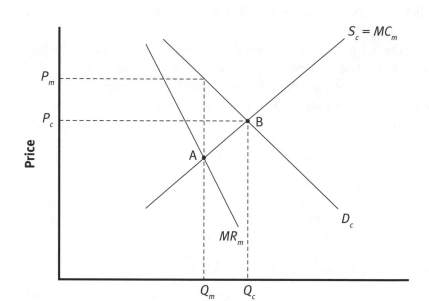

suppliers can induce demand for healthcare. Suppliers could shift the demand
and marginal revenue curves in Figure 6.4 to the slashed curves D_i and MR_i.
The provider with market power could then produce more than the conventional monopoly model would predict (Q'_m), and could charge more as well
(P'_m).

Another important issue is how market power in one market affects behavior in another market. Concentration in a market such as health insurance
may affect the market structure, organization, and performance of hospitals
(Devers, Brewster, and Casalino 2003; Dranove, Simon, and White 2002).
To counter the buying power of insurance companies and to gain economies
of scale, hospitals may become more concentrated (Ginsburg 2005). This
may cause restructuring and affect the labor force and quality of care.

One of the earliest examples of the snowballing effect of concentration occurred in Minneapolis–St. Paul in the 1980s. Health plans began to
concentrate their purchasing power through a series of mergers, to the point
where two large HMOs controlled 90 percent of the HMO market (Christianson et al. 1995). In response, hospital systems and multispecialty group
practices began their own consolidation to regain bargaining power, until
only three hospital networks controlled the bulk of hospital beds (National
Health Policy Forum 1995).

The ultimate effect of such consolidations is difficult to predict; it depends in large part on the relative bargaining power of different market participants, but also on the importance consumers put on factors such as health plan premiums and quality of care.

Given the considerations above, the primary economic questions regarding competition are how it affects outcomes such as quality and quantity of services, and what the costs of achieving these outcomes would be in prices and expenditures. Do more competitive markets compete over price or over services and quality? Do efficiencies in imperfectly competitive markets balance out the higher prices that may occur? What about quality and scope of services in competitive versus concentrated markets? Finally, what impact does market concentration in one healthcare market, such as insurance, have on the behavior in another market, such as hospitals?

Different policies are advisable depending on the answers to these questions. If, for example, hospital mergers in response to HMO penetration are important to the financial stability of the hospital sector and do not result in significantly higher prices, an attempt to increase competition in hospital markets would not be beneficial. If, on the other hand, hospital mergers result in large profit margins and high prices, a more competitive market may be the answer.

FIGURE 6.4: Pricing and Output Decisions by Competitive Firms and Monopolists with Demand Inducement

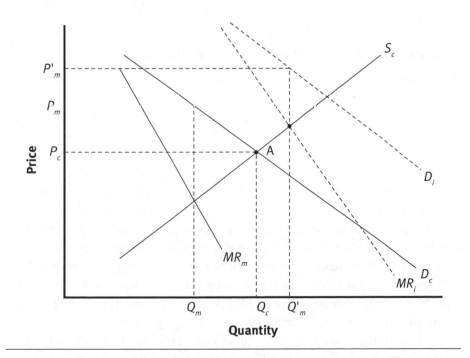

Answers to these questions differ depending on the time period and geographical area. Changes in healthcare markets over time have affected the way healthcare providers compete and produce services, and these changes and responses to them have been more rapid or more acute in certain geographical areas than in others.

The major catalysts in competitive behavior have been the increase in managed care and changes in reimbursement systems. Prior to the managed care growth of the mid-1980s, higher prices were observed in competitive hospital markets due to nonprice competition (Bodenheimer 2005; Feldman et al. 1990). Once managed care implemented selective contracting with hospitals in the 1980s, hospitals had an incentive to lower prices—to gain contracts, and therefore market share (Devers, Brewster, and Casalino 2003). The mid-1980s change from retrospective reimbursement, in which providers are paid their charges after performing a service, to prospective reimbursement, in which payment is arranged before the service, forced providers to keep prices within fixed or contracted ranges (Devers, Brewster, and Casalino 2003).

Greater hospital contracting leverage due to hospital market concentration may be leading to a decrease in managed care bargaining power and higher hospital prices (Cunningham 2001; Devers, Brewster, and Casalino 2003). This is occurring unevenly across the United States, with California and Minnesota healthcare markets in the lead (Zwanziger and Melnick 1996).

Keeping these issues in mind, in the following sections we briefly examine the empirical research regarding the extent of market power and its effects on prices, costs, efficiency, quality, and scope of services in insurance and hospital markets.

Studies of Market Power in Insurance Markets

Early studies found that the entry of additional HMOs into the market significantly lowered their ability to charge higher premiums (Feldman and Dowd 1993; Wholey, Feldman, and Christianson 1995). The findings from recent studies are more ambiguous. Robinson (2004) finds that an increase in profits and prices among insurance companies in 2000–2003 occurred at the same time as consolidations in those companies and increases in market concentration in the industry, as measured by HHI. Kopit (2004), however, contends that Robinson's overall correspondence of profit and premium increases with consolidation does not mean that market concentration *in the relevant local markets* contributed to premium increases in those markets. Even if insurance concentration does lead to higher prices and lower demand, Town (2001, 989) estimates that this could be offset by gains in efficiency. He concludes that "the welfare consequences of HMO mergers turn on the ability of the health plans to realize efficiencies through the merger process."

Few studies have examined the effects of managed care concentration on providers. Roger Feldman and Douglas Wholey (2001) find that between

1985 and 1997, HMOs with a larger share of hospital days in their market area paid lower prices to hospitals. Zwanziger and Melnick (1996) report that high managed care enrollment in California (covering more than 80 percent of the privately insured) and the mergers of several plans allowed managed care to extract large price concessions from physicians and hospitals. Dranove, Simon, and White (2002) find that across the United States higher levels of managed care penetration were associated with a 14 percent decrease in solo physician practices between 1986 and 1995, and a decrease in the number of hospitals from 10.4 to 6.5 between 1981 and 1994. Cuellar and Gertler (2005) conclude that hospitals were more likely to join systems if they had high managed care loads. In contrast, Town and colleagues (2007) do not find a connection between HMOs and hospital consolidation.

Studies of Market Power in Hospital Markets

Studies indicate that in the pre–managed care era, hospital markets with greater competition had higher prices, supporting the nonprice "medical arms race" theory of hospital competition. Using data from 29 metropolitan statistical areas (MSAs) in 1991—a year the authors consider representative of the pre–managed care era—Rivers and Bae (1999) find that costs were higher in MSAs with greater competition. Another study, using national data from 1990, reports that hospitals in multihospital systems were less costly than freestanding hospitals (Menke 1997).

In a review of the literature on competition in hospital markets before and during the managed care era, Daniel Kessler and Mark McClellan (2000, 581) conclude that

> research based on data from prior to the mid-1980s finds that competition among hospitals leads to increases in excess capacity, costs, and prices . . . and research based on more recent data generally finds that competition among hospitals leads to reductions in excess capacity, costs and prices.

Kessler and McClellan (2000) report similar results from their own research: 1990 was the dividing line between higher and lower costs related to competition. Additional studies agree with this assessment. Connor, Feldman, and Dowd (1998) find a shift away from nonprice competition toward price competition nationally due to increased market penetration by managed care companies. The rate of increase in prices in more competitive markets in California was higher in the pre–managed care period, and lower in the managed care period (Melnick and Zwanziger 1988). Price increases were greater over time in merged California hospitals (Melnick, Keeler, and Zwanziger 1999), and in more concentrated California hospital markets (Keeler, Melnick, and Zwanziger 1999).

Most studies using only data from the managed care period find increased costs with higher concentration or mergers. A literature review by

Cuellar and Gertler (2005) reports that mergers and acquisitions from 1990 to 1995 increased prices.[18] Hospitals in networks are associated with higher prices (Burgess, Carey, and Young 2005). Hospitals are more likely to accept prospective payment or retrospective discount as the number of hospitals increases (Gift, Arnould, and Debrock 2002).

Some studies of the managed care period contradict these findings. According to Danger (1997), from 1990 to 1993, nonprofit hospital mergers did not lead to significant price increases. Two studies using data from 1989 into the 1990s find that costs and prices were lower in hospitals that merged (Connor, Feldman, and Dowd 1998; Spang, Bazzoli, and Arnould 2001). A fourth study indicates that price levels in concentrated hospital markets may vary depending on the degree of competition and whether the hospitals are for-profit or nonprofit (Lynk 1995a). In contrast, another study concludes that there is no significant difference between for-profit and nonprofit prices in concentrated markets, but that nonprofits use the higher prices to cover charity care (Simpson and Shin 1998).

The evidence suggests that in the managed care era greater hospital market competition leads to lower prices, and higher concentration leads to higher prices. (However, more research is necessary, especially to tease out issues such as ownership.) These findings can be attributed to the change in hospitals' market behavior in response to the growth of managed care selective contracting. Hospitals had to compete over prices to contract with managed care companies, and this replaced competition over quality and services. Hospitals in more concentrated markets could use their market power to charge higher prices.

The empirical evidence regarding the effects of hospital concentration on quality is tentative. Using data from before the managed care period, one study finds that mortality rates were lower in more competitive markets (Rivers and Bae 1999), another finds them lower in more concentrated markets (Tomal 1998), and a third finds no significant relationship (Rivers and Fottler 2004). In the managed care period, one study indicates that hospitals in markets with higher concentration have lower 30-day mortality in two to three out of five patient conditions (Rogowski, Jain, and Escarce 2007). On the other hand, one study finds that concentration leads to significantly higher rates of adverse outcomes (Kessler and McClellan 2000). Other studies report no relationship between hospital mergers or acquisitions and mortality (Ho and Hamilton 2000), or between hospital consolidation and mortality, adverse safety events, or charity care (Cueller and Gertler 2005). Clearly, the jury is still out on whether more market power in the hospital sectors improves or detracts from quality.

Market Power: Implications for Health Policy

Producers and purchasers in all healthcare markets have some degree of market power, and some, such as hospitals and insurance, have significant market power. What should be done about the market power, however, is not clear. Although the research indicates that prices have been higher in more concentrated hospital markets since the 1990s, it also suggests that concentration may be a survival mechanism that maintains prices at a financially viable level and increases efficiency. If hospitals had not consolidated and prices had not increased, the hospital market may have faced greater instability. Since instability is marked by hospital closings and mergers, it was inevitable that hospitals would concentrate in response to managed care. Because the overall impact of hospital concentration is not yet clear, the best policy may be to monitor the market, collect more data, and regulate the industry in a way that discourages predatory practices and high prices. This would include antitrust discipline where needed.

Policy changes with regard to market power are considered less often for insurance markets. Yet these markets are highly concentrated, and the research suggests that this concentration can result in seller-side (monopoly, oligopoly) and buyer-side (monopsony, oligopsony) power, without the cost savings being passed on to consumers. Other countries with private insurers are much more active in regulating prices charged and practices (e.g., requiring that everyone can obtain coverage at reasonable premiums irrespective of health status) than the United States. We return to these issues later in the book.

Perhaps the biggest policy lesson we can learn from concentration in healthcare markets is that policies must take into account the connections between markets. For example, to pursue antitrust and other pro-competitive approaches in the hospital markets without doing the same in insurance markets could lead to financial instability among hospitals. On the other hand, to break up the insurance systems without also reducing levels of concentration among hospitals could leave insurance companies with less bargaining power with providers, and either fail to reduce premiums or put insurance companies in financial difficulties.

In general, more research is needed to guide policy in this area. There is not enough evidence to promote more competitive approaches, nor is there enough to be complacent in the face of high concentration.

6.3 Cost Shifting

One controversial issue regarding market power in healthcare—especially hospitals—is whether providers can successfully engage in *cost shifting*. This section presents some of the theory of cost shifting, then summarizes evidence and offers some policy implications.

Theory

The term "cost shifting" is a bit of a misnomer. It is not *costs* that are hypothesized to be shifting, but *revenues*. Loosely speaking, cost shifting occurs when a provider (such as a hospital) responds to low reimbursement rates by public payers (such as Medicare or Medicaid) or uncompensated care provided to the uninsured by charging private payers (insurers, managed care companies, or private individuals) more. Essentially, hospitals are trying to compensate for providing care below costs to some patients by raising their charges to others. This sort of behavior may also apply to physicians, but we focus on hospitals since that's where most research and discussion has centered.

Before proceeding, we need to define another economic concept: a *price-discriminating monopolist*. This term was mentioned briefly earlier in Chapter 2. We noted that a price-discriminating monopolist can charge different prices to different customers. This allows the monopolist to make even higher profits by segmenting its markets. Customers who are more price sensitive—that is, who have a higher price elasticity of demand—are charged less, and those who less price sensitive are charged more.

Since the traditional economic model assumes that firms maximize profits, a firm obviously would want to price discriminate if it could. However, this requires (1) some market power, (2) the ability to segment purchasers into those who are willing to pay more and those who will pay less, and (3) the ability to prevent resale—that is, those who are charged less are not able to turn around and sell to those who are charged more. Hospitals offer a good example. Generally they have some market power, since they do not lose their entire market if they raise their prices; they can segment their market according to the insurance statuses of their patients; and people cannot resell hospital services, as they must consume them themselves.

In the case of hospital care, price discrimination would manifest itself a little differently than in the traditional model. For simplicity, assume that there are just two payers for care, Medicare and private insurers. In Figure 6.5, Medicare payment is shown as the horizontal line P_{med}. Regardless of how many Medicare patients are treated by hospitals, they receive the same price or marginal revenue (MR), which would be the DRG price. Private insurers, in contrast, would have the typical downward-sloping demand curve, and a marginal revenue curve below it (D_{priv} and MR_{priv} respectively).

To maximize profits, the hospital would take the patients who provide the highest MR. To understand how the hospital would behave, consider what happens when private patients provide the higher MR versus when public patients do. Following the MR_{priv} curve downward and to the right until point A, private patients are more lucrative. To the right of point A, public patients are more lucrative, since beyond that point, the MR from Medicare, P_{med}, exceeds that from the private market, MR_{priv}. Thus, a profit-maximizing private insurer would treat private insurer patients from the origin to Q_{priv} and charge them at as much as they could, at P_{priv} on the demand curve. This is a higher price than Medicare pays.

One important implication of this is can be seen in Figure 6.6. Suppose that Medicare *reduces* its payment rates to $P_{med'}$. The theory of the price-

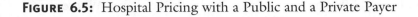

FIGURE 6.5: Hospital Pricing with a Public and a Private Payer

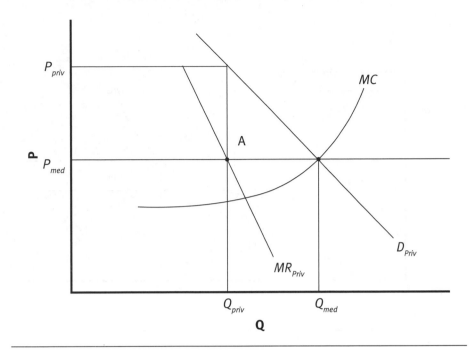

discriminating monopolist predicts that private insurers will respond by charging less, not more, than before: $P_{priv'}$. This is the opposite of what we expect in cost shifting, when private prices rise in the wake of falling public payment rates. Thus, although the ability to price discriminate is necessary for cost shifting to exist, the two theories provide different predictions for hospitals' pricing behavior.

Even if hospitals could engage in cost shifting, why would they? Michael Morrisey (2003) argues that economic theory would allow for the existence of cost shifting—but that a hospital would be smarter to fully exploit its monopoly power in the private market at all times (Morrisey 1994). Paul Ginsburg (2003a, W3-478) succinctly states what is perhaps the key point: "Provider cost shifting requires the ability of providers to raise prices in the marketplace combined with a history of not having fully exploited it."

Why, then, would hospitals not charge the profit-maximizing amount to private insurers in the first place? Perhaps it is the fact that most hospitals are nonprofit. Ginsburg (2003a, W3-475) hypothesizes that nonprofit hospitals, while needing to price high enough to stay afloat, must also meet community needs, including "providing care to the poor, offering the latest medical technology, [and] avoiding delays in physicians' obtaining care for patients." He offers some related evidence, which we cover in Chapter 7. Moreover, Ginsburg contends that we might even see cost shifting among

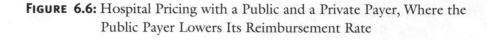

Figure 6.6: Hospital Pricing with a Public and a Private Payer, Where the Public Payer Lowers Its Reimbursement Rate

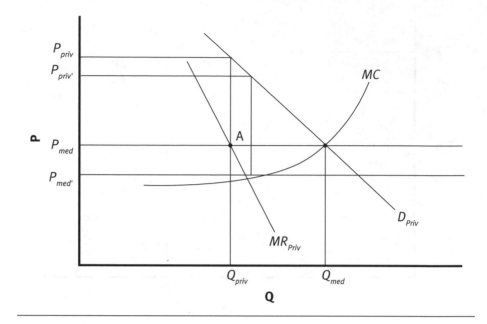

for-profit hospitals for two reasons: They often have to compete with the nonprofits in the community, and they may provide some charity care to engender community support.

There is some agreement that the extent of cost shifting depends on the relative market power of hospitals. In particular, hospitals were more powerful in two, noncontiguous periods: before managed care companies became dominant in the 1990s, and in the 2000s, when the market power of managed care firms waned as hospitals consolidated and consumers became disenchanted with the restrictions of HMOs (Dowless 2007).

Figure 6.7 compares the payment-to-cost ratios of public and private payers, providing descriptive evidence of cost shifting during the two periods in question. A widening between the lines indicates possible cost shifting. The lines show that from the late 1980s to around 1990, the payment-to-cost ratios between public and private payers widened, indicating that hospitals were able to compensate for the underpayment from public payers by extracting higher payments from private payers. Then, between 1990 and 2000, the gap between public and private payment-to-cost ratios narrowed, perhaps because managed care purchasing power prevented cost shifting in the 1990s, or because higher Medicare and Medicaid prices reduced the need to cost shift during this period. At 2000, the trend lines widen again. This could indicate the effect that Dowless theorized—that an increase in hospitals' market

FIGURE 6.7: Aggregate Hospital Payment-to-Cost Ratios for Private Payers, Medicare, and Medicaid, 1981–2005

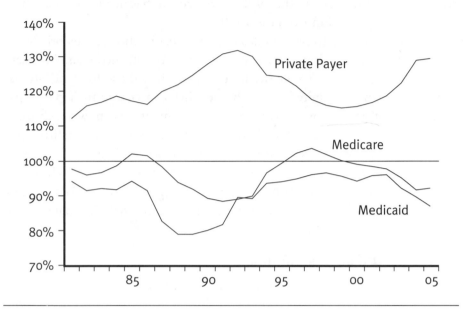

SOURCE: Reprinted with permission from American Hospital Association. 2008. "Trends Affecting Hospital and Health Systems: 2008 Chartbook," Chart 4.6. Chicago: AHA.

power at the end of the 1990s gave them greater power over prices in the private markets, which allowed a return to cost shifting.

Dobson, DaVanzo, and Sen (2006) have arrived at a similar conclusion. They also observe that cost shifting does not need to be dollar for dollar, as hospitals can compensate for low public payments through increased efficiency and decreases in services.

Studies on Cost Shifting

Based on this discussion, one would expect to see the strongest evidence for cost shifting in studies using data from prior to 1990 and after 2000. Some research using data from the late 1980s through the early 1990s does not demonstrate cost shifting (Morrisey 1994; Hadley, Zuckerman, and Iezzoni 1996), while other research does (Zwanziger and Melnick 2000; Clement 1997–1998; Dranove 1988).

There are few studies using data from the 1990s and later. Zwanziger and Bamezai (2006) make a case for moderate cost shifting from 1997 to 2001. A 1 percent relative decrease in the average Medicare price was associated with a 0.17 percent increase in the price paid by private-pay patients. A 1 percent reduction in average Medicaid price was associated with a 0.04

percent increase in private-pay prices. The cost shift per patient day to private payers amounted to a 12.3 percent price increase.

Theory, descriptive evidence, and some empirical evidence suggest that hospitals cost shifted before the 1990s. More research is needed to assess hospitals' ability to cost shift from the 1990s on.

Before moving to policies dealing with cost shifting, let us briefly address the issue of whether physicians cost shift. As with hospitals, Medicare and Medicaid payments to physicians are lower than those from private patients. Physicians are limited as to whether they can charge their public patients an additional amount over the public payment, and how much more they can charge. Therefore, they have an incentive to recoup costs from private patients. They may not do so, however, for several reasons (Rice et al. 1996). They may (1) have reached their profit maximizing price, (2) be under competitive pressures, or (3) be compensating for low public payments by inducing demand. Empirical evidence thus far indicates that physicians do not cost shift (Rice et al. 1996).

Polices Regarding Cost Shifting

One line of thinking is that since lack of competition permits cost shifting in the first place, the way to prevent cost shifting is to make healthcare more competitive by enforcing antitrust laws and by removing barriers to entry and exit such as certificate of need (CON) laws, which regulate the construction of new healthcare facilities in some states.[19] On the other hand, it could be argued that if cost shifting can only occur when suppliers are not fully exploiting their market power, we should not worry about reducing that market power. One could also argue that approaching the problem of cost shifting with respect to market power does not fully address the root problem of cost shifting—underpayment by public agencies compounded by uncompensated care costs—and the need for providers to compensate for these deficits. If these trends continue or worsen, and if hospitals have already "trimmed all the fat" from providing care so that further cost reductions and efficiencies are not possible, preventing cost shifting by promoting competition may only worsen their financial performance.

Altman, Schactman, and Eliat (2006) ask whether U.S. hospitals could go the way of U.S. airlines, where intense price competition has led to a decline in quality and services, financial instability, and bankruptcies. Promoting increased competition in healthcare might reduce inefficiencies and keep prices low. But without cross-subsidization for the low reimbursement from public payers, U.S. hospitals could end up severely cutting costs, eliminating services, and suffering from financial instability. Altman, Schactman, and Eliat (2006) predict that by 2025 the need for hospitals to cost shift will increase, but their ability to do so will be diminished.

So if promoting competition alone won't help, how should we handle cost shifting? There are two clear policies that could eliminate cost shifting.

First, public payers could eliminate the need for cost shifting by paying hospitals enough to cover the costs of an efficiently run organization (Altman, Schactman, and Eliat 2006; Lee et al. 2003). Second, policymakers could remove uncompensated care costs by ensuring that all Americans have access to healthcare. As Needleman (2001, 1128) remarks, "Universal insurance would virtually eliminate the need for private provision of (uncompensated care) services."

6.4 Are There Increasing Returns to Scale?

We touched on the issue of scale economies in healthcare in the discussion on market power, but will discuss it in more depth in this section. Generally, economic markets experience constant or decreasing returns to scale in production. That is, when a firm expands the use of all inputs by a certain proportion, the corresponding increase in output is the same (constant) or less than (decreasing) the increase in input usage. When this is the case, the average costs per item produced do not change (with constant returns) or increase (with decreasing returns) with the expansion. In other words, there are no economies of scale in expanding production, therefore there is no advantage for society to having a monopoly.

If, on the other hand, the average cost of production declines as we move from many small firms that each supply a fraction of the total output to one large firm that supplies all of the output, and if the firm can produce enough to meet demand without production becoming unmanageable, economies of scale exist. (If, however, the firm must expand to the point of production being unwieldy, decreasing returns to scale could occur.) A society might therefore be better off encouraging the monopolization of an industry characterized by economies of scale, regulating the firm to ensure that it does not take advantage of its monopoly power by charging too much, producing too little, or both. In contrast, without increasing returns to scale, there would be little advantage to encouraging monopolies.

In the United States, a case can be made for the existence of increasing returns to scale in the hospital sector, particularly with larger hospitals in more concentrated markets. Stephen Finkler (1979, 270) conducted the classic study of this issue, examining economies of scale in the provision of open-heart surgery in California in the 1970s.[20] He found that the average costs of these surgeries reached their lowest point when hospitals provided about 500 procedures per year, but that only 3 percent of California hospitals provided that many services. Finkler calculated that, in 1975 dollars, the United States could have saved $400 million by *regionalizing* open-heart surgery—that is, by providing such surgery in a select few regional facilities. He further calculated that the resulting incremental travel and other inconvenience costs would have absorbed only 6 to 9 percent of the savings. He also noted that "[h]eart surgery is only the tip of the iceberg."

Lynk (1995b) carried out a similar analysis of cardiac surgeries in four hospitals. Consolidating the services into one hospital reduced the variability of patient demand. This could allow for a reduction in staffing for peak patient loads, an increase in output without increasing inputs, or both. Menke and Wray (1999) examined the effect on costs of closing open-heart surgery units in selected U.S. Veterans Affairs hospitals. Even after accounting for the associated costs of transferring patients between hospitals and transportation expenses, they found that closing one of four underused facilities would reduce costs by 18 percent.

Michigan hospitals exhibited a range of scale economies in a recent study by Timothy Butler and Ling Li (2005). Twenty-three percent were operating under decreasing returns to scale and 32 percent under increasing returns, although 66 percent of these hospitals were technically inefficient (use of inputs was not at an optimum). A study of North Carolina hospitals supports a constant-returns-to-scale environment (Conrad and Strauss 1983).

An analysis of British healthcare trusts suggests that a percentage of healthcare providers in the United Kingdom are also operating under increasing returns to scale (Tsai and Molinero 2002). In this study, 5 out of 27 trusts (18.5 percent) operated with increasing returns to scale, while 6 (22 percent) had decreasing returns. One result of this study, which examined the scale economies of multiple healthcare services, is that a given trust may appear to be operating under constant returns to scale when it is really operating under increasing returns in one service and decreasing in another.

These results do not indicate that the hospital industry as a whole tends toward increasing returns to scale, only that some hospitals do, and only within particular regions. However, a recent national study of U.S. hospitals from 1982 to 1996 made a stronger case for increasing returns to scale (Wilson and Carey 2004). This study used a large sample from the American Hospital Association (AHA) Annual Survey. Increasing returns to scale are found among hospitals from above the median size to the largest size. The authors conclude that these larger hospitals are exploiting economies of scale. Likewise Lynk (2005b) uses AHA Hospital Statistics 1991–92 to examine newborn census and bassinets in all U.S. hospitals. He finds that that excess capacity falls as average census rises. The doubling of newborn census reduces the excess capacity of bassinets by 32.6 percent.[21]

Another aspect of increasing returns to scale in the hospital sector concerns health outcomes from surgery. Most health services researchers agree that hospitals and physicians that have more experience providing surgical services tend to obtain better health outcomes for their patients—the so-called "practice makes perfect" hypothesis. One of the earliest studies of this type found that hospitals that performed more than 200 operations of a particular type per year had mortality rates 25 percent to 41 percent lower than lower-volume hospitals, after controlling for case-mix differences (Luft, Bunker, and Enthoven 1979). A more recent study found that mortality rates for coronary artery bypass operations by high-volume surgeons in high-volume hospitals were 38 percent lower (Hannan et al. 1991). These results indicate increasing returns to scale, in that quality is one of the chief outcomes in the hospital market.

The fact that returns to scale exist in some hospital sectors, and that these sectors experience higher efficiency and possibly higher quality, gives even more reason to construct careful policies with regard to market competition. A more competitive market with many small providers may not be as cost effective or provide as high quality of care as a less competitive market with large providers. Nevertheless, if the hospital industry is allowed to become more concentrated, price regulations or payment structures would be necessary to ensure that the larger providers would not take advantage of their market power by charging higher prices and offering fewer services.

6.5 Chapter Summary

In this chapter, we have attempted to show that the independent and passive role typically attributed to suppliers in competitive markets does not apply to healthcare suppliers. We questioned the validity of three assumptions of the competitive market—that supply and demand are independently determined, that firms do not have market power, and that increasing returns to scale do not exist. We discussed several implications concerning how suppliers' behavior can be influenced if these assumptions are relaxed, and we reported on some evidence that these assumptions may not reflect the reality of healthcare markets. The usual arsenal of demand-side policies are not likely to produce a significant reduction in healthcare expenses, while supply-side policies must be chosen carefully.

Notes

1. One possible exception to this is if physicians have a backward-bending labor supply curve, which is discussed later.
2. For the anti-inducement side, see Feldman and Sloan (1988). For a contrasting opinion, see Rice and Labelle (1989).
3. A few notable studies that find evidence of inducement using physician-population ratios include Evans, Parish, and Sully (1973); Fuchs (1978); Hemenway and Fallon (1985); Cromwell and Mitchell (1986); and Tussing and Wojtowycz (1986). Some studies concluding that demand inducement is not terribly significant include Wilensky and Rossiter (1983); McCarthy (1985); Stano (1985); Escarce (1992); Carlsen and Grytten (1998); Grytten, Carlsen and Skaus (2001); and Grytten and Sorensen (2001).
4. Reinhardt's article also shows that two other ways of examining inducement—output per physician and income per physician—also provide ambiguous results.

5. A review of much of the earlier literature (through the early 1980s) can be found in Gabel and Rice (1985).

6. For a thorough list of different approaches, see Labelle, Stoddart, and Rice (1994).

7. The Bunker and Brown study was not about demand inducement per se, because it was written before the debate started to rage.

8. One possible difference is that health professionals are less tolerant than others of uncertainty with regard to their own health, and therefore demand more services when they are patients in an effort to minimize this uncertainty.

9. For critiques of this research, see the commentaries by Thomas McGuire and Uwe Reinhardt, along with the authors' reply, in the same issue of the journal.

10. For a review of the results of many DRG studies, see Coulam and Gaumer (1991).

11. The American Heart Association has published principles and recommendations for the development, implementation, and evaluation of P4P programs. See Bufalino and colleagues (2006).

12. Game theory, developed by mathematicians such as John von Neuman, Oskar Morgenstern, and John Nash, has been used to model the behavior of oligopolistic markets. In game theory, agents develop strategies that will give them the largest benefits, given the strategies the other agents choose (McKay 1994). The Cournot duopoly equilibrium is another way to model the interactions of firms. Each firm takes the quantity set by its competitors as a given, estimates the remaining demand, and then sets price and output according to that demand (Calem, Dor, and Rizzo 1999; Dranove and Satterthwaite 1992).

13. A document by the Department of Justice states that "only those activities that would harm health care markets and consumers by raising prices, decreasing availability or quality of services, or discouraging innovation face potential antitrust challenge." (Statement of Anne K. Bingaman, Assistant Attorney General Antitrust Division United States Departments of Justice. Submitted to the Committee on Finance United States Senate on Competition and Antitrust Issues in Health Care Reform. May 12, 1994. Available at: www.usdoj .gov/atr/public/testimony/0119.htm.)

14. For details on healthcare antitrust activities and FTC actions, see Pender and Meier (2005).

15. Authors' calculations from Table 103 of Centers for Disease Control and Prevention (2007).

16. In 2005, HCA had 182 hospitals in 22 states, Tenet Healthcare Corporation had 83 hospitals in 13 states, and Ascension Health had 78 hospitals in 20 states *(Modern Healthcare's* Hospital Systems Survey, June 12, 2006).

17. If there is only one price at which all output is sold, the marginal revenue curve must be below the demand curve for a monopolist. This is because if the firm wishes to increase output by one unit, its marginal revenue increases

by an amount less than the market price at which the output sells. This is true, in turn, because the firm must lower the price it receives on all of the goods sold, not just the last one. If, in contrast, a monopolist can charge a different price to all customers (or different classes of customers), then it can reap even higher profits. Such monopolists are called *price discriminators* due to their ability to charge different prices to different buyers.

18. Studies with these results include Vita and Sacher (2001); Krishnan (2001); Young, Desai, and Hellinger (2000); and Capps and Dranove (2004).

19. CON laws exist in 36 U.S. states. The laws require approval by state planning agencies in the construction and development of new hospitals, nursing homes, and other medical facilities, and in the introduction of new medical equipment such as magnetic resonance imaging scanners.

20. Finkler used a methodology called component enumeration to establish exactly what hospital resources were necessary for performing open-heart surgical procedures at the margin.

21. Lynk (1995b) believes that an even stronger case for economies of scale could be made if researchers were better able to control for patient acuity and hospital technology. Since larger hospitals tend to attract sicker patients and use more expensive complex technology, the results of economies of scale studies may underestimate the efficiency of larger hospitals.

THE PROFIT MOTIVE IN HEALTHCARE

In traditional economic theory, the profit motive leads to the production of goods and services in the most efficient manner. Consumers seek the highest quality products and services at the lowest prices, and sellers compete to provide them. Prices are driven down to the level at which profits are attainable only if firms maintain efficient production and a quality acceptable to consumers. This does not mean, however, that the quality of all the products will be the same. If some consumers are willing to pay more for higher quality, a range of products will be produced. At each point on the cost continuum, quality will be maximized.

As we discussed in earlier chapters, this efficient result of market exchange is only possible under certain assumptions: The consumer is able to make informed choices, the seller does not have excessive market power, and there are no significant externalities in production or consumption. Two additional assumptions that we have not yet addressed concern the profit motive:

Assumption 12: Firms maximize profits.
Assumption 13: Profit maximization results in the most efficient production and the highest consumer welfare.

These two assumptions may not always hold in healthcare because of the presence of nonprofit organizations. Nonprofit organizations may pursue goals other than just maximizing profits. For example, they may put more resources into charity care, or they may provide a broad range of services, including less profitable ones. They may also have a commitment to the community that includes education and continuity of care.

In this chapter, we discuss the distinctions between for-profit and nonprofit ownership in healthcare and examine differences in the behavior of the two ownership types. Unlike most of the other chapters, the focus here is almost entirely on the United States. We briefly review the history of ownership in U.S. healthcare markets, and we consider special issues associated with completely for-profit markets, such as pharmaceuticals. We observe recent shifts in the U.S. healthcare system toward commodification and corporatization that are linked to for-profit growth. The chapter ends with a discussion of several policy issues related to ownership in healthcare.

7.1 For-Profit Ownership in Healthcare

The health sector in the United States has always been a mix of for-profit and nonprofit organizations. The proportion of for-profits to nonprofits has changed over time, though, and it varies by setting.

Currently, several healthcare settings have strong private nonprofit sectors, and a substantial number of services are provided by the public nonprofit sector (government-owned entities). In 2006, only 18 percent of U.S. community hospitals (all acute-care general hospitals, excluding federal[1]) were for-profit (Kaiser Family Foundation n.d.). The rest were split between private nonprofit (60 percent) and public nonprofit entities (23 percent). Although the percentage of for-profit community hospitals is relatively low, the current level is the result of a steady increase in their numbers over the past decades (Kaiser Family Foundation 2007b). Figure 7.1 shows that the percentage of for-profit community hospitals doubled over 26 years, increasing from 9 percent in 1980 to 18 percent in 2006 (Kaiser Family Foundation 2007b).

Although nonprofit ownership is strong in areas such as hospital care, in other areas for-profit and nonprofit ownership is more evenly distributed. But the for-profit sector has been growing. In 2000 roughly 40 percent of home care agencies were for-profit, a sevenfold increase since 1980 (National Association for Home Care 2001).[2] Among hospices, for-profit agencies increased fourfold in the 1990s alone (Carlson, Gallo, and Bradley 2004).

For-profit ownership dominates nursing home care, health insurance, ambulatory surgical care, specialty hospitals, and physician services. In 2006, 66 percent of nursing facilities certified by the Centers for Medicare & Medicaid Services (CMS) were for-profit (Harrington, Carrillo, and Blank 2007). As Figure 7.1 indicates, this percentage has been relatively stable over the past two decades. In 2005, 66 percent of all HMO enrollees were in for-profit plans, a five-fold increase since 1980 (Kaiser Family Foundation 2007b; Sanofi-aventis 2006). Another area where for-profit services are strong is outpatient dialysis, in which the number of for-profit units climbed from nearly none in the 1970s to around 54 percent in 1990, then to 80 percent in 2006 (Garg and Powe 2001; Rettig and Levinsky 1991; Szczech et al. 2006; United States Renal Data System 1997, 2006). Approximately half of all ambulatory surgical centers (ASCs) are investor owned; the rest are owned by physicians and hospitals (for-profit and nonprofit) (Frey 2007). Physicians' practices also tend to be owned by physicians in solo and group practices; by physician practice management companies, most of which are for-profit; or by for-profit or nonprofit hospitals and healthcare systems (Burns, DeGraaff, and Singh 1999).

Finally, healthcare product markets are completely for-profit. Investor-owned companies provide a vast array of drugs, technologies, and healthcare products.

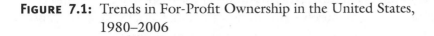

FIGURE 7.1: Trends in For-Profit Ownership in the United States, 1980–2006

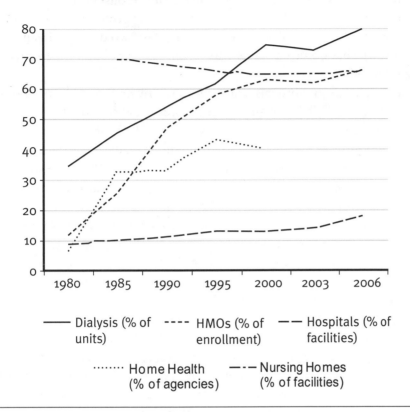

SOURCE: Data sources for dialysis facilities:
(1) Rettig, R., and N. Levinsky. 1991. *Kidney Failure and the Federal Government.* Washington, DC: National Academy Press.
(2) USRDS. 1997. *Annual Report: Atlas of End-Stage Renal Disease in the United States.* Bethesda, MD: National Institutes of Health, U.S. Renal Data System.
(3) USRDS. 2006. *Annual Report: Atlas of End-Stage Renal Disease in the United States.* Bethesda, MD: National Institutes of Health, U.S. Renal Data System.

Data source for home healthcare organizations:
(1) National Association of Homecare. 2001. *Basic Statistics About Home Care.*
www.nahc.org/Consumer/hcstats.html

Data sources for hospitals and HMOs:
(1) Kaiser Family Foundation. 2007. *Trends and Indicators in the Changing Health Care Marketplace,*
www.kff.org/insurance/7031/print-sec5.cfm.
(2) NA. 2006. *Managed Care Digest Series, 2006.*
www.managedcaredigest.com/resources/hmo2006/2006hmo.pdf

Data sources for nursing homes:
(1) Rhoades, J. A., and N. A. Krauss. 1999. *Chartbook #3, Nursing Homes Trends, 1987 and 1996.* Rockville, MD: AHRQ.
(2) Harrington, C., H. Carrillo, and V. Wellin. 2001. *Nursing Facilities, Staffing, Residents, and Facility Deficiencies,* 1994–2000. Washington, DC: NCCNHR.
(3) Harrington, C., H. Carrillo, and B.W. Blank. 2007. *Nursing Facilities, Staffing, Residents, and Facility Deficiencies,* 2000–2006. Washington, DC: NCCNHR.

For-profit healthcare takes two different forms: new start-ups and conversions of existing nonprofits. In home care and specialty hospitals, most growth has been a result of new for-profit organizations attracted to a lucrative business. In the ambulatory care setting, for-profit enterprises have been responsible for nearly all the growth in the past two decades. Insurance industry growth has occurred via new for-profit start-ups and conversions of existing nonprofits.

Among for-profit hospitals, conversions of private and public nonprofit organizations have fueled growth. Financial pressures are thought to play a role in these conversions (Mark 1999). Rosenau (2003, 402) states that in the 1980s and early 1990s "many small, often unprofitable, community hospitals were purchased and reorganized as for-profit hospitals."[3] One study of eight nonprofit hospital conversions found that four out of the eight had been losing money prior to the sale (Mark 1999). Another study of 50 nonprofit hospitals purchased by for-profit chains between 1978 and 1983 found that they tended to be small hospitals that had low profitability, highly depreciated assets, and weak equity (McCue and Furst 1986). Conversions also occur because of administrative goals of acquiring capital, market share, economies of scale, and other advantages (Gray 1997).

Whether the conversion is reactive or proactive, an organization that converts to for-profit status (1) has access to capital from investors, which it can use to make the hospital more efficient and competitive; (2) often becomes part of a system, which increases economies of scale and market share; and (3) faces reduced regulations (Claxton et al. 1997). In addition, inside information about the sale might create personal financial gain for managers at the converting organization by providing an opportunity for them to purchase shares of the stock created by the public offering of the organization at low prices (Claxton et al. 1997). This last result has led to conversions in which the sale price of hospitals and HMOs has been considerably below market value, and raises strong ethical issues.

In summary, although for-profit ownership is not dominant in the hospital sector, it has a stronger presence or completely dominates in other areas of healthcare. Furthermore, the for-profit sector has grown in nearly every area of the health industry over the past few decades. Growth has occurred due to the establishment of new for-profit organizations and the conversion of nonprofit organizations.

Why do we care about the presence and growth of for-profit organizations in healthcare? It is a generally held belief that the differences between for-profit and nonprofit organizations affect the goals, outcomes, and direction of the healthcare delivery system. In the next section we outline the distinctions between for-profit and nonprofit organizations and discuss differences in their behavior. In a subsequent section we review the empirical evidence for differences in performance.

7.2 Differences and Similarities Between For-Profit and Nonprofit Organizations

There are clear legal and organizational differences between for-profit and nonprofit organizations, but behavioral and performance differences are less distinct. The goals for-profits and nonprofits work toward are not exclusive to only one or the other type of organization. Behavior that results from these goals will vary depending on the emphasis placed on a particular goal and the strategies developed to pursue it (Shen et al. 2007). For example, for-profit and nonprofit hospitals may share the goal of providing community services, but each may approach that goal with different emphasis and actions. Market pressures, such as the level of market concentration, market competition, payer reimbursements, and regulation and accreditation, affect both nonprofit and for-profit organizations and may motivate them to perform somewhat similarly (Baker et al. 2000; Shen et al. 2007).

We begin with the legal and organizational differences between for-profits and nonprofits. For-profit organizations are investor owned, may solicit equity capital, and must pay federal corporate income taxes and other state and local taxes. A portion of profits can be distributed to owners and stockholders. Nonprofit organizations, on the other hand, are not owned by individuals or stockholders, must look to donations for equity capital, and do not pay federal corporate income taxes. In many states they do not have to pay property taxes and other state and local taxes. Net income above that necessary to run the organization must be reinvested in the organization or community or redistributed to donors and must not be distributed to any individual or shareholder (Rotarius et al. 2005). The proceeds from a sale or closing of a nonprofit institution may not be paid to individuals (Pauly 1987). Nonprofit organizations may receive tax-deductible private donations, tend to have better access to tax-exempt bonds and other subsidized loans, and are more likely to use volunteers (Reinhardt 2000). Nonprofits are considered public goods or community assets, and depending upon the state, may be expected to provide an amount of charity care at least equal to the tax subsidies they receive (Harrison and Sexton 2004).

Gray (1997) lists some important organizational similarities between for-profit and nonprofit organizations: Both rely on retained earnings and debt for new capital, and payments for services rendered are the major source of revenue for both. Like nonprofits, for-profits may receive tax breaks to stimulate investment during their development. Like for-profits, nonprofits are not exempt from all taxes. They pay payroll taxes, and in some states they pay taxes on hospital admissions, or they make payments to the state in lieu of taxes. Some nonprofits with large payrolls and large numbers of admissions pay more taxes than for-profits (Gray 1997).

The key assumption underlying predictions of differences in behavior between for-profit and nonprofit organizations is that for-profits focus on profit maximization and nonprofits do not. For-profit organizations will minimize costs and exploit market advantages that enhance their profitability. Nonprofits pursue other goals and usually face a break-even constraint.

Economists have developed several theories regarding this difference in goals and its implications for performance differences. These theories may or may not predict the same behavior, and the predictions may be challenged by empirical studies. The *property rights theory* predicts that for-profit organizations, which distribute a share of profits to owners, may pursue cost control at the expense of quality (Grossman and Hart 1986; Shen et al. 2007). In contrast, because nonprofit organizations do not have claimants to profits, they may produce higher quality products and services but with lower efficiency.

According to Newhouse (1970), rather than maximizing profits, nonprofit hospitals maximize *quality*, *prestige*, or both. This is accomplished through the actions of agents of the institutions—administrators and physicians—who are interested in being associated with a high-quality institution that will confer prestige upon them. When prestige is the goal, the organization pursues the best technology and staff. As a result, quality will be high, but efficiency will be low.

Pauly and Redisch (1973) believe that the goals of nonprofit hospitals are to meet *physician needs*—to maintain a high amount of physical, technical, and personnel resources. Attempts to meet this goal will also result in inefficiencies, since there will be unused capacity and unproductive uses of resources.

According to the *trust signal theory*, information asymmetries and consumers' reduced abilities to discern quality give for-profit organizations an incentive to underprovide quality. Nonprofit ownership is a "trust signal" to consumers, who believe that nonprofits are less concerned about making a profit and therefore have less incentive to reduce quality (Frank and Salkever 1994; Hansmann 1980; Shapiro 1983).

Others believe that nonprofit organizations focus mainly on *altruistic* goals, such as reducing unmet needs in the community, fulfilling the demand for public goods, meeting donor expectations, and maximizing the well-being of consumers (Frank and Salkever 1994; Weisbrod 1988; Rose-Ackerman 1996; Ben-Nur and Gui 1993). Nonprofit hospitals "act as social columns" by providing unprofitable services to millions of Americans (Phillips 1999). With these goals, efficiency may or may not be affected, but quality is expected to be high. The primary challenge for nonprofit hospitals, says Phillips (1999), is to maximize efficiency while furthering charitable missions.

One altruistic theory of nonprofit goals and behavior is the *public goods theory*, which suggests that nonprofit hospitals exist to provide public goods that the government does not. Nonprofit hospitals are willing to provide more charity care and other community services than for-profits because of this mission and because they are less concerned about profit margins (Weisbrod 1988).

Some economists and policy experts (Rosenau 2003) theorize that nonprofits should be able to provide services *more* efficiently, because non-profit organizations

- have lower administrative costs (Himmelstein et al. 1999);
- have no taxes on income or property (Sloan 1998);
- benefit from volunteers, receive tax-deductible contributions, have access to subsidized loans, and pay lower salaries to CEOs (Reinhardt 2000); and
- are better at motivating knowledge workers (Drucker 1989).

Still others theorize that for-profit and nonprofit organizations react to market power differently. For-profits take advantage of market power and tend to set prices high, while nonprofits set prices just sufficient to cover charity care or other unprofitable services. Due to their price-setting reaction to market power, for-profits could cause higher hospital expenditures (Rosenau 2003).

Based on the legal distinctions between for-profit and nonprofit and on theories regarding their goals and behaviors, nonprofit behaviors are predicted to differ from for-profit to some degree along the following lines (Needleman 2001; Rosenau 2003):

- Quality is higher.
- They engage in more trustworthy behavior.
- They have a stronger commitment to community service.
- They are more efficient—or they are less efficient, depending upon the theory.
- They use market power differently.

We end this section with a caveat. These theories set for-profit and nonprofit organizations apart as if each type of ownership has completely different goals and behaviors. In reality, goals and behaviors overlap, and the differences are of emphasis rather than extremes. On the one hand, the need to retain a surplus for growth and innovation may motivate efficiency in nonprofits, especially when competing with for-profits (Baker et al. 2000; Rosenau 2003). On the other hand, maintaining quality services and providing charity care may be a goal of for-profits, especially given market competition over reputation and the trend toward more benchmarking and regulating of quality (Marsteller, Bovbjerg, and Nichols 1998). The question is whether the drive to maximize profits, typical of for-profit organizations, is stronger than the goals related to quality of care and community service, typical of nonprofit organizations.

Kuttner (1999) and others believe that for-profit motives dominate hospital care and have transformed hospitals into a commercial market. Due to market pressures and competition, nonprofit hospitals are paying less attention to social responsibilities and more to commercial interests (Mobley and Bradford 1997). Executives from both types of hospitals say that they are facing the same market pressures and are beginning to converge in terms of goals and behavior (Rosenau 2003).

Others feel that although the two sectors have become similar in some aspects, important differences remain (Hollingsworth and Hollingsworth 1987). For example, both sectors provide similar services, but for-profit hospitals have fewer unprofitable services. All hospitals increase prices after a merger, but the amount of the price increase is related to ownership (two for-profits merging leads to the highest price increase), among other things. Hollingsworth and Hollingsworth (1987) believe that these complex relationships explain some of the inconsistent research findings on ownership.

7.3 Research Evidence Regarding Differences Between For-Profit and Nonprofit Healthcare Organizations

In this section we examine the research evidence for differences in performance and outcomes between for-profit and nonprofit healthcare organizations with regard to quality, trustworthiness, community service, efficiency, and use of market power. There are many types of healthcare markets, and this topic has been actively studied for years, so the literature is voluminous. Where possible we use existing reviews to summarize findings. Where evidence is available, we explore differences in performance in hospitals, nursing homes, dialysis centers, and health plans.

Differences in Quality

Several reviews on the topic of ownership and quality have been conducted. One by Needleman (2001) found mixed evidence for higher quality in nonprofit hospitals and stronger evidence for higher quality in nonprofit nursing homes, dialysis units, and health plans. We now look at the research in each of these settings in more detail.

Quality in Hospitals   Some reviews find strong evidence of higher quality in nonprofit hospitals. In five of seven studies linking mortality to ownership type, for-profit hospital ownership was found to be related to higher mortality (Baker et al. 2000). For-profit ownership was also related to adverse events such as urinary tract infections, pneumonia, and pulmonary compromise in the three studies that looked at these factors. This review noted that the differences between ownership types are minimized in markets in which hospitals are more competitive over insurance contracts and price.

Devereaux and colleagues (2002) completed a meta-analysis of 15 studies on the relationship between ownership and mortality in hospitals. The analysis assessed the data collection period, the number of hospitals and patients in the sample, the source of data, mortality results, and whether there were control variables for confounding factors. They found that for-profit hospitals were associated with a statistically significant increased risk of inpatient death. Nineteen additional studies that were not included because they did not meet study criteria also indicated that for-profit hospitals had higher inpatient mortality than nonprofit hospitals.

The latest review at the time of this writing finds mixed evidence for differences among nonprofit and for-profit hospitals with regard to mortality and adverse events. In 2006 Eggleston and colleagues undertook a quantitative review of 31 studies of ownership and patient outcomes between 1990 and 2004. They found that most studies did not demonstrate a significant difference in mortality and other adverse events between for-profit and nonprofit hospitals. The authors concluded that the divergent results were due to different analytic methods, different diseases studied, and different data sources.

In summary, there is some evidence of a difference in quality between for-profit and nonprofit hospitals in terms of higher mortality and adverse events. The evidence is not conclusive, however.

Quality in Nursing Homes

Needleman's (2001) review found strong evidence that quality was higher in nonprofit nursing homes. The nursing home quality literature assesses a variety of resident outcomes and care processes. Nonprofit facilities have more comfortable physical environments, more cohesive relationships, more resident control (Lemke and Moos 1989), and fewer residents with pressure sores than for-profit facilities (Aaronson, Zinn, and Rosko 1994; Grabowski 2001). Nonprofit nursing homes are more likely to be restraint-free (Castle and Fogel 1998) or are less likely to receive restraint deficiencies than for-profit nursing homes (Graber and Sloane 1995).

For-profit nursing homes have been cited for more deficiencies in quality of care, resident rights, and quality of life (Johnson-Pawlson and Infeld 1996; Harrington et al. 2001), and for more serious deficiencies (O'Neil et al. 2003) than nonprofit nursing homes. Residents of for-profit nursing homes feel less responsiveness and empathy from nursing staff (Steffen and Nystrom 1997). Spector, Selden, and Cohen (1998) find that for-profit nursing homes have higher rates of mortality and infections than nonprofit nursing homes.

A number of studies look at nurse staffing in nursing homes. Higher staffing is considered an indicator of quality. Studies find that for-profit nursing homes have lower staffing levels (Aaronson, Zinn, and Rosko 1994; Cohen and Spector 1996; Elwell 1984; Fottler, Smith, and James 1981; Kanda and Mezey 1991; Centers for Disease Control and Prevention 2000).

Some studies, however, find no difference in quality between non-profit and for-profit nursing homes (Munroe 1990; Porell et al. 1998). Zinn, Aaronson, and Rosko (1993) conclude that for-profit ownership is associated with lower-than-expected mortality. Restraint use, catheterizations, and numbers of residents with pressure sores were not significantly different from those in nonprofit facilities. In another study, residents in for-profit facilities were less likely to die within six months but did not have any improvement in functional status (Spector and Takada 1991). Unruh, Zhang, and Wan (2006) report that for-profit nursing homes have higher composite quality indexes, but the same authors find worse quality scores in for-profit nursing homes in another study (Wan, Zhang, and Unruh 2006).

Most studies find that nonprofit nursing homes provide higher quality of care across an array of quality indicators. A few find no difference or higher quality in for-profit nursing homes with some quality indicators. The inconsistency of these studies points to the need for further research in this area.

Quality in Dialysis Units

Needleman (2001) also found strong evidence of higher quality in nonprofit dialysis units, but the studies are not without controversy. Using data from the U.S. Renal Data System (USRDS), Garg and colleagues (1999) found that from 1991 to 1995 for-profit dialysis units had a 20 percent higher mortality rate and 26 percent fewer placements of patients on the renal transplant waiting list than nonprofit units. Using USRDS data from 1995 to 1997, Port, Wolfe, and Held (2000) also reported significant differences between for-profit and nonprofit units: In for-profit units patient mortality was 6 percent higher, and 15 percent fewer patients were placed on transplant lists. However, physicians associated with for-profit dialysis centers criticized Garg and colleagues for having a small, unrepresentative sample, for possible sampling error and selection bias, and for failure to adjust for patient factors (such as age and existence of diabetes) among other reasons (Bander, Lazarus, and Lindenfeld 2000). Garg and Frick (2000) defended their data as reflecting a nationally representative sample and their methodology as sound. They stated that they controlled for more patient factors than studies cited by their critics.

In a follow-up article, Garg and Powe (2001) relate evidence that could explain why mortality rates are different: For-profit dialysis units use less staff and equipment than nonprofit units (Griffiths et al. 1994; Farley 1993); they also are more likely to administer a lower dialysis dose and reuse dialyzers (Held et al. 1991; Agodoa, Wolfe, and Port 1998).

Following this controversy, Devereaux and colleagues (2002) analyzed studies comparing mortality in for-profit and nonprofit dialysis units from 1973 through 1997. The authors found that six of the eight studies they analyzed showed adjusted mortality to be significantly greater in for-profit dialysis units. The Garg and colleagues (1999) study was one of the six. Physicians employed by companies in the dialysis for-profit sector criticized this meta-analysis. They stated that the authors had excluded valid studies that indicated no difference in mortality between for-profit and nonprofit units, while including questionable studies.[4] Devereaux and colleagues defended their study methodology as unbiased (it was blinded, with exclusions on the basis of sound methodological criteria), and their inclusions as proper (Devereaux et al. 2003). One study appearing after the Devereaux controversy did not find any differences in mortality related to ownership (Szczech et al. 2006).

The 2001 review by Needleman found that the number of studies comparing quality in for-profit and nonprofit health plans is small, that the studies are mostly descriptive, and that further study is needed. Keeping that in mind, the evidence we do have suggests that quality is higher in nonprofit health plans. For example, quality measures in the Healthcare Effectiveness Data and Information Set (HEDIS)[5] were higher in nonprofit health plans (Greene 1998; Himmelstein et al. 1999), while disenrollment and appeals were higher in for-profit plans (ProPAC 1994), and patient satisfaction was lower (Landon et al. 2001). In another study, rates of complaints per thousand enrollees were 4.58 in Humana (a for-profit company) and 0.18 in Group Health Cooperative of Puget Sound (a nonprofit company) (Gray 1997). A *Consumer Reports* survey of patient experiences with 37 HMOs found that 12.2 percent of respondents in for-profit plans felt that they did not get the care they needed because the plan discouraged it, while 7.8 percent in nonprofit plans felt this way (*Consumer Reports* 1996).

Quality in Health Plans

A 2001 study by Born and Simon conflicts with Himmelstein and colleagues' 1999 results. Born and Simon found that patients in for-profit and nonprofit HMOs receive similar preventive and chronic-disease care. Their results were criticized by Woolhandler and colleagues (2002) for using a biased and inappropriate data set.

Differences in Trustworthy Behavior

In his seminal 1963 paper, Kenneth Arrow wrote, "virtually all the special features of [the healthcare industry]... stem from the prevalence of trust" (Arrow 1963b, 946). Providers need to exhibit trustworthy behavior because patients' lack of information about their condition and care makes them vulnerable. Trustworthy behavior is defined as actions that indicate that the organization operates in the best interests of its customers and the public. Behaviors typically scrutinized include those that might indicate "upcoding" of patient diagnoses and procedures to higher reimbursement categories, excessive charges for care, and unnecessary treatments or denial of necessary treatments (Needleman 2001).

Several studies in the Needleman (2001) review find that charges are higher in for-profit hospitals and clinics. The review also reports that for-profit hospitals are more likely to upcode Medicare claims, and that nonprofit hospitals in markets with a high proportion of for-profit organizations are more likely to do the same. Several other studies find that, all else being equal, for-profit hospitals have more cesarean sections (Tanio 1989; Stafford 1991) and shorter lengths of stay (Kuttner 1996) than nonprofit hospitals. One finding we mentioned earlier is that for-profit renal centers make fewer referrals for renal transplantation than nonprofit institutions (Garg et al. 1999).

In a nursing home study, the behavior of a large for-profit nursing home chain was observed over time to ascertain how management maximized profits for shareholders (Kitchener et al. 2007). The authors discovered three main strategies for profit maximization: (1) rapid growth through debt-financed mergers, (2) maintenance of low labor costs through low nurse staffing, and (3) acceptance of fraud and abuse sanctions as a cost of doing business. They observed similar strategies among other nursing homes. Such strategies, especially the last two, raise issues of trustworthiness.

Differences in Community Commitment and Service

Studies of differences in community services between for-profit and nonprofit organizations have had conflicting results. One reason is that studies do not always take confounding factors into account. A factor that should be accounted for, but often is not, is the difference in demand for charity care by locality (Claxton et al. 1997; Gray 1997). In areas where the demand for charity care is low, for-profits and nonprofits may provide similar levels of care, but in areas where the needs are high, nonprofits may provide more care.

Another reason for conflicting results is that community benefits are often measured only as "charity care," defined as unpaid services to the poor. This undercounts the value of community commitment and service. A broader view considers several factors, such as levels of all unpaid services (uncompensated care that is charity care plus "bad debt"), losses from serving public program patients, losses from subsidizing community services (burn units, 24-hour trauma, special needs programs), costs of research and education, location in urban areas with large numbers of poor and uninsured people, the degree of commitment to location, and stability in ownership and control (Claxton et al. 1997; Gray 1997). To fully assess differences in community benefits between for-profit and nonprofit hospitals, all these measures should be considered. However, due to the difficulty of obtaining data and quantifying the results, studies generally rely on a subset of the measures. This contributes to incomplete comparisons between for-profit and nonprofit hospitals.

Research comparing community benefits among for-profit and nonprofit hospitals needs to be interpreted in light of the limitations discussed above. Beginning with unpaid service (uncompensated care), a review of the literature by Needleman (2001) indicates that in some states nonprofit hospitals provide significantly more of these services than for-profits, while in other states the difference is small. Some of the difference is due to local demand, as we discussed above. As Norton and Staiger (1994) report, for-profit hospitals often indirectly avoid the uninsured by locating in better-insured areas.

For-profit hospitals are less likely than nonprofits to provide unprofitable services (Gray 1986). Physicians report conflict with administrators over the treatment of indigent persons more often in for-profit hospitals than in nonprofit hospitals (Burns, Anderson, and Shortell 1990; Schlesinger et al. 1987). Nonprofit hospitals admit more uninsured and Medicaid patients than for-profits (Frank, Salkever, and Mullan 1990). Nonprofit hospitals also conduct more hospital-based health promotion services and collaborative health promotion services than for-profit and government hospitals (Ginn and Moseley 2004).

Needleman (2001) finds that for-profit hospitals play less of a leadership role in their communities and view their relationship to the community as commercial. They are more willing to sell hospitals that no longer fit their corporate plans. A descriptive study by Ferris and Graddy in 1999 also finds that more for-profit hospitals than nonprofit hospitals close, suggesting that nonprofit hospitals are more likely to continue providing services when profit margins are reduced.

Based on a review of 20 studies, Claxton and colleagues (1997) conclude that, overall, nonprofit hospitals provide significantly more community benefits than for-profits, and this is most apparent when comparisons are made within states. However, there is wide variation among nonprofit hospitals in how much benefit is provided. Public and major teaching hospitals provide the most community benefits, while a number of nonprofits provide few benefits. When using a reasonably broad definition of community benefits that includes charity care, bad debt, losses from public programs, and the net cost of teaching and research, nonprofit hospitals as a whole contribute significantly more than the cost of their tax exemption. However, many nonprofit hospitals receive more in tax exemptions than the value of the benefits they provide. Morrisey, Wedig, and Hassan (1996, 143) also report that "the vast majority of nonprofit hospitals [in California] provide community dividends in excess of the tax subsidies they receive," but around 20 percent do not cover the value of their tax exemption. If the taxes paid by for-profit hospitals are counted as community benefits, the total benefits provided by for-profit hospitals would exceed those of nonprofit hospitals on average (Claxton et al. 1997). However, the relationship between taxes and community benefits is not clear, so counting the value of taxes as a community benefit does not necessarily seem appropriate.

Differences in Efficiency and Costs

Theoretically, without the incentive of profits, nonprofit organizations should perform worse, or at best no better, than for-profit organizations in terms of efficiency and costs. We would expect for-profit organizations to have shorter patient lengths of stay, to use fewer physical and labor resources, and to have lower costs. The literature, however, suggests that costs are as high or higher in for-profit hospitals. A 1997 study of hospital administrative costs suggests that they are higher in for-profit hospitals (Woolhandler and Himmelstein 1997). A review of 37 studies from 1980 to 2002 reports that 62.5 percent of the studies found nonprofit hospitals to have lower costs, 14 percent found for-profits to have lower costs, and 24.5 percent reported inconclusive results (Rosenau 2003). A meta-analysis by Shen and colleagues (2007) finds little difference in cost related to hospital ownership.

A few studies contradict these results. In 2005, McKay and Deily divided a sample of hospitals into high- and low-performing quartiles for risk-adjusted mortality and cost efficiency and found that more for-profit hospitals were in the high-performing group. Two studies by Jiang, Friedman, and Begun (2006a, 2006b) using data from 1997 and 2001 also found that for-profit hospitals were more likely to be in the high-quality, low-cost quartile.

The findings in nursing homes are quite different. Studies generally show that for-profit nursing homes are more efficient (Anderson, Lewis, and Webb 1999; Chattopadhyay and Heffley 1994; Fizel and Nunnikhoven 1992; Knox, Blankmeyer, and Stutzman 1999, 2001; Nyman and Bricker 1989; Nyman, Bricker, and Link 1990; Rosko et al. 1995; Sexton et al. 1989). The higher efficiency in for-profit nursing homes may be due to the use of fewer physical and labor resources keeping costs lower. Efficiency may appear higher in for-profit nursing homes when in reality quality may be lower to accommodate cost cutting or other efficiency measures (Zhang, Unruh, and Wan 2008). One study that adjusts estimates of efficiency for quality differences finds that for-profit nursing homes are significantly more efficient than nonprofit homes (Zhang, Unruh, and Wan 2008). More studies of efficiency with adequate controls or adjustments for quality are necessary.

Differences in Prices and Financial Performance

Although for-profit and nonprofit hospitals have similar costs and efficiencies, for-profit hospitals tend to have higher profit margins. This appears to be due, in large part, to higher prices. These results are fairly robust across different time frames and study methodologies. A large-scale review by Baker and colleagues (2000) reveals that although costs are similar between for-profit and nonprofit hospitals, for-profit hospitals charge more and are more profitable. Taylor, Whellan, and Sloan (1999) report that payments to for-profit hospitals for congestive heart failure (CHF) were higher than those to government or nonprofit hospitals. Patients with CHF in for-profit hospitals also had higher Medicare payments for subsequent nonhospital care, but did not have better outcomes. Higher profit margins in Virginia for-profit hospitals are thought to be due to higher pricing and cost management such as lower staffing and decreased maintenance (Shukla, Pestian, and Clement 1997).

Using Medicare Provider Analysis and Review files and cost reports from 1985 to 1992, Dafny (2005) finds that hospitals, particularly for-profit hospitals, respond to price changes by upcoding patients to diagnosis codes with the largest price increases. Research by Horwitz (2005) in which more than 30 services were categorized as relatively profitable, unprofitable, or variable, found that for-profit hospitals have higher profits because they choose more profitable services. Government hospitals are most likely to offer relatively unprofitable services. Private nonprofit hospitals often fall in between.

In 2004, Devereaux and colleagues performed a meta-analysis of research from 1964 to 2002 on ownership and payments for care in hospitals. The authors' selection criteria resulted in eight usable studies. Five of the studies found significantly higher payments for care at private for-profit hospitals. Only one of the studies found significantly higher payments for care at nonprofit hospitals. The pooled estimate showed that for-profit hospitals were associated with higher payments for care. Combining estimates across several studies, a meta-analysis by Shen and colleagues (2007) found that for-profit hospitals produce more revenue and greater profits than nonprofits, yet their costs are not significantly different, suggesting that they achieve greater profits by charging higher prices.

Differences in the Use of Market Power

For-profit and nonprofit healthcare organizations are expected to use market power differently (Needleman 2001). For-profit organizations maximize profits by setting higher prices, while nonprofits keep prices lower because they are less concerned about profits, or because they want to maintain charity care and unprofitable services by charging different prices to different payers. This difference is important because of the antitrust implications. If nonprofit organizations do not take advantage of their greater market power due to mergers by raising prices, an argument can be made that nonprofit mergers should be evaluated differently than for-profit mergers.

Several studies find that nonprofit hospitals, like for-profit hospitals, set prices higher following a merger or in more concentrated markets. Melnick, Keeler, and Zwanziger (1999), for example, use California data from 1986 through 1994 and find that regardless of ownership type, after 1986 all hospitals raised prices in response to a merger, and that these merger-related price increases grew over time. Nonprofit and government hospital prices were below those of for-profit hospitals before the merger, but they had the greatest price increases post-merger. A second California study using 1989 data also finds post-merger nonprofit price increases (Dranove and Ludwick 1999). A case study of a merger between two nonprofit hospitals in California had similar results (Vita and Sacher 2001). Another study of nonprofit behavior in California indicates that nonprofit hospitals set prices higher in more concentrated markets (Simpson and Shin 1998). Finally, Young, Desai, and

Hellinger (2000) looked at pricing patterns in relation to degree of market concentration for three types of nonprofit hospitals: independent, member of a local hospital system, and member of a nonlocal hospital system. All three had higher prices in more concentrated markets. Nonprofit hospitals that were members of nonlocal systems had the highest prices.

7.4 Issues with Specialty Hospitals

Specialty hospitals are a fairly recent development in the health services market. The U.S. Government Accountability Office defines a specialty hospital as a hospital in which two-thirds or more of inpatient claims are in one or two major diagnostic categories, or two-thirds of the inpatient claims are for diagnostically related surgical groups (Blackstone and Fuhr 2007). Specialty hospitals typically serve cardiac, orthopedic, or general surgical patients. For the most part they are investor owned, with individual physicians sharing a small part of ownership (usually 1–2 percent per physician, with total physician ownership of 50 to 80 percent) and national for-profit companies or local nonprofit hospitals sharing the rest (Guterman 2006). They are small, averaging 52 beds for cardiac, 16 for orthopedic, and 14 for surgical patients (Medcare Payment Advisory Commission 2005). Many do not have emergency departments. Most are located in only a few states that do not have certificate of need (CON) laws (60 percent are in South Dakota, Kansas, Oklahoma, and Texas). In 2006 there were around 100–120 specialty hospitals in the United States (Morrisey 2006). Their growth slowed during a moratorium on physician investment in specialty hospitals from the end of 2003 through August 2006.

Specialty hospitals may provide services efficiently by concentrating them in one institution. The services may also be of high quality because the providers have gained experience performing a high volume of the same procedures. There is evidence that this "focused factory" approach produces higher quality at lower costs (Blackstone and Fuhr 2007).

Another positive aspect of specialty hospitals is that patient satisfaction tends to be high. Patients often believe that the nursing staff is more knowledgeable and has more specialized skills than nurses in community hospitals. They also like the fact that there is better scheduling and fewer cancellations because there are no conflicting emergency procedures (Blackstone and Fuhr 2007). Finally, the better hours, scheduling, and equipment typical of specialty hospitals may lead to similar changes in community hospitals because of the competition between the two types (Blackstone and Fuhr 2007).

On the other hand, there are concerns with the growth of specialty hospitals. One of the biggest is that they take better-paying patients away from community hospitals; for example, cardiac specialty hospitals attract a high proportion of Medicare patients needing cardiac surgeries, which are in the high diagonsis-related group (DRG) reimbursement range. Because some DRGs, such as general surgical and cardiac, have higher profit margins on average than other DRGs, hospitals that serve only patients in these DRGs will have higher profits than those that serve all types of patients (Blackstone and Fuhr 2007).

Profitability also differs *within* DRGs depending upon patient severity. Blackstone and Fuhr (2007) calculate that for patients with the least severity, DRG reimbursements for coronary bypass grafts with cardiac catheterization are 47 percent *more* profitable than the average DRG, but for the most severe patients they are 21 percent *less* profitable than the average DRG. Since sicker patients tend not to be treated at specialty hospitals because they are a greater risk and need the more extensive facilities of a general hospital, specialty hospitals are able to exploit insufficient severity adjustments of the DRG payment system to their advantage.

At the same time, specialty hospitals tend to treat fewer nonpaying uninsured and lower-paying Medicaid patients than community hospitals in the same market (Blackstone and Fuhr 2007; Guterman 2006). Cardiac specialty hospitals treat mostly Medicare patients, while orthopedic and surgical specialty hospitals treat mostly patients with private insurance (Guterman 2006).

Specialty hospitals can earn higher profits from caring for a patient population that is better insured and/or is less severely ill within given DRG categories. For example, cardiac specialty hospitals that treat patients with more profitable DRGs and that have a less severe patient population can be up to 9 percent more profitable than the average community hospital in their market area because of this between- and within-DRG selection bias (Blackstone and Fuhr 2007). Based on 2002 data from 48 physician-owned specialty hospitals (12 heart, 25 orthopedic, and 11 surgical), MedPAC (2005) found that annual returns to specialty hospitals were often greater than 20 percent of their initial investment, and their average all-payer margin was 13 percent, compared with 3–6 percent in community hospitals. The difference could not be attributed to greater efficiency.

Specialty hospitals obtain most of their higher-paying patients by capturing market share from community hospitals. As we discussed in the preceding chapter, community hospitals use better-paying patients to cross-subsidize poorer-paying patients, not only those without insurance, but those on Medicaid, who pay the lowest amount of all insurers, and those on Medicare who fall into the lower-paying DRGs. When competition from specialty hospitals reduces the number of better-paying patients in community hospitals, the financial stability of community hospitals could be affected. So far, a negative effect has not been demonstrated (MedPAC 2005), but few studies have been conducted.

Physician self-referral is another major issue with specialty hospitals. Since physicians own the hospitals, they gain financially when additional tests or procedures are done, and this incentive may negatively affect their clinical decision making. Studies have shown a significant increase in the frequency and expense of services when the ability to self-refer exists (Blackstone and Fuhr 2007; Mitchell 2007). Although the Stark Act restricts physicians' abilities to self-refer, specialty hospital self-referrals are exempt through the "whole hospital" exemption. This exemption was made under the assumption that individual physician ownership would be small in an organization as large as a hospital, such that physicians' benefits from self-referrals would be minimal. It is problematic to apply this to specialty hospitals, however, because physician ownership in those hospitals is more significant.

When physicians have admitting privileges at community hospitals and ownership in a specialty hospital, referral patterns are of particular concern. It is then in the financial interests of physicians to refer the most stable, higher-paying patients to their own hospitals, while admitting the sicker, lower-paying patients to the community hospitals (Blackstone and Fuhr 2007). Although to our knowledge empirical evidence for this behavior is lacking at this time, community hospitals have become concerned about it and some have taken to revoking physician admitting privileges when the physicians are owners of nearby specialty hospitals. In turn, physicians have been suing hospitals for antitrust restraint of trade violations (Blackstone and Fuhr 2007).

7.5 Commercial Healthcare Sectors: Pharmaceuticals

The increase in demand for medical services, brought about in the 1960s by the enactment of Medicare and Medicaid and the growth of employer-based insurance, encouraged the rapid and extensive development of commercial markets supplying products for medical applications, most notably medical devices, supplies, technology, and pharmaceuticals (Weisbrod 1991). These sectors of healthcare are completely for-profit.

The products of these purely commercial markets have revolutionized healthcare in positive and negative ways. The changes for the good are the great strides in the early diagnosis and treatment of illnesses, reducing the discomfort and time required to recover from illnesses or surgery, and successful treatment of conditions that in the past would have been lethal or crippling. The use of anesthesia with less severe side effects, such as headaches and nausea, and less invasive surgical instruments and procedures has drastically reduced recovery time from surgery. An operation that once would have required several days in the hospital can now be done on an outpatient basis with a much faster return to normal activity (Kozak, McCarthy, and Pokras 1999). These changes, in turn, have led to growth in sectors such as ambulatory care centers, dialysis centers, home care, specialty hospitals, and others already mentioned in this chapter. Outpatient surgeries increased by 32 percent between 1992 and 2001, and the number of freestanding ASCs increased by over 140 percent (Morrisey 2006). Other examples of extraordinary improvements in medical care include cancer "cures," organ transplantation, open-heart surgery, and ever more accurate and informative diagnostic imaging such as computed axial tomography scans, magnetic resonance imaging, and positron emission tomography scans.

On the negative side, these products tend to deal with illness and injury rather than prevention and health promotion. In the long run, the products and the procedures that go with them are expensive compared to basic public health and health promotion measures (Levi, Segal, and Juliano 2008). For example, a recent study estimated that a $10-per-person, per-year investment in community-based prevention programs (e.g., improving physical activity and nutrition, preventing smoking) could save $18 billion annually in healthcare costs within ten years (Levi, Segal, and Juliano 2008). The authors' explanation for the cost savings is that low-cost basic health promotion improves the health and quality of life of individuals so that fewer expensive health services are needed.

The dual effects of the commercial healthcare sector may have something to do with the twin paradoxes of the U.S. healthcare system: (1) high healthcare expenditures despite shorter hospital lengths of stay and other efficiencies in the delivery of healthcare, and (2) less than satisfactory outcomes despite high expenditures and medical advances. Obviously other issues are involved in these paradoxes, some of which we discuss in Chapter 10. Whether and to what extent the commercial markets have played a role in these paradoxes are questions for further study.

One example of a commercial market in healthcare is the pharmaceutical industry. This market has generated controversy because of problems surrounding the safety and efficacy of drugs and spending on drugs. Drug expenditures, for example, are often listed as a contributor to our high healthcare costs. To aid in understanding these important issues with pharmaceuticals, the following subsections present a short primer on the pharmaceutical industry. The first subsection begins with the regulation, development, and costs of drugs. Subsequent subsections discuss the marketing, safety, and effectiveness of pharmaceuticals. The final subsection addresses spending on pharmaceuticals.

Regulation, Development, Testing, and Costs of Pharmaceuticals

The development and testing of pharmaceuticals is highly regulated by the Food and Drug Administration (FDA). The FDA oversees the new drug application process, the clinical trials periods, and the post-trial marketing. New drug discoveries must be judged to be potentially beneficial and safe enough to be accepted for clinical trial. They then pass through several phases of clinical (human) trials that further assess their safety and efficacy.

This regulatory climate emerged over time. After deaths from elixir sulfanilamide in the 1930s, the Food, Drug, and Cosmetic Act (FDCA) was passed in 1938. This act required for the first time that drugs receive FDA approval before being marketed. Approval depended on safety and adequate labeling, but the FDA did not specify which drugs needed prescriptions and which could be sold over the counter (OTC) (Donohue 2006). Further regulations in 1951 established that some drugs had to be prescribed because it would not be safe to allow consumers to self-medicate with them. Then, following the thalidomide birth defects in the early 1960s, the Kefauver-Harris Amendments to the FDCA expanded the FDA's authority over prescription drugs. New prescription drugs had to meet high scientific standards (Donohue 2006). The testing and clinical trial periods were made more rigorous and longer.

New drug development can be summarized as follows (Dimasi, Hansen, and Grabowski 1991): Chemists and biologists research potential new chemicals and compounds that could have pharmacologic properties. When one is developed that is considered a potential new drug, it is tested in vitro for its pharmacological activity and toxicity. If it continues to hold good potential it is then tested on animals. If, after that, the chemical is still considered a potentially viable drug, the company files an Investigational New Drug Application with the FDA. Unless a hold is placed on the potential drug, the company can begin clinical testing 30 days after filing. In Phase I, tests are performed on a small number of volunteers to obtain information about toxicity, safe doses, and other chemical reactions in the human body. In Phase II, the drug is tested on a larger sample of patients that the drug is intended to help. Phase III testing is a set of large-scale studies that test whether there is adequate, statistically reliable evidence of improvements in outcomes or control of symptoms. Frequently, animal testing continues during these phases. If the company believes that there is enough evidence for approval, a New Drug Application is filed. Once the FDA approves it, the drug can be marketed. Post-FDA approval trials can also be conducted (Phase IV testing), but are not required. Often, pharmaceutical companies use Phase IV trials to test the drug for other uses (Angell 2004).

The entire development process from discovery research to FDA approval can be long and costly. The Pharmaceutical Researchers and Manufacturers of America (PhRMA) estimates that it takes 15 years from the time a drug is discovered until it reaches patients (Pharmaceutical Researchers and Manufacturers of America 2004).

New drug development and sales are protected by patents, which, in the United States, give the holder the exclusive right to make and sell the drug for 20 years. Since patents are usually obtained during the development period, up to five years of patent time expended during the development phase can be used to extend the patent period after drug approval, to a maximum of 14 years of post-approval marketing (U.S. FDA 2008). A patent gives the holder an effective monopoly for the period of the patent, but advocates for the pharmaceutical industry say that patents are necessary in order for drug companies to financially recoup the costs of research and development (R&D). Once patent protection is lost, other producers can market biologically equivalent versions of the drug (generic drugs). Drug companies may then seek new patents on variations of the original drug (Angell 2004). This latter practice is often challenged by generic drug manufacturers.

There is disagreement over the development process for new drugs. Some believe the process is not rigorous enough to prevent unnecessary injuries and deaths due to pharmaceuticals, while others think it is unnecessarily rigorous and lengthy, delaying or even preventing the introduction of needed drugs. There is probably truth to each position in that there may be times when the process fails to prevent an ineffective or dangerous drug from being marketed and times when a needed safe drug is delayed.

There is also a difference of opinion as to how costly the development process is. Pharmaceutical companies say that the costs of R&D are quite high, therefore justifying high drug prices and high profit margins needed to sustain the ongoing R&D costs. A 2003 study by Dimasi, Hansen, and Grabowski supports the high-R&D-cost claim, estimating R&D costs at $802 million per new drug, including expenditures on failed projects and opportunity costs (Dimasi, Hansen, and Grabowski 2003).

Others say that there is little objective evidence regarding new drug costs, and that the highest estimates of costs tend to be those obtained from pharmaceutical-supported studies with data provided by the companies themselves (Light and Warburton 2005; Light 2007). Light (2007) criticizes the 2003 Dimasi, Hansen, and Grabowski study for focusing on self-originated new molecular entities (NMEs). NMEs are totally new drugs that are much more expensive to develop. They constitute only 35 percent of the new drugs approved by the FDA. Only 62 percent of these are self-originated. Therefore, the $802 million per new drug estimate pertains only to 22 percent of new drugs, while other new drugs cost less to develop and test (Light 2007). The study also excluded drugs receiving financial support from the government for R&D (for example, studies performed with federal grant money at universities), which would lower the costs (*Public Citizen* 2001). Another criticism of the study is the inclusion of "opportunity costs"[6] (Light 2007). Actual costs (without opportunity costs) were $403 million. Finally, the use of pre-tax costs that are tax deductible is criticized (Light 2007). Around 34 percent of R&D costs can be deducted from taxes. All of the above adjustments bring the estimate down to $240 million for the drugs used in the study. According to one critic, the average cost of bringing a drug to market is probably well under $240 million (Light 2008).

Dimasi, Hansen, and Grabowski (2003) reply that their data were checked against several other data sets, and that their results were validated by the Office of Technology Assessment. They justify their pre-tax figures by pointing out that tax structures change over time, so tax-adjusted figures can misrepresent the actual production costs. They justify the use of NMEs because many of the non-NME new drugs are additions to drug product lines, not entirely new drugs, and don't reflect the expense of developing a new drug. Dimasi and colleagues also state that their $802 million in costs excluded government grants toward the drug development.

The debate over pharmaceutical costs is far from over. Perhaps the most important point to take away is that cost estimates tend to be "constructed realities that one can reconstruct by using different assumptions, data, or calculations" (Light 2008, 325).

Marketing of Pharmaceuticals

Marketing pharmaceuticals to consumers was common in the first half of the twentieth century, when drug companies were able to assign most medications to OTC status (Donohue 2006). When regulations were established in 1951 removing the pharmaceutical companies' ability to decide OTC status and requiring certain drugs to be made available by prescription only, pharmaceutical companies abandoned consumer marketing and targeted those who had the power to prescribe—physicians (Donohue 2006).

This changed again in the 1980s when a few companies began to market directly to consumers (DTC). At the time, the FDA had no stipulations against DTC advertising. But by 1983, the agency became concerned that DTC advertising would lead patients to:

> pressure physicians to prescribe unnecessary or unindicated drugs, increase the price of drugs, confuse patients by leading them to believe that some minor difference represents a major therapeutic advance, potentiate the use of brand name products rather than cheaper, but equivalent, generic drugs, and foster increased drug taking in an already overmedicated society. (Donohue 2006, 676)

Following a two-year moratorium on DTC advertising, the FDA required DTC advertisements to meet the same requirements as those directed to physicians. The ads needed to contain "a true statement" as to the side effects, contraindications, and effectiveness of the drugs (Donohue 2006, 671).

In 1997 the FDA removed the requirement that DTC ads provide a detailed description of side effects and effectiveness. Instead, drug advertisements only need to list major risks and provide sources of further information (PHARM Committee 2004). Since then, DTC advertising has exploded. Forty percent of pharmaceutical advertising expenses in 2005 went to DTC marketing, and most of the spending for some drugs is on DTC (Donohue 2006). Only two countries in the world, the United States and New Zealand, fully allow drugs to be advertised directly to consumers (PHARM Committee 2004).

There are two takes on the value of DTC drug advertising. Proponents believe that the advertising provides information to consumers and empowers them (Holmer 1999, 2002). Critics say that DTC advertising can be deceptive, that it encourages patients to take costly medications that they do not need, that it puts stresses on the patient–physician relationship, and that it, along with marketing to physicians, promotes the "medicalization" of healthcare (Angell 2004; Chandra and Holt 1999; Donohue 2006; Mintzes 2002). Physicians are mostly opposed to DTC advertising, whereas consumer groups are divided on the practice (Donohue 2006).

Surveys of consumers show that DTC advertising does affect their behavior. Of consumers who had seen an advertisement in 2002, 33 percent spoke with their physician about the medication, 30 percent of those asked for a prescription, and 79 percent of those received the prescription (Donohue 2006).

Of course, a substantial amount of marketing is still aimed at physicians. The major issue with marketing to physicians is the practice of pharmaceutical companies "courting" physicians with gifts and other financial benefits so that they prescribe the company's medications. The danger is that physicians will be influenced to make choices that are not scientifically based, that are not the best for treating the condition, and that are more costly than alternatives.

These concerns are justified by some evidence. For example, physicians who accept free meals or travel from drug companies are significantly more likely to request additions to hospital drug formularies (Chren and Landefeld 1994) and have higher prescription rates of the sponsor's medication (Wazana 2000). They also appear to be less likely to choose medications on the basis of evidence of effectiveness. In a 2001 article, Goodman points out that diuretics and beta-blockers have been shown to be effective antihypertensive medications in controlled clinical trials, and have been recommended for initial therapy. Yet from 1992 to 1995 the number of prescriptions written for these medications decreased by 50 and 40 percent, respectively, whereas prescriptions for calcium channel blockers (such as Norvasc) increased by 13 percent. The recommendations for diuretics and beta-blockers continue, but calcium channel blockers are still the top-selling antihypertensive drugs. Norvasc, for example, is among the top five best-selling drugs in the world. The large proportion of prescriptions for calcium channel blockers does not seem to be based on evidence, since there has not been conclusive empirical evidence indicating superiority to the other medications, and a recent meta-analysis suggests they are inferior (Pahor et al. 2000). Is their popularity based on low prices? No; they are much more expensive. So, "in short, they are less effective, more expensive, and the most heavily prescribed. How do we explain this?" (Goodman 2001, 232).

Safety of Pharmaceuticals

Despite extensive regulations requiring evidence of the safety of new drugs, it remains a concern. In several cases, drugs that had been marketed for months or even years were found to have harmful side effects. Examples are the cardiovascular incidents that occurred with Vioxx, cardiovascular incidents and gastro-esophageal injury with Celebrex, suicides or attempted suicides of children and adolescents using Paxil, muscle wasting and kidney toxicity with certain anticholesterol medications, and liver toxicity with Strattera, an attention deficit disorder drug (Lurie 2005; Brody 2007).

In some drugs, such as Vioxx, the side effects have been prevalent and harmful enough for the drugs to be removed from the market altogether. With other drugs, such as Strattera, the serious side effects have occurred in only a few people, so the FDA has simply required the company to issue warnings, including warnings on the labels.

Of particular concern is that with some of these drugs—for example, Vioxx—the pharmaceutical company knew of the dangers, repressed the studies (or portions of studies) bearing these assessments, published studies (or portions of studies) supporting their claims of safety, and marketed the drug anyway (Brody 2007). These business practices violate notions of transparency of information and ethical and fair trade practices.

Effectiveness of Pharmaceuticals

We have already mentioned that some of the older medicines seem to be as effective or better than newer ones while costing much less. Research by Heidenreich and McClellan in 2001 found that 71 percent of the increase in 30-day survival following acute myocardial infarction between 1975 and 1995 was due to low-cost treatments such as aspirin, beta-blockers, and angiotensin-converting enzyme (ACE) inhibitors. The greatest single effect was that of cheap, over-the-counter aspirin, which contributed 34 percent to the increase in survival.

Another questionable pharmacological advance involves the Cox-2 inhibitors, medications marketed for pain relief, particularly from arthritis. These medications have never been proved to be more effective pain relievers than many OTC nonsteroidal anti-inflammatories (NSAIDs) (Lurie 2005).

A serious concern regarding effectiveness is that a number of new drugs are minor variations of existing ones. These are the so-called me-too drugs. Most do not offer significant therapeutic gain over existing drugs, so unless they compete with existing drugs to lower price, the expenses involved in developing them are largely a waste. In some cases the me-too drugs are introduced at lower prices, but later the prices are raised (Lexchin 2006). Angell (2004) writes that some me-too drugs are developed by the same company that produced the original drug to help extend the monopoly rights that would otherwise end when the patent on the original drug ends. The author gives the example of Nexium, which was AstraZeneca's nearly identical replacement for Prilosec. Other me-toos are developed by competitors to get a piece of a profitable market. Lipitor, for example, was the third me-too statin drug, all of which have basically the same action in the body. Angell (2004, 1451) points out that there is no reason to believe that one me-too drug is better than the other since they are rarely compared in clinical trials. Instead, they are tested against a placebo, "so all we know is that they are better than nothing." It is possible, she continues, that with each successive me-too, the effect is worse than the one before.

Spending on Pharmaceuticals

Spending on prescription drugs is the fastest growing component of U.S. health costs. Spending increases peaked at 16 percent annually in 2000 (KFF 2007a), fell to 6 percent between 2004 and 2005 due to Medicaid cutbacks and the increased use of generics, then rose again in 2006 to 8.5 percent due to Medicare Part D's drug benefits (Catlin et al. 2008; KFF 2007a). The increases in spending appear to be due to three factors: drug prices, utilization, and changes in the types of drugs being used (KFF 2007a).

The first component of spending is the price of prescription drugs, which increased around 7.6 percent a year from 1994 to 2006 (for a total increase of over 100 percent) (KFF 2007a). Prescription prices were three times generic prices in 2006. Prices vary depending upon the payer. Those paying out of pocket pay full retail price, whereas those with public or private insurance coverage will pay negotiated prices.[7] The price of a prescription drug is a combination of R&D costs, production costs, marketing and administrative costs, taxes, and profit. Higher prices for prescription drugs are also the result of monopoly power due to patents. In addition, the argument has been made that high prescription drug prices in the United States are partially due to lower prices negotiated by the governments of other countries.

As we discussed earlier, claims that the costs of R&D are a considerable component of the price of a drug are common. Others have deconstructed these arguments and estimate the proportion of R&D costs to be lower than those claims. As a proportion of sales, the pharmaceutical industry reports that about 18–19 percent of drug sales are invested in research (Pharmaceutical Research Manufacturers of America 2004). The National Science Foundation believes that the amount is lower, reporting that 1999 data indicate that companies invest only about 12.4 percent of gross domestic sales on R&D (Light and Lexchin 2005). The 12.4 percent matches an estimate from investment bank Deutsche Banc Alex. Brown that 13 percent of revenues are spent on R&D (Reinhardt 2001b). This estimate is based on data from the eight largest pharmaceutical companies in the world. Tax deductions bring the after-tax proportion of sales that goes into R&D down even further (Light and Lexchin 2005). Thus, it appears that R&D is not the most significant contributor to the price of drugs.

Remaining contributors to high drug prices are production, marketing, administration, taxes, profits, and possible cost shifting due to lower foreign prices. Reinhardt (2001b) cites a report by Deutsche Banc Alex. Brown that 27 percent of the revenues of the eight largest pharmaceutical manufacturers in the world were spent on production in 1998. But even more—35 percent—was spent on marketing and administration (Reinhardt 2001b).[8]

According to records from the top seven U.S. pharmaceutical companies, marketing and administration costs range from 25 to 33 percent (averaging 32 percent), more than is spent on R&D (Families USA 2005). Within the marketing category, DTC advertising has become a larger and larger proportion of marketing costs, going from $166 million in 1993 to more than $4.2 billion in 2005 (Donohue 2006). Deutsch Banc estimates that 7 percent of revenues go to taxes (Reinhardt 2001b).

Deutsche Bank provides a figure of 18 percent for the profit margin of drug companies, an amount corroborated by other estimates. Profits of pharmaceutical companies were estimated by *Fortune* magazine to be 18.6 percent of after-tax revenue in 1999, the highest profit margins of all companies in the Fortune 500 (Reinhart 2001b). In 2004, the top seven U.S. pharmaceutical companies reported profits of 18 percent (Families USA 2005). Pharmaceutical companies also rank in the top of the *Fortune* 500 for their return on assets. By all estimates pharmaceutical profits on the average constitute a higher percentage of sales than the costs of R&D, and they are among the highest profit margins of any industry in the United States. It should be noted that the monopoly power due to patents may play a role in maintaining these high profit margins.

Finally, high U.S. prescription drug prices are partly attributed to low foreign prices. It is argued that prescription drug prices in other countries are not enough to cover R&D, so prices must be higher in the United States to make up for the shortfall. However, Light and Lexchin (2005) report that they cannot find evidence to this effect. An economic explanation is that pharmaceutical companies are exploiting their monopoly power to price discriminate by charging segmented national markets whatever price the markets will bear. Since the United States does not regulate the price of pharmaceuticals (other than drugs bought directly by the Department of Veterans Affairs and the Department of Defense), whereas other countries do, the U.S. market will generally bear higher prices. Adjusting for prices negotiated with insurance and managed care, Danzon and Furukawa (2003) find some evidence of lower prices in Canada, the United Kingdom, and other foreign markets, compared to the United States. However, drug prices were higher in Japan than in the United States.

The quantity of prescription drugs purchased in the United States is the second component contributing to rising drug expenditures. From 1994 to 2005 the number of prescriptions purchased increased at a rate much higher than that of U.S. population growth; a 71 percent increase compared to a population growth of 9 percent (Latham 2003). In 2000, Americans had an average of nine prescriptions per person. DTC advertising may be partially responsible for the increase in drug utilization. There is little research evidence as to whether this is the case, however. The aging of the population is likely one of the reasons, since older people tend to use more drugs (Latham

2003). An increase in prescription drug insurance coverage may be another reason for higher prescription drug use. And finally, some of the increase in pharmaceutical expenditures comes from the substitution of pharmaceuticals for other medical interventions, thus reducing expenditures elsewhere (Latham 2003).

The third component of increasing expenditures is changes in the types of drugs being purchased. New drugs tend to increase drug expenditures if they are used in place of older, less expensive medications; if they supplement existing drugs; or if they treat a condition not previously treated with drug therapy (KFF 2007a). Sometimes new drugs are introduced at lower prices than existing drugs if they have other competitors. Prices also decrease when brand-name drugs lose patent protection, due to competition with generic substitutes (KFF 2007a). There is some evidence that physicians are switching patient prescriptions to the new, more expensive, medications, but there are no estimates as to how much this has affected pharmaceutical expenditures (Latham 2003).

7.6 Commercialization of Healthcare

Some point out that the growing for-profit influence in U.S. healthcare has dramatically moved it in a more commercial direction. These changes go by several names, including commercialization, commodification, corporatization, and medicalization (Budetti 2008; Conrad and Leiter 2004; Kuttner 2008; Starr 1982).

Commercialization or commodification is the provision of healthcare as a commercial product that is bought and sold. It is characterized by the production of products and services for profit, with supply determined by profitability and demand determined by ability to pay. Signs that healthcare is becoming commodified include an antiregulatory, promarket climate; the conversion of nonprofit organizations to for-profit corporations; the development of completely for-profit sectors; the predominance of commercial products in the provision of healthcare; the medicalization of health (defined below); the erosion of public health and of public and private insurance coverage; and the promotion of individual health savings accounts, discussed in Chapter 4 (Budetti 2008; Callahan 1999).

Corporatization is the development of large, integrated organizations that manage and deliver health-related products and services, which in turn provide sellers with more market power (Starr 1982). As healthcare providers develop contractual relations with or become employees of these corporations, they can lose some of their professional independence (they become "deprofessionalized").

Medicalization is the conceptualization of human conditions as illnesses, abnormalities, or disorders, and treating these conditions with various degrees of medical intervention (Budetti 2008; Conrad and Leiter 2004). Indications of medicalization are high proportions of the population identifying fairly normal life experiences as disorders, and a heavy reliance on pharmaceuticals and other medical interventions to treat these problems. Wrinkles or balding with aging are examples. These used to be accepted as just part of getting older. Now, there is a tendency to see them as unacceptable problems that should be dealt with surgically or medically. Medicalization and commodification feed off of each other in that the provision of healthcare products and services for profit is better served by a public that believes that they have many medical problems that can be fixed if they just consume enough healthcare commodities.

There are some indications of these transformations in the United States. Federal requirements for CON laws were abolished in 1986. Since then, an antiregulatory climate has continued. Hospitals and health plans are converting to for-profit, and, as we discussed earlier, for-profit organizations have grown in healthcare sectors such as nursing homes, ambulatory surgical care, and managed care. Even in markets where the percentage of for-profit organizations is low, such as hospitals, their existence in the local markets encourages nonprofits to behave more like for-profits (Kuttner 1999). Health plans, hospitals, and nursing homes have consolidated into large integrated companies. The pharmaceutical and medical device industries have grown and benefited from healthcare that focuses on the application of their products and technologies in the diagnosis and treatment of illnesses. DTC prescription drug advertising promotes the medicalization of health in order to sell more drugs (Budetti 2008). Managed care measures and hospital restructuring have led healthcare providers to feel that they are less able to make their own professional decisions and that they do not have time to provide quality care (Serow et al. 1993; Smith and Walshe 2004).

Commercialization encourages expansion of services that generate revenues and provides few incentives for those that do not generate revenues. As the consumption of medical products and services expands, healthcare expenditures increase. The high costs limit the healthcare system's ability to meet public health needs and provide basic health promotion and illness prevention (Budetti 2008). National health expenditures in the United States are greater than $2 trillion, but only 3 percent is used for public health (Budetti 2008). National, state, and community healthcare planning become more difficult as the multiple healthcare markets—insurance, hospitals, nursing homes, pharmaceutical companies, and others—function as separate, competing, profit-making markets rather than operating in a cooperative way to coordinate the most efficient, efficacious, and equitable healthcare.

Kuttner (2008, 549) believes that our inability to contain medical costs in the United States is due mainly to "our unique, pervasive commercialization." He cites "the dominance of for-profit insurance and pharmaceutical companies, a new wave of investor-owned specialty hospitals, and profit-maximizing behavior even by nonprofit players" that raise costs due to "profits, billing, marketing, and the gratuitous costs of private bureaucracies [that] siphon off $400 billion to $500 billion of the $2.1 trillion spent" (549). The for-profit environment allocates resources to profit opportunities rather than health needs, which results in unnecessary medical care for some, inadequate treatment for others, and a reduction in basic public health and health promotion measures. As a result, costs for healthcare are much higher than they would be if resources had been rationally allocated based on effective education and therapies for identified true health needs (Kuttner 2008).

As Kuttner relates, numerous studies have shown that the use of clinically proven screenings such as mammograms, the provision of childhood immunizations, changes to diet and exercise, and the use of standard protocols to treat chronic conditions such as diabetes, asthma, and high cholesterol can improve health and reduce costs later on. But these are not profitable, or are the least profitable healthcare services, so they are not emphasized in the U.S. healthcare system. Kuttner (2008, 550) writes,

> Great health improvements can be achieved through basic public health measures and a population-based approach to wellness and medical care. But entrepreneurs do not prosper by providing these services, and those who need them most are the least likely to have insurance.

Furthermore, as healthcare becomes a profitable commodity, a sector of powerful commercial interests devotes itself to expanding the commercial system and to resisting attempts to slow or reverse that progress. Lobbyists for the pharmaceutical and health plan industries, for example, have marshaled concerted resistance to most iterations of a universal healthcare system, which these industries see as reducing their respective market power (Budetti 2008). The political power of the health insurance industry was a significant factor in the defeat of the Clinton health plan proposal in the early 1990s. The political clout of the pharmaceutical industry played a significant role in the formulation of the Medicare Part D legislation, which relies entirely on private insurers and prevents the government from using its purchasing power to obtain medications at a reduced price for beneficiaries (Angell 2004).

An example of commercialization and medicalization can be seen with the marketing of Paxil. When Paxil was introduced for the treatment of depression, it was preceded by Prozac and several other selective serotonin reuptake inhibitors (SSRIs), so the drug faced much competition in the "depression market." GlaxoSmithKline (GSK) decided to expand beyond the "depression market" to the "anxiety market." It targeted "social anxiety disorder" (SAD) and "generalized anxiety disorder" (GAD), conditions the psychiatric community considered to be debilitating. Once the FDA approved the use of Paxil for these conditions, GSK spent millions of dollars to raise the public awareness of SAD and GAD. GSK infomercials created an impression that shyness and worry are signs of these medical disorders, that the medical disorders are common, and that Paxil is the way to treat them (Conrad and Leiter 2004). "Marketing diseases and then selling drugs to treat those diseases is now common in the 'post Prozac' era" (Conrad and Leiter 2004, 163).

The Paxil marketing strategy has been successful for GSK. Paxil is one of the three most widely recognized prescription drugs, after Viagra and Claritin (Conrad and Leiter 2004). Has it been beneficial for those who have taken the medication for these conditions? Has it reduced healthcare costs? Would other, nonpharmaceutical therapies for these conditions have produced better results with lower costs? For the most part, research is lacking, so we have no definitive answers to these questions.

The misallocation and waste of resources is exemplified in a popular book by Abramson (2004), *Overdo$ed America: The Broken Promise of American Medicine*. In it he relates that in the United States there are three times as many angioplasties, two times as many statin prescriptions, and three times as many bypass operations per capita as the Organisation for Economic Cooperation and Development average, yet the United States ranks seventeenth in industrialized countries for death rates from heart disease. Cross-national comparisons such as these are detailed in Chapter 10.

7.7 Policies in Response to the Profit Motive in Healthcare

This chapter raises policy issues with regard to the profit motive in healthcare. Should the growth of for-profit organizations be encouraged? What should be done about specialty hospitals? What policies could improve the pharmaceutical market? Should anything be done about the increasing commercialization of the healthcare system? While economic analysis does not provide definitive answers to these questions, it can point to some possible policy alternatives.

Should the Growth of For-Profit Organizations Be Encouraged?

Empirical findings indicate that, generally speaking, nonprofits are better or no worse than for-profits in nearly all aspects of performance. One area where nonprofits perform better is the quality of patient care in hospitals, nursing homes, and other healthcare markets. They also tend to excel in trustworthiness and community benefits. They tend to perform similarly to for-profits in terms of efficiency, with the exception of nursing homes, where for-profits have higher efficiency. However, in contrast, for-profits tend to perform better financially, although this may be at the expense of payers and consumers, since it appears to be a reflection of higher prices and a more profitable selection of location, services, and patients.

These findings suggest that we should be cautious about encouraging for-profit growth, whether through conversions or through the development of new organizations. Regarding hospitals, some researchers believe that the evidence "strongly supports a policy of not-for-profit healthcare delivery" (Devereaux et al. 2004, 1823). Others list arguments for and against encouraging hospitals to convert from nonprofit to for-profit status (Gray 1997). Reasons for encouraging conversions are that the new for-profits could do the following:

- Increase tax revenues
- Put charitable assets to potentially more productive uses
- Enhance access to needed capital
- Facilitate consolidation and capacity reductions in the presence of excess supply

The reasons conversions should not be encouraged include the following:

- It is difficult to estimate the value of nonprofit organizations. Conversions can cause private gain and social loss.
- Conversions could leave communities without adequate protection of their interests, since neither the trustees of the converting organization nor the purchasers are responsible for the effects of a conversion on the community, and there are no standard mechanisms for deciding what the impact could be.
- There could be a substantial loss of social benefits from the care formerly provided by the nonprofit organization.
- The tax exemption of the nonprofit organization could provide a regulatory lever that policymakers could use to attach a variety of conditions.

One issue is whether the positive aspects would outweigh the negative in a given conversion. If the hospital converts, will the increased taxes the state now receives be enough to cover the increased costs to the state for charity care? Will people needing charity care have somewhere to go? What will happen to the quality of care, community services, and the provision of unprofitable services that had been provided by the nonprofit hospitals? This would depend on the degree to which the community is involved in the conversion, and whether the conversion is closely monitored and regulated by state and local governments.

In the past, conversions have not been well regulated and there has been a tendency for community benefits to decline following conversion (Needleman, Lamphere, and Chollet 1999). When conversions are pursued in the future, state governments will need to ensure that alternatives to the nonprofit hospital, such as Medicaid expansions and other state assistance, will help meet public policy goals. Policies need to be established so that when a conversion occurs, the value of the nonprofit organization is preserved within the community, private benefit from the conversion is prevented, and community benefits such as charity care and service obligations are maintained in some form (Claxton et al. 1997; Gray 1997). Quality of care and scope of services should also be monitored and maintained.

A policy of complete opposition to hospital conversions may not be advisable, because sometimes a conversion may be the best strategy for a hospital's survival, and it may help to maintain essential services in a community. However, as Claxton and colleagues (1997) suggest, conversions should be an option rather than a necessity. Policies and regulations need to facilitate access to alternatives to equity capital and reexamine regulatory constraints on nonprofit hospitals. With these policies in place, a conversion could be avoided.

Promoting a mix of for-profit and nonprofit entities in given markets could possibly bring out the best of both ownership types (Marsteller, Bovbjerg, and Nichols 1998; Schlesinger and Gray 2006). The nonprofit emphasis on quality, trustworthy behavior, and community benefits may influence for-profits to improve in those areas, while the for-profit emphasis on efficiency may influence nonprofits to improve in that area. Finding the right mix is important because it is possible that a strong for-profit influence in healthcare markets could have negative effects on quality, scope of services, community service, and trustworthy behavior among nonprofits (Horwitz 2005). More research on the impact of for-profit ownership on nonprofit behavior and the best mix of ownership is needed. As Gray (1997) points out, we have no evidence about the consequences of the conversion of most or all of the nonprofits in a particular market or the development of an entirely for-profit market.

It may be important to actively encourage the nonprofit sector in markets currently dominated by for-profit institutions (e.g., nursing homes, dialysis, specialty hospitals) (Schlesinger and Gray 2006). Government policies can encourage nonprofit ownership through federal income tax exemptions and tax incentives or subsidies at the state or local level. States with CON laws could use those laws to regulate growth on the basis of ownership, ensuring the desired ownership mix for the state and locality. Government oversight would be needed to make sure that the incentives and regulatory controls are achieving access and performance goals.

In summary, we know that nonprofit ownership in healthcare compares favorably to for-profit, yet this knowledge does not lend itself to specific policy prescriptions. The best policy is to be cautious about promoting further for-profit growth, to monitor the outcomes of for-profit conversions and growth, to evaluate ownership mix on a specific market basis, and to continue to support nonprofit ownership through federal, state, and local tax exemptions, subsidies, and CON laws.

What Should Be Done About Specialty Hospitals?

There are two major policy issues with regard to specialty hospitals. First, there is the issue of specialty hospitals selecting the more profitable patients. This makes it more difficult for full-service hospitals to maintain a healthy financial status and reduces their ability to cross-subsidize unprofitable services and under- and unreimbursed care. Second, there is the issue of physician self-referral, which gives specialty hospitals an unfair advantage in patient referrals over full-service hospitals, and can lead to unnecessary care through physician-induced demand.

One way to deal with both of these issues is to restrict the growth of specialty hospitals. The moratorium that was placed on specialty hospitals from November 2003 to August 2006 could be reinstated (Guterman 2006). The moratorium could be (as it was in the past) applied in two ways: (1) by prohibiting the building of new specialty hospitals or (2) by prohibiting physicians from referring their patients to their own new specialty hospitals (Murer 2006). While these measures do not eliminate competition from existing specialty hospitals, they do restrict their growth, and they protect communities that do not yet have specialty hospitals.

The problem with this approach is that it denies the positive qualities of specialty hospitals: efficient provision of services, high quality through the "focused factory" effect, and high patient satisfaction. It might be preferable to take a softer, more market-based approach, by allowing the development of new specialty hospitals while regulating them. The following regulations that CMS issued after the end of the specialty hospital moratorium in 2006 could be maintained: disclosing physician investment and compensation arrangements to CMS; informing patients that the hospital is owned by physicians; and providing emergency care to patients regardless of ability to pay if the hospital has the ability to do so (Murer 2006).

There are other ways to deal with the issues. Cherry-picking of better-paying patients would be less of a problem if existing reimbursement systems did not have distorted financial rewards. The DRG categories that provide greater net revenues, such as those in the cardiac surgery categories, need to be adjusted to reduce the variance in net revenue between those DRGs and others (Guterman 2006). Adjustments for patient acuity also need to be brought more in line with the actual resources used to care for those patients (Guterman 2006). In 2007, CMS began these changes. The old charges-based DRG weighting system was replaced with a cost-based system that is being phased in over three years (KFF 2006). Adjustments to the acuity system began in 2008. It remains to be seen what effect these changes will have on specialty hospital Medicare reimbursements and whether other payers will implement similar adjustments.

Several policies would reduce the conflict of interest associated with physician ownership. One recommendation is to amend the Stark Act to place greater restrictions on physicians' abilities to self-refer. This could be accomplished by disallowing physician ownership of specialty hospitals altogether, or by reducing the proportion of assets that could be owned by a single physician or the overall group of physicians per facility (Blackstone and Fuhr 2007). There could also be more oversight of physician referrals and profits.

What Policies Could Improve the Pharmaceutical Market?

Pharmaceutical industry practices raise concerns in terms of marketing, safety, effectiveness, costs, and expenditures. What policies could improve these practices?

DTC advertising faces little regulation at this time, other than limited requirements to inform consumers about the major effects and side effects of the drug. The effects that the drug has on the many conditions it is marketed for may not be adequately reported. Reporting the relative effectiveness of the drug compared to others for that condition is also not required. Hollon (1999, 382) notes that the information provided by pharmaceutical companies with DTC advertising is "of suspect quality." Additional regulation of DTC advertising could require stricter disclosure of the drugs' effects, side effects, and interactions; whether it has been tested on the condition it is advertised as treating; and how it compares to other drugs for that condition.

Marketing practices involving drug companies giving physicians gifts and financial incentives have largely been left to physician discretion. An argument can be made that the best course would be to continue to allow physicians to decide their relationship with pharmaceutical marketers, while encouraging consumers to hold physicians accountable for meeting their needs. Public pressure can be used to encourage physicians to refuse gifts, honoraria, travel, consulting, and other incentives that would influence their judgment (Kassirer 2007). On the other hand, Brennan and colleagues (2006) suggest that self-regulation will not be enough to protect the interests of patients. They recommend more stringent regulation that would eliminate or modify gifting, pharmaceutical sample giveaways, medical education offerings, physician travel funding, speaking engagements, and consulting and research contracts.

To ensure drug safety and efficacy, careful, scientifically rigorous, independent research in the development and testing of drugs is essential. Drugs that are brought to market should be found to be safe and effective for the specific conditions for which they are being marketed. If efforts at drug safety and efficacy are to be voluntary, pharmaceutical companies must have the integrity to fund sound research without interference or influence, and to abandon products that are shown to be unsafe or ineffective. The growing influence of pharmaceutical companies over the design and reporting of clinical trials (Angell 2004) and the fact that some have actively suppressed negative results and marketed unsafe drugs and drugs with questionable or untested efficacy (Cafferty 2005) does not bode well for voluntary improvements in honesty and integrity. Additional regulations that require independent research, transparent results, stricter requirements for proof of efficacy, and research on comparative efficacy may need to be developed. Other approaches would be to require greater consumer information in DTC advertisements, and to add liabilities above those brought forward by consumers (Spence 1977).

Price control of pharmaceuticals is a recurring topic among consumer advocacy groups, but it is a controversial economic policy. On the demand side, lower prices would lead to lower out-of-pocket costs for consumers, and this would improve access to needed medications. However, if the demand for drugs is elastic, it is possible that the expanded access could lead to overall drug expenditures that are as high as or higher than before. There are relatively few studies of the price elasticity of demand for pharmaceuticals. One study of the demand for pharmaceuticals across countries and time found that overall, prescription drugs are fairly elastic (Alexander, Flynn, and Linkins 1994). Another study by Goldman and colleagues (2006) found demand of privately insured patients to be inelastic for specialty prescription drugs for conditions such as rheumatoid arthritis, kidney disease, multiple sclerosis, and cancer. Therefore it is unclear whether lower prices would lower overall expenditures on medications.

On the supply side, would the control of drug prices contribute to a reduction in the supply of new prescription drugs? Whenever price controls are suggested, the pharmaceutical industry states that R&D would be negatively affected and that consumers would miss out on many new drug opportunities. Empirical research on the pharmaceutical supply reaction to price control is not conclusive. One thing that might happen, at least for a time, is that pharmaceutical companies would attempt to increase the volume of sales of existing drugs (Reinhardt 2001b). Another possibility is that R&D could initially *increase* to compensate for lost revenue through the sale of new drugs. Eventually, lower profit margins could lead to a drop in R&D (Reinhardt 2001b). However, since profit margins are in the double digits for pharmaceutical companies, a small to moderate drop in profit margin might not have a strong effect on R&D.

Elimination of the cap on prescription drugs that can be bought abroad would be an approach that would *change* existing regulations. Currently, U.S. residents can buy 90 days worth of drugs for personal use from other countries, such as Canada. By allowing U.S. consumers to buy larger or unlimited quantities of prescription drugs from abroad (including, possibly, through Internet sales) the segmentation of, and the price discrimination between, the U.S. and Canadian markets would be lessened. This could force a reduction in U.S. drug prices. One problem with this approach concerns whether the safety of the imported medications could be guaranteed. Another problem is the potential increase in prices of the imported drugs due to higher demand. The higher price could affect U.S. residents and those in the countries exporting the drugs.

A final policy concern is the enormous political influence of the pharmaceutical industry. It has the largest lobby in Washington, DC (there are more pharmaceutical lobbyists than members of Congress), and it is a large campaign donor. As a result, laws continue to be advantageous to pharmaceutical companies. Patent laws, brand-name marketing rights, essentially free public funding for research, insufficient oversight of research, and lack of price controls all favor pharmaceutical companies over the public (Angell 2004). The Medicare prescription drug legislation in 2003, for example, prohibited Medicare from using its purchasing power to bargain for lower prices. Campaign finance reform could reduce some of this special interest advantage.

We have mentioned several additional regulatory steps that could be taken. Increasing regulation is always a concern, because there can be unintended results; we address this issue in chapters 3 and 10. Lee and Herzstein (1986) summarize the arguments against over-regulation of drugs as follows:

- R&D and the introduction of medically needed drugs could be slowed.
- Pharmaceutical production could decline due to companies leaving the market.
- From a macroeconomics perspective, unemployment could be higher and exports lower.

We do not know that any one or more of these would be the result, however, since these are not empirically tested arguments. Additional targeted regulations, such as requiring additional research to show efficacy compared to other drugs or greater oversight of marketing practices, could have little negative effect on the supply of pharmaceuticals and a positive effect on health outcomes and healthcare costs.

The best approaches to these issues are not yet known. However, it is premature to write off additional pharmaceutical industry regulation as having a negative effect on demand or supply. We concur with Angell (2004, 1453), who believes that the excesses of the pharmaceutical industry in particular "are perhaps the clearest example of the folly of allowing healthcare expenditures and policies to be driven by largely unregulated market forces and the profit-making imperatives of investor-owned businesses."

What Should Be Done About the Commercialization of U.S. Healthcare?

Commercialization is hypothesized to negatively affect health promotion, public health, access to healthcare, health outcomes, and healthcare costs.

But the commercialization process seems to be inexorable. Should something be done about this, and if so, what?

Suggested answers to this question, especially evidence-based policy solutions, have been few. The first step should be to conduct additional, targeted research on the processes involved in commercialization and its impacts on the healthcare system. Clearer policies may emerge from this research.

In lieu of specific, evidence-based policies, some broad policy measures can be sketched out at this time. Assuming that we will not be able to eliminate the profit motive and commercialization from healthcare, according to Kaveny (1999, 220), we must be sure that healthcare remains "incompletely commodified." This can be accomplished by encouraging the non-market aspects of healthcare. Health promotion and public health need to be promoted. When physicians and nurses speak of corporate constrictions on their ability to provide adequate care, we should study their situations and explore possible changes. When we identify negative effects of the profit motive in a service or product, we should search for policies that ameliorate those effects. As we mentioned in the previous section, in some healthcare sectors, a shift in ownership mix toward more nonprofit organizations should be encouraged. Further regulations in sectors such as the pharmaceutical and medical device industries may also be required.

A demand-side policy could assist in achieving the goal of incomplete commodification: comprehensive, government-funded and organized, universal healthcare. A universal healthcare system could ensure effective and efficient provision of healthcare, writes Kuttner (2008, 550), "because everyone is covered and there are not incentives to pursue the most profitable treatments rather than those dictated by medical need."

7.8 Chapter Summary

Although for-profit organizations are a small part of some healthcare sectors, such as hospitals, they have grown in all areas of healthcare delivery, and they predominate in sectors such as nursing homes, ambulatory surgical centers, and specialty hospitals. The pharmaceutical industry is an example of a completely commercialized sector. Since nonprofit healthcare organizations appear to perform better than for-profit organizations in terms of quality, trustworthiness, and community service, and perform no worse than for-profit organizations in terms of efficiency and market power, a mix of ownership that ensures health-related policy goals should be explored. Some healthcare markets, such as specialty hospitals and the pharmaceutical industry, may need further regulations in order to operate optimally. The precise impacts of the commercialization of U.S. healthcare and the methods for responding to this development require further research and policy discussion.

Notes

1. The federal government operates hospitals serving active military and their families, veterans, and Native Americans. These federal hospitals in 2007 represented around 4 percent of all U.S. hospitals, and 6 percent of all beds. The Department of Veteran Affairs hospitals and clinics is one of the largest health systems in the world (see American Hospital Association 2007a).

2. In Figure 7.1, as of 2006 the percentage of home care agencies that are for-profit peaked in 1995. The reduced growth since then was most likely due to the effects of the 1997 Balanced Budget Act, which reduced payments for home care, resulting in the closure of many home care agencies, and making the industry much less lucrative for investment.

3. Nonprofit hospitals began having financial difficulties when the Medicare DRG prospective payment system, which reduced payments to hospitals, was implemented in 1983. The Balanced Budget Act of 1997, which reduced payments from Medicare even more, put more pressure on them (Harrison and Sexton 2004).

4. See *Journal of the American Medical Association* 289 (23): 3087–91.

5. HEDIS measures quality of care, access to care, and member satisfaction with the health plan and doctors that allows comparison between health plans in these areas.

6. "Opportunity costs" or the "costs of capital" are the estimated profits that could have accrued had the company put the money into bonds or an equity fund instead of R&D.

7. In the United States, those without insurance coverage for prescription drugs (the "cash payers") pay the most, those who purchase drugs directly (the Department of Veterans Affairs and the Department of Defense) pay the least (around 58 percent of what cash payers pay), managed care plans and hospitals in managed care arrangements pay around 75 percent of cash payers' prices, and hospitals and nursing homes pay 91–95 percent (Latham 2003).

8. According to Reinhardt (2001b), the percentage of revenue spent on marketing might be lower since some of the costs in this category might actually be part of R&D.

THE HEALTHCARE WORKFORCE

The most important component of any healthcare system is the people who deliver the services—the healthcare workforce. Without the human resources to gather information, use technologies, make decisions, and provide care and compassion, the physical resources available for healthcare are useless.

The healthcare workforce is a set of interconnected labor markets, the products of which are substitutes for or complements of one another in healthcare delivery. To some degree these markets respond predictably to wage changes, with the quantity supplied increasing and the quantity demanded decreasing when wages or salaries rise, and the opposite occurring when wages or salaries fall. But supply-side factors such as long educational periods for professionals or demand-side factors such as market power, regulations, and financial constraints may prevent, delay, or attenuate the typical adjustments. Age, family responsibilities, and working conditions also factor into supply responses, while demand for workers depends on societal demand for healthcare, which in turn depends on socioeconomic, political, and demographic factors. Because of all these factors, workforce imbalances are common. In the market for registered nurses, for example, shortages are chronic. In this chapter we find that assumptions introduced in prior chapters, specifically whether supply and demand are independently determined (Assumption 9), and whether firms have market power (Assumption 10), also need to be addressed in relationship to healthcare labor markets.

The current and future adequacy of the healthcare workforce is an important issue for economists. To address it, they employ relevant theory, conduct empirical studies of labor market participation, and use forecasting models to project future supply and demand. They investigate the reasons for maldistributions and shortages and suggest policies that could improve the situation. Another important issue for economists is how the supply of and demand for healthcare workers affects access, quality, and costs.[1]

Although this chapter focuses on the United States, the healthcare workforce is an international issue. Several countries may experience personnel shortages or surpluses simultaneously. For example, several nations are currently experiencing a registered nurse shortage. One country's demand for healthcare personnel may affect the supply of another. The demand for physicians and registered nurses in the United States has led individuals in those professions from several nations to immigrate to the United States. This could create a drain on the healthcare systems of the emigration countries. The factors influencing supply or demand may be similar or may differ among countries. In short, dealing with issues related to the healthcare workforce requires an international perspective.

Section 8.1 provides a brief introduction to the U.S. healthcare workforce. Section 8.2 covers economic theory on labor markets. Sections 8.3 through 8.5 assess the current and future adequacy of the healthcare workforce, with a discussion of forecasting methods and models in Section 8.4. Section 8.6 explores the effect of workforce imbalances on access, quality, and costs. The chapter concludes with a discussion of public and private policies for reducing imbalances.

8.1 A Picture of the U.S. Healthcare Workforce

The healthcare workforce made up 10.4 percent of the total U.S. workforce in 2007 (Bureau of Labor Statistics 2008). In addition to being a large part of the total workforce, the healthcare sector spans a diverse set of roles and scopes of practice. Table 8.1 lists some healthcare occupations, along with the educational requirements, number employed, median hourly wages, and mean yearly income for each in 2007.[2] As the table indicates, a significant number of healthcare workers are licensed professionals who are college graduates, or who, at a minimum, have had postsecondary educational training. Entry into some of these professions, such as physician and physician specialty practices, advanced practice nursing, and physical therapy, requires advanced degrees and long educational periods. For example, the educational period for physicians is anywhere from 11 to 16 years, depending on the specialty. Advanced practice nurses (APNs) currently require a master's degree in nursing, but in the future they may require a doctorate of nursing practice (Whitcomb 2006).

Physicians, registered nurses (RNs), and physician assistants (PAs) typically provide overall direction and medical care for patients. Physicians, who can be doctors of medicine (MDs) or doctors of osteopathy (DOs),[3] can practice in the three generalist (primary care) areas of family practice, internal medicine, and pediatrics, or in specialties such as obstetrics, general surgery, neurology, neurosurgery, cardiology, cardiac surgery, radiology, and psychiatry. Generalists are usually the first contact the patient has with the healthcare system, and they tend to remain the patient's long-term provider.

APNs and PAs in the family practice, community health, and pediatric areas play similar roles to those of primary care physicians. APNs, such as nurse practitioners (NPs), practice independently or with limited physician oversight in 43 states, can prescribe some drugs in 49 states, and can order some tests, diagnose conditions, and refer patients to other providers in many states (Friedman 2008). An APN can also have a specialized practice as a nurse anesthetist, nurse midwife, or clinical nurse specialist (Whitcomb

TABLE 8.1: Educational Requirements, Employment, Wages, and Income of Healthcare Occupations, 2007

Occupation	Education	Employment	Median Hourly Wage	Mean Annual Income
Healthcare Professionals				
Chiropractors	2–4 yr UG + 4 yr + license	27,190	$31.68	$81,390
Dentists[1]	2–4 yr UG + 4 yr + residency + license	100,520	$66.17– > $70	$147,010– $185,340
Dieticians and Nutritionists	2–4 yr UG + license	52,800	$23.56	$50,030
Optometrists	2–4 yr UG + 4 yr + license	24,900	$45.09	$101,840
Pharmacists	2–4 yr UG + 4 yr + license	253,110	$48.31	$98,960
Physicians and Surgeons[2]	2–4 yr UG + 4 yr + 3–8 yr internship and residency + license	550,220	$67.64– >$70	$145,210– $192,780
Physician Assistants	2–4 yr UG + 2–4 yr training + license	67,160	$37.72	$77,800
Podiatrists	2–4 yr UG + 4 yr + 2–4 yr residency + license	9,320	$53.13	$119,790
Registered Nurses	2–4 yr UG + license	2,468,340	$28.85	$62,480
Occupational Therapists	2–4 yr UG + masters + license	91,920	$30.67	$65,540
Physical Therapists	4 yr UG + masters + license	161,850	$33.54	$71,520
Respiratory Therapists	2–4 yr UG + license	101,180	$24.07	$50,930
Speech-Language Pathologists	2–4 yr UG + masters + license	103,810	$29.18	$63,740
Laboratory Technicians and Technologists	2–4 yr UG + license	309,160	$16.48– $24.87	$36,110– $52,410
Dental Hygienists	1–4 yr UG + license	168,600	$31.12	$64,910
Emergency Medical Techs and Paramedics	1–2 yr training + license	201,200	$13.66	$30,870
Licensed Practical and Vocational Nurses	1–2 yr training + license	719,240	$18.24	$38,940
Athletic Trainers	2–4 yr UG + license	14,790	NA	$40,720

TABLE 8.1: *Continued*

Occupation	Education	Employment	Median Hourly Wage	Mean Annual Income
Healthcare Nonprofessionals				
Nursing Aides, Orderlies, and Attendants	HS diploma (+ certificate in some settings)	1,390,260	$11.14	$23,920
Occupational Therapist Assistants and Aides	Varies	32,770	Varies	Varies
Physical Therapist Assistants and Aides	Varies	102,470	Varies	Varies

SOURCES: Data from Bureau of Labor Statistics (2008).

UG = Undergraduate.

HS = High school.

[1] Includes general dentists, oral surgeons, orthodontists, and all other dental specialists.

[2] Includes anesthesiologists, family and general practitioners, internists, obstetricians and gynecologists, pediatricians, psychiatrists, and surgeons.

2006). PAs are licensed to practice medicine with physician supervision. They may perform examinations, diagnose, order tests and treatments, and prescribe medications.

RNs without advanced degrees tend to work in institutional settings such as hospitals, nursing homes, doctor's offices, or home care. In hospitals they usually specialize in particular settings such as intensive care, emergency room, operating room, medical-surgical, obstetrics-gynecology, or pediatrics.

The other professional occupations listed in Table 8.1 tend to focus on particular parts or functions of the human body. Chiropractors, for example, specialize in body alignment, particularly the back. Physical therapists focus on body movement, coordination, strength, and function. Respiratory therapists treat respiratory and cardiovascular problems.

The relationships among these professions are complex. Primary care and specialty medical providers use the expertise of many of the other professionals, such as nurses and various therapists and technicians, to help them diagnose and treat their patients. From an organizational standpoint, these relationships require a degree of collaboration and teamwork. To what degree this has been achieved in many healthcare settings is an ongoing issue. From an economic standpoint, these relationships reflect *complementarities*, which we will discuss further in later sections.

On the other hand, the relationships between some of the health professionals can be more competitive than collaborative. Primary care physicians and NPs, for example, compete over patients in the primary care markets and over independence in their practices. PAs and NPs compete with each other in their roles as physician-extenders and substitutes for primary care physicians. Chiropractors compete with physicians and physical therapists for the care of patients with alignment problems. From an economic standpoint, these relationships reflect *substitution*. The question is whether these occupations are good substitutes in terms of quality of care, patient outcomes, and resource usage. This is an issue for patients, who want to receive the highest quality of care possible; payers such as insurance companies, who are concerned about costs and welcome cost-effective substitutes to physicians; and practitioners, who are concerned about the quality of patient care and inroads into their profession.

The unlicensed nonprofessional healthcare workers listed in Table 8.1 are fewer in number of occupations and in number of people employed, but they play important roles in healthcare delivery. They assist the professional workforce with tasks that don't necessarily require attention from a licensed professional. These workers provide the less-skilled care, such as personal care, that patients require.

Unlicensed nonprofessionals usually have a high school education and may or may not receive additional formal training and certificates. Employers have recently been making greater use of the nonprofessional workforce—for example, nursing assistants. This is due in part to shortages in the professional occupations, but also to employer cost-cutting. To some degree, the nonprofessional workforce has substituted for the professional workforce (Robinson 1988a). As the role of the unlicensed workforce broadens and the acuity of patients in hospitals and nursing homes rises, the use of workers with a lower educational level and minimal training is becoming an issue.[4] RNs in particular are concerned about the effect of the nonprofessional workforce on quality and on the nursing profession.

Wages, salary, and incomes vary enormously among healthcare occupations. Physicians are among the highest paid, while nursing assistants are among the lowest. The figures listed in Table 8.1 can be deceptive, however, as a given occupation may have a wide range of salaries and income. Physician incomes in particular range from an average of less than $150,000 per year for primary care practices to more than $500,000 per year for some specialties, such as cardiac surgery (Friedman 2008). Minimum and maximum salaries are even more extreme.

The large income range among occupations is partly related to the amount of time and money invested in education. A cursory examination of Table 8.1 suggests a positive correlation between education and income. Income differences are also related to the degree of the practitioner's autonomy. For example, physicians who are in practice by themselves can charge what the market will bear for their services, although this is often limited by how much insurance companies and other payers are willing to pay. Nursing assistants, on the other hand, are employees of hospitals, nursing homes, and other organizations. Their income is determined by the wages their employers offer and can be kept low if the organizations have significant power over the labor market.

Lower wages in occupations such as nursing assistant may be a manifestation of what England, Budig, and Folbre (2002, 455) call the "relative pay of care work" in which workers in "caring" occupations are paid less than those in other occupations even after controlling for education, employment experience, and the characteristics of the occupation. England and colleagues hypothesize that this is due to the association of care with women and mothering, low productivity in the care sector, and the fact that workers receive positive intrinsic rewards from the job ("compensating differentials"), among other factors.

Taking a closer look at two of the occupations, Table 8.2 shows trends in the number of physicians and RNs employed per 100,000 U.S. residents since 1970. Note that these numbers do not necessarily reflect available supply (the numbers of workers and professionals desiring to work at prevailing wages and salaries) or effective demand (the number of workers and professionals that provider institutions desire to employ at prevailing wages). Total supply could be larger because of individuals who aren't actively working but who still desire to work, while demand could be larger because there are vacancies in the places of employment. What the numbers do reflect is the active supply of persons actually working given the existing demand for those persons at the prevailing wages and salaries. The number of active physicians per 100,000 people shows a steady upward trend over time and has more than doubled since 1970. While the number of active physicians has increased, the table shows that the percentage of physicians who are practicing in primary care has dropped over the years. The number of active RNs per 100,000 has also more than doubled since 1970, but the increase leveled off in 1995. The number actually dropped for a few years before reaching 1995 levels again in 2005.

Is the current healthcare workforce adequate? What about in the future? If there are imbalances, why hasn't the market equilibrated supply and demand? The next four sections explore these questions by examining theories about the labor market, discussing forecasting models and empirical evidence regarding supply and demand, and reviewing projections regarding future supply and demand.

8.2 The Economics of Labor Markets

In economic theory, the labor of individuals is bought and sold in markets like other commodities. People supply labor in exchange for money that they can then use to buy goods and services. Employers demand labor to produce goods and services. As with product markets, perfectly competitive labor markets have downward-sloping demand curves and upward-sloping supply

TABLE 8.2: Active Physicians and Registered Nurses (RNs) in the United States, 1970–2005

	Physicians/100,000 Population	% Primary Care*	RNs/100,000 Population	Nursing Graduates
1970	122	37.3	368	43,103
1980	183	35.2	560	75,523
1990	221	33.5	717	66,088
1995	238	33.2	794	97,052
1996	243	33.6	NA	94,757
1997	248	32.6	NA	76,523
1998	247	32.7	NA	71,392
1999	245	33.0	789	68,709
2000	246	32.9	776	NA
2001	250	34.6	NA	NA
2002	254	**33.1	NA	NA
2003	266	NA	NA	NA
2004	263	**33.1	788	NA
2005	269	**33.1	800	NA

SOURCES: (1) Data from *Health United States. Chartbook on Trends in the Health of Americans.* Years and tables: year 2003, tables 101, 102, and 103; year 2004, table 102; year 2005, table 105; year 2006, table 104; year 2007, tables 108, 109, and 110: www.cdc.gov/nchs/products/pubs/pubd/hus/2010/2010.htm. (2) Data from National and State Population Estimates. U.S. Census Bureau. www.census.gov/popest/states/NST-ann-est.html; (3) Data from Inglehart et al. (2008).

* As a percent of active physicians in primary care (family practice, internal medicine, and pediatrics).

**Obstetricians were added to the primary care categories in 2002, so to maintain continuity of the table, these figures were derived by subtracting obstetricians from the primary care total.

NA = not available.

curves. Figure 8.1 shows this relationship with a familiar-looking market supply and demand graph. In this case, the horizontal axis represents the quantity of labor demanded and supplied in the labor market, while the vertical axis represents the wage level (analogous to price in the product market). Demand curves (D_L) are downward sloping because as wages and salaries increase, employers will demand fewer workers or fewer hours of work. Supply curves (S_L) are upward sloping because as wages and salaries increase, more workers will be drawn into the labor force and the hours of work will increase, at least up to a point.[5] The relationship of supply and demand to the price of labor (wages or salary) leads to the equilibrium point where supply and demand intersect. At that point, there will be Q_0 quantity of labor demanded and supplied at W_0 wages.

This familiar market graph depicts what happens in the aggregate but not what happens at the individual firm level with regard to demand or at the

Figure 8.1: The Market for Labor

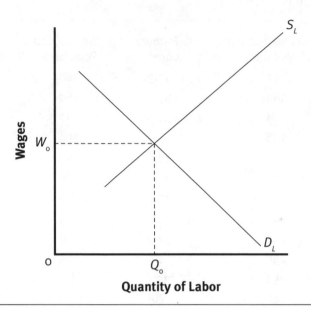

individual worker level with regard to supply. To understand the choices re-garding the quantity of labor demanded and supplied that lead to this market result, we turn to a discussion of demand and supply at the individual level.[6]

Demand for Labor in the Short Run: The Marginal Product of Labor

The production process model consists of two inputs and two time periods. The inputs are represented by labor and capital. Labor is the physical and mental work performed by humans in production. Capital consists of the physical structures and equipment used in production. (Technology, often as-sumed to be a part of capital, is actually a mechanism that contributes to the level of utilization of both labor and capital.) The time periods are classified as the short run and long run. The short run is the period of time during which only the labor input can be changed. In other words, major changes to build-ings and equipment are not feasible. The long run is defined as the period of time during which both labor and capital inputs can be changed. The exact amount of time for the short and long run varies by industry.

The primary input decision for the firm in the short run, therefore, is the amount of labor to demand. In the product market, quantity demanded is a direct result of price. Demand in the labor market is determined not only from the price of labor, but also from the demand for the product that the labor produces. That is, the demand for labor to produce a product is partially derived from the prices and demand in that product market. So the first labor demand consideration for an employer is the level of demand and the prices for the product the firm produces.

Once an individual firm knows the demand for and the prices that it can charge for its product or service, and once it has the capital and technologies it needs for production, it must determine the type and quantity of labor that will be needed for production. If we assume that the product and labor markets are perfectly competitive, the price of the product and the wage of labor have already been determined by their respective markets. Under these conditions the firm will hire workers for the number of hours at which their labor contributes to revenue equal to that of their employment costs (modeled as wages, but actually wages and benefits).

Generally, economists think about this decision in terms of marginal relationships—what happens when you change the amount of something by one unit. The additional physical good or service produced by an additional laborer is termed the *marginal product of labor* (MP_L), and the additional amount of revenue from additional labor is called the *marginal revenue product of labor* (MRP_L).

The marginal product of labor depends on the relationship of labor to capital and the available technologies. Labor and capital interact in such a way that the amount used of one affects the amount needed by the other. To some extent, additional capital can be introduced without the need to hire more workers, and more workers can be hired without the need for more capital. Beyond a certain point, however, adding more of one input without changing the other will result in a decrease in the marginal product, also known as *diminishing marginal productivity*.[7] In the short run, because capital is fixed, at some point employing more labor will result in the diminishing marginal productivity of labor.

Introducing a few formulas, the marginal product of labor is the change in total items produced (ΔQ) given the change in one unit of labor (ΔL):

$$MP_L = \Delta Q / \Delta L \qquad (8.1)$$

The marginal revenue product of labor is derived by multiplying the marginal product of labor by the marginal revenue of the product. Since under perfect competition the price of the product is determined by the interaction of many buyers and sellers in the market and does not go down or up when one firm sells more or fewer items, the price at which the firm sells the product is the same as the marginal revenue it receives for the product. So the marginal revenue product of labor is the marginal product times the price of the product:

$$MRP_L = MP_L \times MR = MP_L \times P \qquad (8.2)$$

In a perfectly competitive market, workers' wages are determined by the interaction of many workers and employers, outside of the demand or supply of any one firm or worker. The equilibrium level of employment will be that at which the wage of the last worker hired is equal to the marginal revenue product of that worker:

$$W = MRP_L, \text{ or}$$
$$W = MP_L \times MR, \text{ or} \qquad\qquad (8.3)$$
$$W = MP_L \times P, \text{ and finally, rearranging terms:}$$
$$W/P = MP_L$$

The following is an example of an equilibrium level of employment: A firm employs 50 workers on a product line. Each worker receives a uniform wage and benefits package that has a value of $20 per hour. The product they make sells for $10 per item. The marginal product of the fiftieth worker hired is three items per hour with a marginal revenue product of $30. Since the wage of the worker ($20) is lower than the marginal revenue product ($MP_L \times MR = 3 \times \$10 = \$30$) the employer should not stop hiring. By hiring more workers, the firm could produce more without the labor costs rising higher than the additional revenue. The employer should stop hiring when the marginal product of the additional labor is two per hour and the marginal revenue product is $20 per hour (where $W = MP_L \times MR$, or $20 = 2 \times \$10$.)

Demand for Labor in the Long Run: The Capital-Labor Decision

As we discussed, holding capital fixed eventually leads to diminishing marginal productivity of labor. This relationship is most relevant in the short run, when a firm is able to change the amount of labor but not the amount of capital. In the long run, however, a firm can make major changes in investment, and can add (or subtract) machines and expand (or contract) the facility. For this reason, the levels of both capital and labor are flexible in the long run. So the question in the long run is the optimum combination of capital and labor that minimizes costs and maximizes profits.

The exact amounts of capital and labor used in production will be influenced by the technologies available and the relative prices of the two factors. For this simplified analysis, economists use a production function model and graph. The model equates the output quantity (Q) to a function of capital (K) and labor (L) inputs:

$$Q = f(K,L) \qquad\qquad (8.4)$$

This model assumes that if wages increase relative to the price of capital, capital will be substituted for labor, and vice versa. The substitutability of capital for labor implies, however, that the proportions of capital and labor are not fixed. In some cases, labor and capital must be used in fixed proportions. For example, the number of operating rooms (ORs) and the number of circulating nurses must be used in the same proportions (in this case one-to-one). For each OR, a circulating nurse is needed to manage the operations.

An additional circulating nurse will not substitute for one less OR, nor will an extra OR substitute for one less circulating nurse.

Figures 8.2a, 8.2b, and 8.2c graphically represent the capital-labor function using quantities of labor on the x-axis and quantities of capital on the y-axis. Isoquants reflect combinations of quantities of the two factors, with the slope of the isoquant indicating the marginal rate of technical substitution. The shape of the isoquants will differ based on the degree of substitutability of capital and labor. The more substitutable the two factors are, the straighter the curves. The isoquants in Figure 8.2a are convex curves, presenting capital and labor as partially substitutable (*imperfect* substitutes). The relationship between labor and capital is typically modeled in this way. If the two factors are *perfectly* substitutable, the isoquants will be straight downward-sloping lines as in Figure 8.2b. In the figure, the firm is using a combination of K_1 and L_1, but it could have used any combination of K and L on that isoquant just as efficiently. The less substitutable the two factors are, the more L-shaped the isoquants become, as in Figure 8.2c. In this figure, K_1 and L_1 are the only combination of capital and labor to be used for an optimum level of output.

Figure 8.2a also includes an isocost line (the downward-sloping straight line), which shows how many units of each input the firm could purchase, given their prices and the total money available for inputs. The slope of the isocost line indicates the relative costs of each of the two inputs. Given the information reflected in the isoquants regarding the relative productivity of

FIGURE 8.2A: The Labor-Capital Decision in the Long Run: Imperfect Substitutes

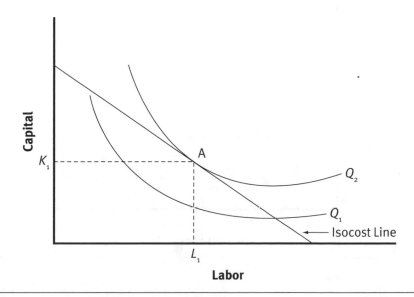

FIGURE 8.2B: The Labor-Capital Decision in the Long Run:
Perfect Substitutes

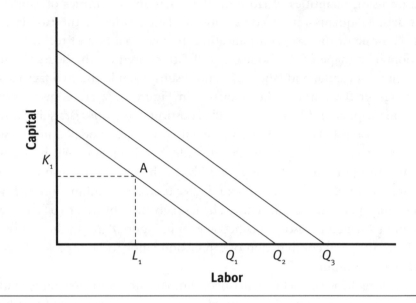

FIGURE 8.2C: The Labor-Capital Decision in the Long Run:
Perfect Complements

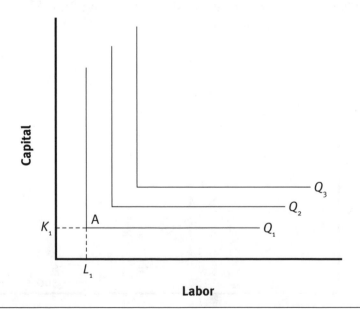

labor and capital and the information reflected in the isocost line about their relative costs, a firm can decide how much of each to use. That amount is determined by the point at which the isocost line is tangent to the isoquant at the desired level of production, as indicated in the figure.

Figure 8.3 shows what happens when wages rise, increasing the costs of labor relative to the costs of capital: The isocost line swings down to the left along the labor axis. This is because the hours of labor a firm can purchase at a particular level of total expenditures decreases. This results in a reduction in the amount of labor used from L_1 to L_2 (at point B). The level of production with the new combination of labor and capital falls from Q_2 to Q_1 because of the overall greater expenses of production.

Demand for Labor: Labor Substitutes and Complements

Capital is not the only production factor that can be substituted for labor when wages change. If the wages for a particular type of worker go up, employers may be able to reduce their demand for that labor resource by substituting other types of labor. This is termed *labor-labor substitution*. The typical substitution occurs when the wages of skilled labor go up. Other skilled, semiskilled, or unskilled labor may be substituted for some of the work originally performed by the higher-paid skilled labor so that fewer of those workers need to be employed. Examples in healthcare are the substitution of NPs

---

FIGURE 8.3: The Change in the Long-Run Demand for Labor Due to a Wage Increase

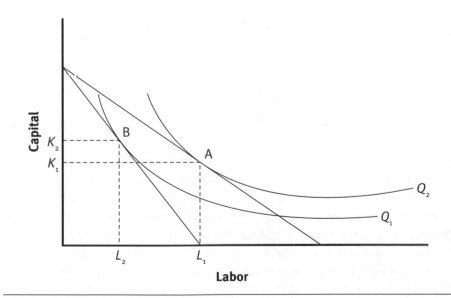

and PAs for primary care physicians, or the substitution of licensed practical nurses (LPNs) or nursing assistants for RNs.

The economic model for labor-labor substitution is similar to the model for capital-labor substitution. The only differences are that both of the inputs in the model are the different types of labor, and that the employer *can* make changes in the combination of these inputs in the short run. As with the capital-labor relationship, this model has isoquants reflecting the combination of the two types of labor inputs to produce a given level of output, isocost lines, and an equilibrium point at which the level of production and the amounts of each type of labor are determined. As with the capital-labor relationship, the degree of substitution is indicated by the shape of the isoquant line.

Different types of workers with different skill levels and occupations not only substitute for each other but also complement each other. When labor inputs are perfect complements, their proportions are fixed, as shown by the L-shaped curves in Figure 8.2c. In healthcare, RNs, LPNs, and NAs are often thought to be complementary nursing labor inputs in that each contributes different tasks to the care of a patient. However, the fact that an increase in RN wages can lead to a simultaneous reduction in demand for RNs and an increase in demand for nursing assistants leads some economists to believe that there is some degree of substitution among nursing occupations in the production function for nursing care (Eastaugh 2007; Spetz et al. 2006).

Deriving the Labor Demand Function and Curve

Factors contributing to the demand for labor include demand for the product, wages of workers, costs of capital, and wages of labor substitutes and complements. In functional form:

$$D_L = f\ (D_P,\ W_L,\ P_K,\ W_S,\ W_C) \qquad (8.5)$$

where D_L = demand for labor, D_P = demand for the product, W_L = wages of the labor input, P_K = costs of capital, W_S = wages of labor substitutes, and W_C = wages of labor complements.

We can graph this demand function as a linear relationship between wages and demand for labor if all other factors are held constant. The shape and slope of the demand curve can be determined from the labor-capital trade-off discussed above, by holding the price of capital constant and varying the price of labor. Points L_1, L_2, and L_3 in the upper graph in Figure 8.4 indicate the amount of labor a firm will demand at a given wage, going from a higher to lower wage, if the price of capital does not change. When we plot those points on a separate graph, we arrive at the typical labor demand curve, as indicated in the lower graph in Figure 8.4, with progressively higher amounts of labor demanded (Q_1, Q_2, and Q_3), at successively lower wages (W_1, W_2, and W_3). Individual labor demand curves can be summed to derive the aggregate curve shown Figure 8.1.

FIGURE 8.4: Derivation of the Demand for Labor

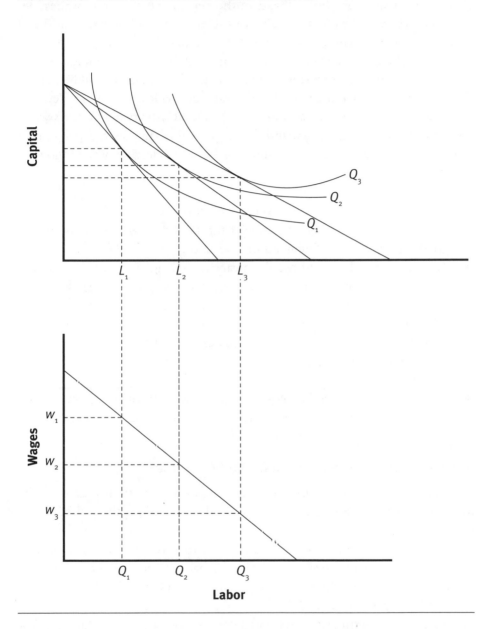

Elasticity of Demand for Labor

The aggregate demand curve depicted in Figure 8.1 could have been sloped more steeply or more shallowly, reflecting different responses of firms to wage increases or decreases. When wages change in the labor market, employers typically change the quantity they demand in response to the higher or lower wages. Elasticity of demand for labor is the percentage change in demand for labor in response to the percentage change in wages. Since demand for labor and wages is generally inversely related, the elasticity of demand for labor is negative and is represented by a downward-sloping line. If the percentage change in demand for labor is less than the percentage change in wages, demand is *inelastic*—the absolute value of the elasticity will be between 0 and 1, and the demand curve generally will be steeper than 45 degrees.[8] If the percentage change in demand for labor is greater than the percentage change in wages, demand is *elastic*—the absolute value of the elasticity will be greater than 1, and the demand curve will generally be shallower than 45 degrees. Unitary elasticity (when the absolute value of the elasticity is 1) occurs when the percentage change in demand for labor is the same as the percentage change in wages. Elasticity of demand for labor is a reflection of the following conditions:

- The extent to which an employer can substitute capital or other labor for that labor input. The greater the substitutability of the labor input, the greater the elasticity of demand for the labor.
- The extent to which a firm can transfer the change in labor costs to the product the labor produces. If, for example, the product has elastic demand in relation to prices, higher labor costs cannot be transferred to the price of the product without a drop in sales. So the employer's response to higher labor costs will be to reduce demand for labor. In other words, if the demand for the product is elastic, the demand for labor will be elastic.
- The percentage of product costs that are due to labor costs. The higher the percentage of costs that are due to labor, the more elastic the demand for labor.

Supply of Labor: Participation in the Workforce

The previous subsection addressed several important decisions regarding the demand for labor. We will now discuss the three decisions that relate to the supply of labor: (1) whether to work in a particular occupation and setting, (2) how much to work, and (3) how much to invest in the skills needed to work. The first two decisions deal with participation in the workforce, whereas the last deals with the development of "human capital."

It is important to understand why people decide to work in certain occupations and settings. Wages and benefits have a strong influence. For example, if the salaries and incomes in physician specialties are much higher than those in family practice, this will draw more individuals to specialty practice than to family practice. Other factors influencing the decision include how interesting, difficult, stressful, or dangerous the work is. Individual demographics also influence occupational choices. Someone with small children may look for an occupation that allows him to work from home, whereas a single person may be more attracted to a job that involves many hours at an office or travel.

Beyond the physical limitations of how many hours in a day a person can work, the amount of time an individual spends at work is directly affected by wages and salaries. In general, holding all else constant, the higher the wages paid to an individual, the more hours of work he will contribute. But this positive relationship between wages and hours may not hold when wages climb above a certain point. Economists have noted that the labor supply curve may be backward bending for some individuals: It is positively sloped at low wages, but negatively sloped at high wages. This means that these individuals work less as wages get progressively higher. We mentioned this phenomenon in our discussion of physician-induced demand in Chapter 6. There, we suggested that the physicians with the highest salaries might work less as wages rise or work more when wages fall.

The main theory to explain this phenomenon is that the individual has achieved an income target, and other activities in that person's life, such as family or community involvement, education, or recreation, become more desirable than the additional income the person could make by working more. Economists lump these non-income activities into one factor labeled "leisure" and model the labor participation choice facing all individuals the *labor-leisure trade-off*. This decision involves a pure trade-off between working and making income on the one hand, and having leisure time during which no income is made on the other. If we think of income and leisure as sources of satisfaction and utility and assume that an individual wants both, we can model the choice between them using a *utility model*. The demand for leisure model is an application of the utility model discussed in Chapter 2, and takes the functional form of:

$$U_i = f(I_i, L_i) \tag{8.6}$$

where I = income, L = hours of leisure per day, and i = an index for each individual.

The hours of work can also be calculated as the difference between the total discretionary hours not needed for bodily maintenance and the hours used in leisure. To illustrate, if we arbitrarily assume that there are 14 discretionary hours per day, the hours of work are $14 - L_i$.

Graphically, the demand for leisure model (also known as the labor-leisure model), shown in Figure 8.5, uses indifference curves and budget lines as in Figures 8.2a–c. But in place of capital and labor, we graph income on the vertical axis and leisure on the horizontal axis. Another difference is that on the horizontal axis we can count the number of leisure hours, moving out from the origin to the point at which the budget constraint is tangent to an indifference curve, *or* we can count the number of hours of work going from the outer end of the axis (the maximum discretionary hours per day) to the same point.

Point A in Figure 8.5 indicates that this individual originally demands 6 hours of leisure (8 hours of work) and makes $100 per day. When this individual's wages rise, indicated by an upward rotation of the budget line in Figure 8.5, he decides to reduce his leisure by 2 hours (increasing work by 2 hours) in order to make an additional $100 in income, thus ending at point C, with 4 hours of leisure per day (and 10 of work). His income goes from $100 to $200 per day.

Arriving at point C in the graph is a result of two responses to an increase in wages: (1) A higher wage gives the individual a higher income, which can be used to work less (increase the hours of leisure) while still making the same or higher income, and (2) a higher wage will encourage the individual to work more in order to increase his income still more (he will give up leisure because the opportunity cost of leisure is higher now). The first response is the *income effect*; the second is the *substitution effect*. In Figure 8.5, the income effect is indicated by a parallel shift in the original budget line and the move from A to B, where the hours of leisure increase from 6 to 8 (the hours of work decrease from 8 to 6). The substitution effect is indicated by the move from B to C, where the hours of leisure decrease from 8 to 4 (the hours of work increase from 6 to 10). The net result of the income and substitution effects in this case is for the individual to arrive at C, with a two-hour decrease in leisure (a two-hour increase in work) and a $100 increase in income.

In this case, the substitution effect outweighs the income effect, producing a net reduction in leisure from 6 to 4 hours and a net increase in work from 8 to 10 hours. However, if the income effect had been stronger than the substitution effect (which would be reflected in the shape and position of the indifference curves), the net result would have been an increase in hours of leisure and a decrease in hours of work. When the income effect outweighs the substitution effect, the individual may have reached his target income level. This effect will be indicated by a backward-bending supply curve.

Deciding how much to work involves factors beyond just wages and income. People may receive enjoyment from their jobs that leads them to work long hours. They also make decisions about how much to work based on family needs such as child-rearing. Job characteristics and working conditions also enter into the equation.

On the demand side, most employers do not offer workers the opportunity to increase their hours of work on a regular hourly basis. Full-time employment tends to be a fixed 40-hour week with some opportunity for unscheduled overtime. Alternatively, workers are offered a part-time option with a fixed number of hours per week. In many occupations, overtime is discouraged, frowned upon, or even forbidden. In these cases, higher wages will not bring more labor hours into the market because the quantity is fixed on the demand side. This interconnection between supply and demand in the labor market indicates that the two are not completely independent, suggesting that the labor market is not perfectly competitive.

FIGURE 8.5: A Wage Change Leading to Increased Hours of Work

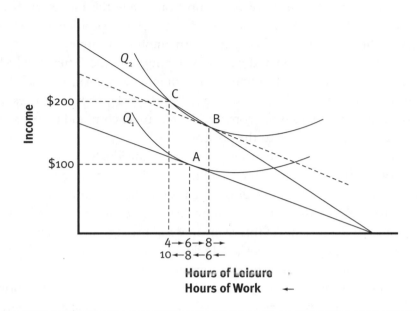

A final consideration is that individuals may be paid a salary, in which case their choice of hours is less directly determined by income. Income still influences the hours of work indirectly, since the more someone works the more successful that person will likely be at her job and the greater chance she will have of maintaining or increasing income.

Supply of Labor: Human Capital Development

Another labor supply decision is how much time and money one should spend on developing one's human capital by increasing one's level of education, training, and skills. Human capital enhancement makes it possible to work at more desirable jobs and earn higher incomes. The skills and knowledge needed for human capital development are acquired through investments by individuals themselves (college and other training), by society (the public education system and higher education subsidies), and by employers (on-the-job training and educational subsidies).

Economic theory holds that individuals will invest in their own human capital development as long as the expected marginal benefit from the investment (in terms of higher income and a more desirable job) is greater than the marginal costs. In figuring this equilibrium point, all costs of the investment, including the opportunity costs, must be included. For example, young people attending college frequently must postpone earning an income. Older adults attending college often must scale back on their hours of work or take lower-paying jobs.

In figuring the amount that should be invested in human capital, an individual must also take the time frame into account. Usually, the *costs* of human capital development are borne up front while the monetary *benefits* in terms of enhanced income are reaped later. This is problematic when it comes to the value of money over time. An amount of money at hand now (say, $100) can be invested and will be worth more in the future (say, $110 in a year), and conversely, the same amount of money in the future (say, $100 a year from now) is worth less now (say, $90). In order to make the estimation of costs and benefits more comparable over time, costs and benefits in all years need to be *discounted* to the present value.[9]

Theoretically, when choosing a career, individuals consider the net benefit of their potential investment, subtracting their discounted educational and opportunity costs from the discounted additional amount of money they will be making over their lifetime. Individuals will consider medical school, for example, if the benefits of future income and prestige are greater than the educational and opportunity costs. Choice of primary care or specialty fields in medicine is also influenced by this consideration.

This decision regarding human capital development can be formalized by calculating its return on investment (ROI), also called the rate of return. The ROI is the net financial benefit from an investment, expressed as the ratio of the amount gained from the investment (or lost, if gains are negative) over the amount invested. Since the amount spent on education and the amount gained from that investment occur over a period of time, the formula for ROI incorporates the present value (PV) of those amounts. The ROI, therefore, is the present value of the financial benefit from the education minus the present value of the costs of education, divided by the present value of the costs of the education[10]:

$$ROI = \frac{PV(\text{financial benefits from education}) - PV(\text{costs of education})}{PV(\text{costs of education})} \tag{8.7}$$

The following is a simplified example: Upon graduation a physician makes $85,000 more per year for 40 years than she would have if she had not had the medical education. Her educational costs were around $100,000 per year times ten years. At an interest rate of 5 percent, the PV of the 40 years of additional income is $895,387. The PV of the educational costs for the first 10 years is $772,170. The ROI is ($895,387 − $772,170)/$772,170 = 15.96 percent.

Deriving the Labor Supply Function and Curves

Wages (or salaries or income); desire for leisure; the age, sex, and marital status of an individual; family needs; human capital investments; and other considerations all play into the labor supply function of an individual. In functional form:

$$S_L = f(W_L, LE, DEM, H) \qquad (8.8)$$

where S_L = supply of labor, W_L = wages, LE = desired number of leisure hours, DEM = demographics (involves several separate variables), and H = human capital investment.

This supply function can be graphed as an upward-sloping linear or curvilinear relationship between wages and supply if all other factors are held constant. The shape and slope of the supply curve can be determined from the income-leisure trade-off discussed above.

Elasticity of Labor Supply

Elasticity of labor supply is the percentage change in labor supply in response to the percentage change in wages. Since labor supply tends to increase with an increase in wages, elasticity is positive and is represented by an upward-sloping line. The determination of elasticity of labor supply is analogous to that of labor demand, except that it will usually have a positive value.

In the case of the backward-bending supply of labor, the elasticity will become negative at the point where an individual approaches his target income level and begins to work less as his wages increase. This is demonstrated in the backward-bending supply curve, shown in Figure 6.2: The lower part of the curve up to the bend (points A and B) represents labor supply at lower wage levels, where an increase in wages induces more hours of work (and elasticities are positive); the "bend" in the supply curve indicates the point at which higher wages no longer induce more hours of work; and the upper part of the curve above the bend (points C and D in the figure) represents labor supply at higher wage levels, where an increase in wages leads to fewer hours of work (and elasticities are negative).

Labor Market Equilibrium, Shortages, and Surpluses

In a perfectly competitive labor market, there should be no extended labor surpluses or shortages. A surplus of labor exists when more workers or hours of labor are being offered than demanded at the given wage. A shortage of labor exists when there is a greater demand for workers or hours of labor than is supplied at the given wage. The market should correct for any temporary imbalances in the short run through an increase or decrease of the wage, which will bring demand and supply in line. Section 2.3 covered the perfectly competitive market equilibrium. However, the unique characteristics of labor markets in general, and healthcare labor markets in particular, make it difficult to apply competitive theories to these markets.

Unique Characteristics of Labor Markets

All labor markets share some unique characteristics that make viewing them as perfectly competitive markets questionable. A perfectly competitive labor market would have the following characteristics:

- Workers in a given occupation or profession are identical with respect to skills and productivity, and jobs offered by firms for each occupation or profession are identical with respect to working conditions and wages.
- Workers and firms have perfect information about each other and the wages and job opportunities in the market.
- Workers can easily enter the market, and can easily and without cost change jobs within the market.
- Workers do not belong to unions, and firms do not collude or dominate the buyer side of the market.
- Demand and supply are independent, and are determined through flexible wages.

The first consideration is that labor and jobs are not homogeneous. The amount and quality of labor differ from worker to worker. Some workers are healthier and take fewer sick days than others, and some are more productive than others given the same tasks and resources to complete the tasks. Jobs are just as heterogeneous as labor. For the same job, some places of employment provide many fringe benefits, while others provide few benefits. Some places of employment are characterized by work overload or inattention to safety, while other places maintain acceptable levels of workload and take safety precautions.

Labor and job heterogeneity are problems for employers and workers, because it is expensive (in time and money) to obtain information about employees and jobs. As a result, workers with different productivity may be paid the same wage, and workers with the same productivity may be paid different wages. There may be no uniform equilibrium point.

The third requirement for a perfectly competitive labor market—easy entry into and mobility within the occupation—is also not characteristic of the labor market. Entry into certain occupations is difficult due to educational and professional requirements. Labor mobility within the occupation is affected by the costs of job searches mentioned above. In addition, mobility is reduced due to the nature of the labor market transaction, which differs from that of the product market. In the product market the transaction between buyer and seller is impersonal and is completed quickly, as when we obtain a pair of shoes by paying a stranger for them and walking away with the shoes. But in the labor market, the transaction is a *relationship* between employee and employer rather than a brief exchange of money for a product or service. Some labor relations are characterized by a formal contractual relationship that specifies the expectations of one or both parties, while others are relatively informal. These relationships lead to less labor mobility than would exist in a competitive market. On-the-job training may also lead to lower job mobility, since it builds firm-specific human capital that may not be transferable to other jobs. In the United States, employer-based health insurance also leads to less job mobility if workers stay at their jobs in order to keep their health insurance coverage.

Fourth, market power can exist in the labor market on both the buyer and seller sides. On the buyer side, workers in a geographical area may have only a few employers from which to choose. This gives rise to the demand for labor being controlled by a few companies or one company (oligopsonies or monopsonies). On the seller side, workers can form unions that allow them to exert market power. If firms can keep wages lower than the equilibrium wage, or workers can keep wages higher than the equilibrium wage, shortages or surpluses may ensue from these "sticky" or "rigid" wages.

Finally, there are differences *within* labor markets. The supply and demand characteristics described in this section fit nonprofessionals and professionals who are not self-employed. However, they do not necessarily apply to professional self-employed markets (such as many of the healthcare professional markets). For example, self-employed professionals do not face typical demand-side restrictions such as limits on hours of work or monopsony-controlled wages. However, due to managed care and public insurance controls, they do face some demand-side limits, such as fixed reimbursement and pressures on their time and practice. The supply responses of self-employed professionals are also similar to the responses of those who are not self-employed. (For example, they have choices with regard to human capital development and how much to work.)

Additional Characteristics of Healthcare Labor Markets

The characteristics of the labor market typify the healthcare labor market, with some additional distinctions. The demand for healthcare labor is derived from the demand for healthcare, which depends on the number of insured, the amount of out-of-pocket payments, the health and age of the population, healthcare technology, utilization patterns, and other factors. Healthcare payment systems, which tend to pay fixed prices for healthcare services, also influence demand. Negotiated insurance contracts and fixed prices paid by government agencies leave provider institutions such as hospitals with little flexibility to increase wages and benefits in response to shortages until contracts or government payment rates change. This may lead to a sluggish wage response to workforce imbalances. For example, when there is a shortage of RNs, hospitals cannot just raise the price of their services (even a little) to increase wages and benefits and draw more RNs into the workforce until contracts are renegotiated with insurance companies or government payment rates increase. Fixed prices that result in low provider profit margins may also reduce institutional demand for healthcare labor.

Another demand-side consideration is that monopsony or oligopsony power appears to be common in hospitals. Many geographical areas contain only one or a handful of hospitals. These few hospitals are the only places of employment in the area for many workers (Robinson 1988b; Staiger, Spetz, and Phibbs 1999). The market power of hospitals could result in wages that are rigidly lower than equilibrium wages, which could contribute to shortages of certain healthcare professionals, such as nurses.

The nonwage factors that determine supply are significant for healthcare professionals. The choice of geographical location, for example, is critical to practitioners such as physicians. Urban areas are preferred due to their greater professional, social, and cultural attractiveness. As a result, there are significant imbalances of physicians along geographical lines (Forrest 2006).

Another important supply distinction is that professional requirements make it difficult to enter professions such as medicine and nursing. The requirements include long educational periods, limits on the number of students that can enter the educational system, and licensing (Cooper and Aiken 2001). These factors contribute to significant lags in the correction of workforce imbalances. Once a shortage of doctors or nurses is discovered, for example, it takes years to increase faculty and resources in the educational system, matriculate, and graduate additional students.

Future expectations of demand, supply, and wages or income also affect the healthcare workforce. When an occupation or a specialty within an occupation is predicted to move into an oversupply situation, concern about future unemployment or lower incomes will influence career choices, and new entrants will decrease (Berkowitz 2004). In the late 1990s, for example, it became known that there was an oversupply of anesthesiologists and that some were having difficulty finding work. Admissions to training programs dropped for several years. Following that there was a shortage of anesthesiologists (Berkowitz 2004). The opposite happens when shortages are predicted. Many see the occupation as a career opportunity and enter into the educational system, resulting in a surplus in that occupation a few years later. These supply overreactions contribute to yo-yo shortages and surpluses in those professions.

The concept of need versus demand comes into play with healthcare labor markets. This is an important distinction that is often blurred. Demand is an *economic* measure of how much of a good or service would actually be bought at a given price. It is based on the willingness to pay for a good or service relative to all other goods and services being offered. Need, on the other hand, is a normative view about how much *should* be consumed of a good or service regardless of the price. It is usually determined through expert opinion. The quantity needed can be higher or lower than the quantity demanded. For example, if experts believe that there is a need for more prevention services than the market currently provides, they will forecast a greater need for primary care physicians compared to forecasts based on market demand for primary care physicians. In contrast, due to factors such as fixed reimbursements and monopsony power, the number and type of healthcare

FIGURE 8.6: Demand, Need, and Supply of Healthcare Labor

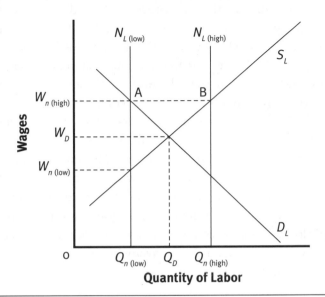

workers demanded by healthcare institutions may be lower than what experts believe is needed to provide quality care. For example, hospital or nursing home administrators may demand RN-to-patient or -resident ratios that are lower than those recommended by experts for the needs of the patients or residents.

The distinction between need and demand in the healthcare labor market is represented graphically in Figure 8.6, which is based on a classic model developed by Jeffers, Bognanno, and Bartlett (1971). Demand for healthcare labor is the downward-sloping line D_L. The need for healthcare labor is represented by two vertical lines, indicating that price has no influence on the quantity. $N_{L\,(low)}$ represents a low level of need as perceived by experts, while $N_{L\,(high)}$ represents a high level of need. If needs are high, the intersection of supply with need will require a greater quantity of labor $(Q_{n\,(high)})$ than that of the market-based, supply-demand equilibrium (at Q_D). Higher wages $(W_{n\,(high)})$ will be needed to induce the additional labor participation compared to the market equilibrium wage (W_D). If needs are low, the intersection of supply with need will lead to a lower quantity of labor $(Q_{n\,(low)})$ and wages $(W_{n\,(low)})$ than that of the market equilibrium.

The distinction between demand and need in healthcare labor markets comes into play because it also exists in the healthcare service market, from which the demand (or need) for healthcare labor is derived. For example, individuals may demand fewer healthcare services than experts would say they really need because they cannot afford them, or they may demand more because they have been induced by the supply side (physician services, pharmaceuticals) to consume more.

These differences in quantity demanded and needed for healthcare carry directly over to the healthcare workforce. If demand for certain healthcare services is higher (or lower) than need, the demand for the corresponding labor will likely also be higher (or lower). This distinction is especially important because assessments of the adequacy of the current and future healthcare workforce are not always based on demand.

We have discussed several ways in which labor markets in general, and healthcare labor markets in particular, differ from product markets. These different characteristics may be played out in disequilibriums between supply and demand or between supply and need. As we mentioned, shortages or surpluses can develop and can even become recurring or chronic. For convenience, we refer to the question of equilibrium or disequilibrium as the "adequacy" of the healthcare workforce given demand or perceived need. This issue of healthcare workforce adequacy is extremely important, and it is the focus of the next three sections.

8.3 Is the Healthcare Workforce Adequate at This Time?

Having neither shortages nor surpluses in the healthcare workforce is important. A shortage will negatively affect access to and quality of care, while a surplus could lead to overutilization of healthcare and high costs (for example, if physicians induce demand) (Garber and Sox 2004). Having an adequate amount does not just mean having the correct amount in general, or having enough of one type (say, physicians). It means having the demanded amount (or the needed amount, if planners are attempting to match supply to need) in each occupation, in each geographical area, and in every healthcare setting. Just because there are enough physicians on a national per capita basis doesn't mean that they are distributed efficiently or equitably on a geographic basis or that there are enough of them in all medical settings. The same applies to RNs, who may choose to work outside of hospitals in settings such as home care, or may work in non–patient care settings such as insurance. Some go on to get advanced practice degrees and work as practitioners in community settings or in educational or management roles in institutional settings. As a result, institutional direct care settings such as hospitals may experience a shortage of patient caregivers even when overall RN supply is sufficient.

Assessing the demand and supply of the healthcare workforce is complicated. It may not be enough to consider how many professionals and workers are demanded in the marketplace; an expert perspective on how many are needed may also be a factor. From the economic perspective, a certain number of workers will be demanded at any given wage or salary. From a healthcare planning perspective, more or fewer than the number demanded may be needed in order to provide high-quality, cost-effective care.

Should healthcare workforce planners use demand or need as their benchmark? This question is debated whenever the adequacy of the healthcare workforce is discussed. It may be that the best way to deal with this issue is to estimate both demand and need.

Supply estimates are more cut-and-dried than demand estimates. Supply for nonprofessionals is determined by the number of workers actively participating in the occupation, including those who are employed and those who are looking for work in the occupation. Supply for professionals is a bit different. It includes all those with a license to work in that profession (Bureau of Health Professions 2006a). However, for various reasons some of those licensed in the profession may not be actively participating in it. If they are working or looking for work in the profession, they are considered to be part of the active workforce. If they are working outside the profession or are not looking for work in the profession, they are considered to be inactive, or nonparticipants.

The reason that the measure of the supply for professionals includes an inactive portion is that these individuals can be considered a reserve to draw from if market and other conditions change. This professional reserve is important, because drawing from the general population to increase the number of active participants involves a long lag period due to licensing and education requirements.

To assess healthcare workforce adequacy, demand (or need, or both) must be compared to supply. If the two are equal, the workforce is in equilibrium. If demand or need is estimated to be greater than supply, there is a shortage. If supply is greater than demand or need, there is a surplus, or oversupply.

Because of these issues, controversy over current healthcare workforce adequacy is substantial. In the following two subsections we outline some of the issues regarding the physician and nursing workforces in the United States. The third subsection raises the issue of ethnic and racial disparities in the healthcare workforce.

Current Physician Supply

Since 2000, some state medical societies, hospital associations, and researchers have claimed that physician shortages already exist or will soon (Iglehart 2008). Their evidence includes difficulties in obtaining access to care (Goodman and Fisher 2008). Other analysts believe that we may need a small increase in U.S.-trained allopathic physicians to meet population growth and to decrease our reliance on international medical school graduates (IMGs). However, they also believe that educating and training many more allopathic physicians would be unnecessary and expensive, since nonphysician providers and osteopathic doctors supplement this supply (Wilson 2005).

Another consideration is whether there is an overall shortage, or if a shortage exists only in some areas (perhaps with surpluses in other areas) due to uneven distribution of physicians. There is substantial evidence that current perceptions of physician shortages may be partially due to primary care shortages and geographical imbalances (Forrest 2006; Wilson 2005). Recent figures show a drop in primary care trainees from 23,800 in 1995 to 22,100 in 2006 (Friedman 2008). Less than 45 percent of primary care residencies were filled in 2006, and 56 percent of these were filled by international medical graduates (Friedman 2008). Table 8.2 shows that the percentage of physicians who practice in primary care is the lowest it has been since 1970.

Physician supply varies between U.S. hospital-referral regions by more than 50 percent, and the variation does not appear to be related to healthcare needs (Goodman and Fisher 2008). For example, the supply of cardiologists has been found to be unrelated to the incidence of myocardial infarction (MI) (Wennberg 2000). Macon, Georgia, is in the top quartile for acute MIs, but is in the lowest quartile of supply of cardiologists, whereas Arlington, Virginia, has a low rate of MIs but high supply of cardiologists. Neonatologists also are not necessarily located in regions where there is higher incidence of low-birthweight newborns (Goodman et al. 2001, 2002). Primary care physicians in particular are distributed unevenly (Goodman and Fisher 2008).

Current RN Supply

In contrast to the uncertainty about the adequacy of the physician workforce, reports of unfilled RN positions (such as vacancy rates) leave no doubt that there is a nursing shortage. As with physicians, the shortage has distributional components related to practice setting and geography. The shortage is primarily of direct patient care RNs (those in nonsupervisory, noneducational roles who provide care to patients) in settings such as hospitals, nursing homes, home care, physician's offices, and ambulatory care centers (Pindus, Tilly, and Weinstein 2002; Unruh and Fottler 2005). Data from the quadrennial RN Sample Survey indicate that the percentage of RNs employed in direct patient care areas peaked at 72 percent in 1992, and fell to 62 percent by 2000 (Unruh and Fottler 2005).

Hospitals have been hit hardest, with vacancy rates peaking at 13 percent in 2001 (Buerhaus, Auerbach, and Staiger 2007), then dropping to 8.1 percent by 2007 (American Hospital Association 2007b). The percentage of RNs working in hospitals (in direct patient care, supervisory, and advanced practice roles) peaked at 68 percent of RN supply in 1984 and declined to 56 percent by 2004 (Bureau of Health Professions 2006a). Seago and colleagues (2001) note that hospitals reporting shortages tend to be in the South, in counties with a high percentage of nonwhite residents, a high percentage of Medicaid or Medicare patients, and high patient acuity. In a study of Nebraska hospitals, the shortages were much more severe in rural areas (Cramer et al. 2006).

Federally funded community health centers (CHC) report RN vacancy rates just under those of hospitals. In 2005, vacancy rates in CHCs were 10.4

percent (WWAMI 2006). The CHC shortages are highest in isolated small rural areas and urban areas and lowest in large and less isolated rural areas (WWAMI 2006). In contrast, RN shortages overall tend to be more acute in rural areas compared to urban areas (Zigmond 2007).

On the other hand, shortages generally have not been reported in non–patient care settings such as insurance, regulatory agencies, and others. The only non–patient care area reporting RN shortages is nursing education faculty. From 1980 to 2004 the percentage of RNs employed in nursing education declined from 3.7 to 2.4 percent of the RN workforce (Bureau of Health Professions 2006a). This decline in RN faculty contributes to the overall nursing shortage by creating bottlenecks in the educational process. An American Association of Colleges of Nursing 2007 survey of colleges of nursing found that 71 percent of schools pointed to faculty shortages as a reason for not accepting all qualified applicants into entry-level nursing programs (American Association of Colleges of Nursing 2008).

Disparities in the Healthcare Workforce

Compared to their proportion in the general population, African Americans, Latinos, and American Indians are severely underrepresented in the health professions (Grumbach and Mendoza 2008). Public health is the only setting in which the proportions of these minorities approaches that of the population. Baccalaureate nursing programs have made the most progress recently, increasing underrepresented minorities from 12 to 18 percent between 1990 and 2005 (Grumbach and Mendoza 2008). Allopathic and osteopathic medicine programs and pharmacy programs have had no increase in diversity between 1990 and 2005. Dentistry programs have shown a little increase in that time period.

Grumbach and Mendoza (2008) write that these minorities are underrepresented because they miss out on educational opportunities starting as early as kindergarten and continuing through their primary education. "By high school, more than one in five Latinos and one in ten African Americans have dropped out of school, compared with one in seventeen white students" (Grumbach and Mendoza 2008, 416). The authors make the case for improving diversity on the basis of civil rights, the improvement in healthcare delivery, and the better business case due to improved customer service and competitive advantage.

8.4 Forecasting Future Healthcare Workforce Adequacy

In addition to assessing the present adequacy of the healthcare workforce, it is important to have some idea about future adequacy. Knowing what future demand and supply could look like is essential to ensuring that the future healthcare workforce will be adequate. If shortages or surpluses are predicted, changes in demand and supply can be made to avoid those situations. In this sense, healthcare workforce forecasting is an important policy tool. Without an idea of what the future will look like, policies may do nothing to make things better, and they may even make things worse. With a forecast, careful policies can steer supply of and demand for the workforce in needed directions.

If assessing current healthcare workforce adequacy is complicated, trying to predict what the situation will be like in the future is even more so. Predictions will only be accurate if the assumptions used to make them hold true. For example, predictions of large increases in demand for healthcare providers are based on one or more of the following assumptions: The population will continue to grow at a strong pace; as the population ages, more healthcare per capita will be consumed; per capita wealth and income will be at current levels or higher; and people will have insurance or otherwise be able to afford healthcare. If any of these assumptions fails, the predicted increases in demand may not come to pass. The same is true of supply. Growth in supply is dependent on increases in the number of new entrants and retention of existing participants. If there are future bottlenecks in the educational system, fewer individuals attracted to the profession, or more individuals retiring early or leaving because the working conditions are difficult, supply will be much smaller than predicted.

There are several ways to make forecasting as accurate as possible:

- Include as many factors that influence healthcare workforce demand and supply as possible.
- Use accurate data regarding past and current patterns of these factors.
- Use models that incorporate realistic assumptions about supply and demand.
- Do not predict too far into the future (the further out one predicts, the less accurate the prediction).
- Use simulations to show what could happen under different scenarios.

We provide more detail about the factors that influence healthcare workforce demand and supply and forecasting models in the following subsections.

Factors Affecting Demand for Labor

Three main factors determine healthcare labor demand (these follow directly from the demand function developed in Section 8.2): (1) the demand for healthcare, (2) healthcare delivery system design and financing (including reimbursement rates, wages, labor substitution, and productivity), and (3) institutional and market characteristics such as ownership and market power (Kirch and Vernon 2008; Maynard 2006; Spetz and Given 2003; Unruh and Fottler 2005).

A few examples of these factors can be found in the demand for RNs, in which key factors are (1) the population demand for healthcare, particularly for hospital care, since the primary place of employment of RNs is hospitals; (2) wages; (3) reimbursement systems and rates; (4) ownership status; and (5) market power.

Managed care reduced demand for hospital care through reductions in admissions and lengths of stay (Spetz 1999). The DRG-based prospective payment system (PPS) had a similar effect on demand for hospital care. As the number of patient days in hospitals fell, fewer RNs could have been demanded. However, as these healthcare demand changes occurred, the patient population in hospitals became much more acutely ill, and patient turnover increased dramatically (Unruh and Fottler 2006). There is some evidence that *more* RNs per patient were needed to maintain the same workload and quality of care (Unruh 2002; Unruh and Fottler 2006).

Studies of the effect of managed care penetration on the demand for RN staffing in hospitals have been inconclusive. One study found that managed care is related to slower employment growth for RNs in hospitals but greater growth in nonhospital settings (Buerhaus and Staiger 1996). Other studies have not found managed care penetration to have significant effects (Brewer and Frazier 1998; Mobley and Magnussen 2002).

Wages have not produced much of a demand response. When wages for RNs go up, hospital demand for RNs does not fall much. Spetz and Given (2003) reason that this is because hospitals reduced their nursing staffs as much as possible during the mid-1990s, and therefore cannot function safely with fewer nurses. The authors also remind us that hospitals face regulations regarding staffing, and many face union contracts. Hospitals may be reluctant to staff lower because it may affect the quality of care.

Reimbursement systems and rates affect demand for RNs by reducing the amount of revenue healthcare institutions have to spend on labor, thereby reducing demand for labor. One study found that pressure from PPS results in somewhat lower staffing in hospitals (Mobley and Magnussen 2002). Another study found that the Balanced Budget Act of 1997, which reduced Medicare reimbursement rates to hospitals, was related to reduced RN staffing in non–safety net hospitals that had financial pressures (Lindrooth et al. 2006). Lower PPS payments have been found to be related to lower nurse staffing in skilled nursing facilities (Unruh, Zhang, and Wan 2006; White 2005).

There is some evidence that for-profit status is related to lower RN staffing. Several studies find that for-profit hospitals (Mark and Harless 2007; Seago, Spetz, and Mitchell 2004) and nursing homes (McGregor et al. 2005) use fewer RN positions or hours.

The research regarding market power suggests that hospitals have monopsony power. Earlier studies showed that RN wages are lower when there are fewer hospitals or when markets are more concentrated (Hurd 1973; Link and Landon 1975; Robinson 1988b). A more recent study that utilized additional control variables found a monopsony effect only in the short run (Hirsch and Schumacher 1995). Staiger, Spetz, and Phibbs (1999) investigated the response of wages and RN supply to legislated increases in wages at Veterans Administration (VA) hospitals. They found that a 10-percent wage increase at VA hospitals produced a 2 percent increase in wages in hospitals within 15 miles of the VA, but only a 1 percent increase in hospitals 15 to 30 miles from the VA. This indicates that a more competitive hospital environment is related to higher and more flexible RN wages. The authors also found that the labor supply curve facing an individual hospital is very inelastic, which indicates that hospitals can set wages. They conclude that one reason for the weak effects found in the Hirsch and Schumacher study is that the monopsony power may be exercised on effort (workload) rather than wages. In other words, the hospitals pay competitive wages but keep workloads high. Currie, Farsi, and Macleod (2005) also found that takeovers of hospitals by large hospital chains in California in the 1990s resulted in an increase in the effort of RNs, as indicated by an increase in the patient-to-nurse ratio.

Factors Affecting Labor Supply

The main factors determining labor supply are the following (these follow directly from the supply function developed in Section 8.2): (1) the demographics of the healthcare labor force, such as age, gender, race, ethnicity, marital status, and family income; (2) the educational system capacity and number of graduates; (3) migration and emigration of the workforce; (4) employment conditions such as wages, working conditions, and job location; (5) the return on educational investment; and (6) the economic system (for example, a recession may bring more nurses back into nursing) (Antonazzo et al. 2003; Maynard 2006; Spetz and Given 2003; Unruh and Fottler 2005).

We will discuss several of these supply factors as they relate specifically to physician and RN supply.

Factors Related to Choosing Medicine and to Choice of Physician Practice

Some of the important factors in the choice to become a physician and the choice between primary or specialty care are the cost of medical education, the salary and income obtained from medical practice, and the ROI from that choice. The average medical school graduate in 2007 had $140,000 of debt (Friedman 2008). This amount will be more or less depending upon the type of physician practice. In 2007, the average family physician earned $147,516 annually, the average cardiovascular surgeon $558,719, and the average neurosurgeon $438,426 (Friedman 2008). Using 1997 data, Weeks and Wallace (2002) found that the hours-adjusted internal rate of return[11] on the educational investment for primary care physicians is 16 percent, compared to 18 percent for procedure-based medicine (surgery, obstetrics, radiology, anesthesiology, and medical subspecialties), 22 percent for dentistry, 23 percent for law, and 26 percent for business.

This comparison has two implications. First, physicians do not do as well financially as comparable professionals. Their ROI is lower than that of dentists, lawyers, and businesspeople. Second, specialists do better than primary care physicians. "Students can still anticipate relatively poorer returns on their educational investment when they choose a career in primary care medicine as compared with careers in procedure-based medicine or surgical specialties, business, law, or dentistry" (Weeks and Wallace 2002).

Friedman (2008) finds additional reasons for choosing specialty over primary care. The first observation is that medical educational culture places a higher value on specialty practice and therefore discourages students from going into primary care. The second observation is that primary care is less prestigious. A primary care physician is less likely to become a medical school dean or achieve other positions of leadership, to get a research grant, or to have opportunities for consulting. The third observation is that the desire for "a life" leads individuals to specialty practice, where there are fewer hours and less or no on-call work, work at night, or rotating shifts.

The growth of managed care was expected to increase the demand for primary care physicians relative to specialty physicians because of HMO requirements for patients to see a primary care physician before going to a specialist. Public and private reimbursement systems were to reduce the income disparity between primary care physicians and specialists through changes in reimbursement (Ginsburg 2003b). Medicare replaced a reimbursement system based on customary charges with the Resource-Based Relative Value Scale, which reimburses physicians through set fees based on the amount of work the physician performs and other practice expenses. Private insurance also began to pay physicians through resource-based systems. However, these reimbursement changes did not eliminate the disparity (Ginsburg 2003b). The supply response to the demand and reimbursement changes should have been an increase in the number of primary care physicians and a decrease in the number of specialty physicians. However, the percentage of primary care physicians has remained stable since the 1980s (see Table 8.2). By the end of the 1990s, HMO penetration had not affected the numbers of primary care or specialist physicians, but higher HMO growth was leading to smaller increases than before in the numbers of specialists and total physicians (Escarce et al. 2000).

Studies have found that gender, race, and age are related to the choice to practice in underserved urban or rural areas. Women and African Americans more often practice in underserved urban areas, whereas men and underrepresented minorities other than African Americans more often practice in rural areas (Freeman, Ferrer, and Greiner 2007). Growing up in a rural area

Factors Related to Physician Choice of Geographic Location

and planning to enter family practice are strongly associated with the choice to work in a rural area upon graduation from medical school (Brooks et al. 2002; Freeman, Ferrer, and Greiner 2007). Individuals who enter medical school at an older age are also more likely to become primary care physicians and work in underserved areas. Age may be a factor because the younger generation wants a good work-life balance.

Educational factors also influence choice of location. Medical schools that have rural curricula and rotations and a positive attitude toward rural practice are more successful in producing physicians who practice in rural areas (Brooks et al. 2002; Rabinowitz et al. 2008; Rourke 2008), while those that emphasize family practice have more graduates in family practice (Brooks et al. 2002). Scholarships and loan repayment programs tied to rural practice upon graduation also increase rural supply (Friedman 2008).

The difference between urban and rural communities and work environments may contribute to physician practice patterns. Urban areas are more attractive to healthcare professionals because of their "social, cultural, and professional advantages" (Dussault and Franceschini 2006). They have better transportation, more opportunities for career advancement, less professional isolation, more employment opportunities for the healthcare professionals and their spouses, better educational access for children, and more cultural amenities and leisure and recreational activities (Brooks et al. 2002; Dussault and Franceschini 2006; Rourke 2008). Rural areas have less specialty support and longer hours of work (Brooks et al. 2002). Finally, lower financial reimbursement in rural areas contributes to the imbalance between rural and urban supply (Brooks et al. 2002).

Factors Related to Physician Dissatisfaction

Dissatisfaction among physicians has several causes. Since dissatisfaction can lead to leaving the profession, these factors are important to consider in forecasting the future physician workforce.[12] These factors include:

- Managed care. Many physicians do not like the administrative paperwork, limitations on referring patients to specialists, financial incentives that could affect clinical decision making, pressures to have a high workload, and limitations on which drugs they can prescribe (Zuger 2004).
- Malpractice. Some physicians have difficulties finding malpractice insurance and paying premiums, and many face high rates of lawsuits (Zuger 2004).
- Discrepancies. The differences between what patients demand and what physicians can actually accomplish, physicians' standards of care and the care that they actually deliver, and how they used to practice medicine and what they must do today can cause frustration (Zuger 2004).
- Lack of time to accomplish necessary tasks. High workloads leave physicians concerned about their ability to provide adequate attention to patients. To add to the distress, the additional administrative tasks involved

with quality improvement and patient safety efforts (such as pay for performance) take away from the time physicians spend with patients (Landon, Reschovsky, and Blumenthal 2003; Mechanic 2003; Zuger 2004).

- Nonmedical responsibilities. Performance of tasks such as administrative paperwork required by insurance companies, government agencies, and courts are seen as a burden (Zuger 2004).
- Erosion of professional autonomy. Utilization review, mandatory use of drug formularies, patient demands, and government regulations diminish physicians' ability to make their own decisions (Landon, Reschovsky, and Blumenthal 2003; Mechanic 2003; Pescosolido 2006).

There are several demographic factors related to working in nursing and the amount of hours an RN chooses to work. Most studies find that as RNs get older, participation in the workforce declines, hours of work decrease, or both changes occur (Askildsen, Baltagi, and Holmas 2003; Buerhaus 1991; Philips 1995). RNs with children in the home work fewer hours (Ezrati 1987; Laing and Rademaker 1990) and may have lower workforce participation rates (Laing and Rademaker 1990). Additional household income is negatively related to both participation and hours of work (Antonazzo et al. 2003; Laing and Rademaker 1990; Link 1992).

Factors Related to RN Supply

The educational system has been a significant factor in RN supply. Current estimates place RN educational system capacity below that needed to maintain adequate supply. There is a severe shortage of educators and clinical settings as evidenced by the turning away of qualified degree applicants (American Association of Colleges of Nursing 2008).

Average wages for RNs tend to be lower than those in other female-dominated professions, and the returns to a baccalaureate education are negative compared to those for an associate degree (Booton and Lane 1985; Chiha and Link 2003; Nowak and Preston 2001). Higher wages should have a positive effect on the choice to work in nursing; however, empirical studies do not show this clearly. Several studies find that wages have a positive effect (Bentham 1971; Ezrati 1987; Parker and Rickman 1996; Philips 1995; Schumacher 1997; Skatun et al. 2005). Other studies find no effect (Chiha and Link 2003; Laing and Rademaker 1990; Link 1992).

Several studies find that the elasticity of RN supply response to wages is small (Askildsen, Baltagi, and Holmas 2003; Philips 1995; Skatun et al. 2005), meaning that a large increase in wages would be needed to induce an increase in the number of RNs (conversely, a large drop in wages would be needed to cause RNs to leave nursing). A 2003 examination of the historical relationship between wage increases and growth of RN supply estimated that inflation-adjusted wages must rise 3.2 to 3.8 percent per year to induce a supply growth of 6.2 percent per year and create equilibrium in the labor market by 2020. Between 2003 and 2016, wages would have to cumulatively rise 55 to 69 percent, with total spending for RNs more than doubling (Spetz and Given 2003).

The effect of wages on hours of work in nursing is also questionable. Some studies find that higher wages are related to more hours of work (Buerhaus 1991; Chiha and Link 2003), while some do not (Ezrati 1987; Laing and Rademaker 1990). Other studies show a backward bend in the relationship between hours of work and wages (Link and Settle 1981, 1985). Many studies are not set up to capture nonlinearity in supply, which may explain the inconsistent results among these studies.

Working conditions, such as staffing levels, workload, degree of autonomy, scheduling, overtime, and professional development, may influence the decisions to work in nursing and how many hours to work (Buerhaus et al. 2006; Unruh and Fottler 2005). A few studies show a strong relationship between work environment and retention of RNs. In a survey by Stone and colleagues (2006), 17 percent of the RNs reported their intent to leave the profession within one year. Over 50 percent of these RNs cited working conditions as a major reason. Control over their practice setting and professional collaboration were important factors in their intent to leave the profession (Stone et al. 2006). In another study, the primary professional reasons for leaving nursing are salary, inadequate staffing, scheduling, lack of administrative support, and lack of time for patient care (Fottler and Widra 1995).

RNs' intent to quit nursing can be related to how satisfied they are with their jobs (Larrabee et al. 2003). The top factors creating dissatisfaction are inadequate staffing, high workload, high work pressure, high job demands, and lack of time to do adequate work. Adequate staffing, balanced workload, and the ability to provide quality patient care are high on the list of satisfiers (Aiken et al. 2002; Demerouti et al. 2000; Dunn, Wilson, and Esterman 2005; Geiger-Brown et al. 2004; Khowaja, Merchant, and Hirani 2005; Shaver and Lacey 2003; Sheward et al. 2005). Other factors include the following:

- Rewards, appreciation, and respect (Khowaja, Merchant, and Hirani 2005)
- Supervisor support (Khowaja, Merchant, and Hirani 2005)
- Empowerment/ability to voice opinion (Trovey and Adams 1999)
- Relationships with physicians (Spence-Laschinger, Shamian, and Thomson 2001)
- Quality of patient care (Spence-Laschinger, Shamian, and Thomson 2001)

Finally, immigration to and emigration from the United States of qualified RNs affect supply. There is currently a large net immigration of RNs to the United States, resulting in a larger U.S. supply than would be available otherwise. The 2000 estimate of the number of RNs in the United States who received their nursing education abroad was 219,000. In 2005 alone,

15,000 foreign-educated RNs passed U.S. licensing exams (Aiken 2007). In that year, the United States surpassed all other countries in the importation of nurses.

Forecasting Models

The model used to forecast labor supply and demand will determine which of the factors just discussed are included in the analysis and how they are related to each other. Forecasts of healthcare workforce demand and supply use different models, each of which produces different results. Underlying these different approaches are fundamental *assumptions* about the status and evolution of the U.S. healthcare system. For example, models that assume that current spending is reasonable (or that even more is needed) tend to predict future physician deficits, whereas models that assume that spending or utilization could be reduced through changes in healthcare delivery tend to predict future physician adequacy or surplus. It is difficult to know which assumptions will hold in the future. In this section we introduce some of the models that are used to forecast the future adequacy of physician and RN supply given demand.

Healthcare workforce forecasting models include the Graduate Medical Education National Advisory Committee (GMENAC) models for the physician workforce beginning in the early 1980s, the Council on Graduate Medical Education (COGME) models for the physician workforce, and the Bureau of Health Professions (BHPr) models for physicians and RNs (Blumenthal 2004; Greenberg and Cultice 1997; McNutt 1981). In 2002, Cooper and colleagues developed a model that links the demand for healthcare services to the growth of the economy. The authors observe that over a 40-year period, for each 1 percent increase in gross domestic product (GDP), overall healthcare spending has increased 1.5 percent on average and spending on physicians by 0.75 percent. They therefore assume that for every 1 percent increase in GDP, demand for physicians will grow by 0.75 percent (Cooper et al. 2002; Cooper 2004). The Cooper model includes other assumptions related to patient acuity, population growth, physician work effort, and the use of NPs as substitutes.

Cooper's model has the advantage of being simple and of recognizing the important link between overall economic demand and healthcare demand. The model's projection can be a guidepost for future demand for physicians if changes in delivery are not made.

Critics of the Cooper model believe that by projecting existing rates of utilization/GDP into the future, Cooper and colleagues do not deal with the needs of patients or the appropriateness of care and ignore the possibility that up to 50 percent of healthcare could be unnecessary or inappropriate (Barer 2002). Critics also argue that supplier-induced demand could contribute to the overuse of services (Barer 2002; Garber and Sox 2004). As Reinhardt (2002, 166) says, "On that hypothesis, the nation's physician supply . . . has a life of its own and during the past three decades has dragged up per capita use of physician services in tow." Another criticism is that this model does not include prices of healthcare and wages of healthcare workers as a determinant. Therefore, there is no limit to the amount of healthcare services that can be demanded (Garber and Sox 2004).

A model developed by Goodman and Grumbach (2008) takes into account changes in the healthcare system that could lead to a much lower demand for physicians. Their approach is to set performance goals for the system and consider how those goals would be furthered by investment in more physicians versus other investments. With this approach historical utilization patterns are not taken as a given.

We end this section with a final caveat regarding forecasting models. No one model will provide an absolutely accurate prediction of the future. All models have limitations due to the multiple interacting factors that determine demand and supply, the unpredictability of future interactions and their impact on demand and supply, and the degree of accuracy of model assumptions and structure. Based on the complexities and uncertainties involved in modeling, it is good to heed Dovey and colleagues (2002, 95), who advise that it is better to use models to "monitor and adjust rather than as a definitive prediction from which policy changes with profound effects might arise."

8.5 Will the Healthcare Workforce Be Adequate in the Future?

This section discusses predictions of the future adequacy of the physician and nursing workforces based on the forecasting models described in the section above.

Forecasts of Future Physician Adequacy

Between 1980 and 1996 the GMENAC, COGME, and BHPr models predicted future physician surpluses (Cooper 2004; Snyderman, Sheldon, and Bischoff 2002). Since 2000, thinking has changed. The 2005 COGME forecast projects a *shortage* of 85,000 to 96,000 physicians by 2020 (approximately 8.5 to 10 percent of the current workforce), and recommends expanding the workforce by 3 percent by 2020 (COGME 2005). In 2006 the Bureau of Health Professions projected a shortage ranging from 55,000 to 150,000 by 2020, with a shortage of specialists making up the largest portion (Bureau of Health Professions 2006b).

These predictions have been bolstered by forecasts from Cooper and colleagues that predict significant shortages in the future (Cooper et al. 2002; Cooper 2004). Given a growth in GDP of around 2 percent per year, researchers predict a growth of 1.1 to 1.5 percent per year in the demand for physician services. They predict a physician shortage of approximately 6 percent in 2010, and 20 percent by 2020 (Cooper et al. 2002). The correlation between GDP and specialty physicians is even stronger, so this model predicts that the demand for specialty services will increase much faster than that for primary care services (Blumenthal 2004).

Other estimates that take the growth of physician substitutes and complements into consideration raise doubts about physician shortage predictions. Although the number of new physician graduates each year has been stable for the past few decades, the number of NPs, PAs, and IMGs has grown considerably. Of the 35,000 new medical care trainees in 2006, only around one-half had an MD or a DO from the United States, 32 percent were NPs or PAs, and 17 percent were doctors who had trained outside the United States (Weiner 2007). A needs-based model estimates that better workforce distribution could possibly eliminate the need for large increases in physicians overall (Dovey et al. 2002; Goodman and Grumbach 2008).

Some feel that we do not know enough about future changes in the supply, demand, and price of healthcare to be able to predict the future adequacy of the physician workforce with confidence.

> In short, we've barely begun to do the necessary homework before we start building new medical schools. Even when we have done our homework, increasing the supply of physicians gradually, in small increments—ones that would not require major new investments in capital or teaching personnel—is a prudent strategy. (Garber and Sox 2004, 734)

In summary, there is little agreement about the future supply of physicians. According to David Blumenthal (2004, 1780), "The debate about the physician workforce is back."

Forecasts of Future RN Adequacy

Forecasts of the future RN workforce have been made using the BHPr models for RNs (Bureau of Health Professions 2002).[13] These models predict that from 2000 to 2020, RN demand will grow 40 percent but supply will increase only 6 percent (Bureau of Health Professions 2002). By 2020 the gap between the number of RNs demanded and the number supplied will be 29 percent. When the BHPr results are weighted for population growth, Unruh and Fottler (2005) find that RN demand per U.S. resident is projected to grow 18 percent in this time period, while supply per resident will fall 11 percent. The BHPr forecast and its weighted estimates indicate that increasing demand and lagging supply will be major contributors to the projected gap.

A series of articles by Buerhaus and colleagues assess how some of the predictors of RN supply will affect RN demand and supply in the future (Buerhaus, Staiger, and Auerbach 2000a, 2000b, 2008; Buerhaus et al. 2006). The aging of the RN workforce is a major factor in future supply, because a greater proportion of the workforce will be retiring (Buerhaus, Staiger, and Auerbach 2000a). Stressful work environments may further contribute to supply attrition (Buerhaus et al. 2006). Given the past growth in demand for RNs of around 2 to 3 percent per year, compared to a much slower projected growth for RN supply, the authors estimate that the deficit of RNs will grow to 16 percent by 2025 (Buerhaus, Staiger, and Auerbach 2008).

Other factors pointing to a future supply deficit include the educator shortage and the stagnant growth of new RN graduates (American Association of Colleges of Nursing 2008). This reduced inflow combined with increased outflows from retiring RNs and those leaving the workforce due to workplace issues make estimates of future RN supply look grim. The interaction between physician and RN supply and demand will also affect supply. If, for example, RNs are used to fill the gap in physician primary care in the future, this will exacerbate the RN shortage (Friedman 2008).

8.6 The Effect of Healthcare Workforce on Access, Quality, and Expenditures

An adequate supply of qualified healthcare professionals and nonprofessionals is essential to providing quality care at a reasonable cost. In this section we review studies that have been conducted on the effects of physician and RN supply on access to care and the quality and costs of care.

Effects of Workforce Supply on Access to Care

The literature on access to healthcare services suggests that the geographical supply of physicians and RNs affects access to healthcare. Rosenthal, Zaslavsky, and Newhouse (2005) find that residents of metropolitan areas have better access to physicians. The further one lives from an urban center, the lower the physician-to-population ratio becomes and the farther one must travel to get care. Geographical maldistribution creates pockets of medically underserved communities while other communities have excess supply (Forrest 2006). According to Forrest (2006, 1062), "Market forces have failed to supply physicians where they are needed. Large numbers of uninsured Americans lack access to care, and as many as 50 million live in communities that the federal government designates as health professional shortage areas."

Primary care shortages also affect access. Friedman (2008) reports that federally designated "primary care shortage" areas are growing. In a 2004 survey of federally funded CHCs, 13.3 percent of family physician positions, respectively, were vacant, 20.8 percent of obstetrician and gynecologist positions were vacant, and 10.6 and 9 percent of RN and NP positions were vacant. Rural CHCs had a higher percentage of vacancies and took longer to fill them (Rosenblatt et al. 2006).

Shortages of healthcare personnel are also affecting plans to improve access to care. Rosenblatt and colleagues (2006) found that workforce shortages are limiting the expansion of CHCs that provide care to underserved populations. The state of Massachusetts does not have enough primary care physicians to meet the healthcare demand from the residents who are newly insured under the state's universal coverage program initiated in 2007 (Friedman 2008). As Friedman (2008) notes, "Waits for an appointment are very long—like over a year for a physical examination" (1).

Nurse practitioners are taking up some of the slack. The number of NPs nationwide has grown from 30,000 in 1990 to 115,000 in 2008 (Friedman 2008). Approximately 250 primary care centers are run by NPs.

Effects of Workforce Supply on Quality of Care

With regard to physician services overall, a few studies indicate that more may not be better. Patient satisfaction with care, perceptions of access to care, and outcomes are no better in regions with more physicians per population (Goodman and Fisher 2008). Medicare beneficiaries in areas with high physician supply do not report better access to physicians or higher satisfaction with care (Fisher et al. 2003a, 2003b). Quality indicators, such as use of beta-blockers after myocardial infarction, are not higher in areas with more physicians (Fisher et al. 2003a, 2003b). Additionally, there is no relationship between overall physician supply and the stage of breast cancer at diagnosis (Ferrante et al. 2000).

There appears, however, to be a difference between primary care and specialty care on the health of the populace. Studies show a positive relationship between the numbers of primary care physicians and population health, and a negative relationship between the numbers of specialty physicians and population health. Several studies indicate that higher primary care physician-to-population ratios are associated with longer life expectancy; lower age-adjusted mortality; lower mortality from heart disease, stroke, and cancer; lower neonatal mortality; and lower incidence of low infant birth weight (Shi 1994; Shi et al. 2003a, 2003b, 2004). The supply of primary care physicians at the county level is related to detecting colorectal cancer at an earlier stage (Roetzheim et al. 1999). The supply of primary care is also related to early detection of breast and cervical cancers (Ferrante et al. 2000; Campbell et al. 2003). Adults with a primary care physician have lower five-year mortality and 33 percent lower annual healthcare expenditures (Franks and Fiscella 1998). Finally, primary care is associated with a more equitable distribution of health compared to specialty care (Starfield, Shi, and Macinko 2005).

In contrast, a higher specialist physician-to-population ratio is associated with lower life expectancy and higher age-adjusted mortality, higher mortality from heart disease and cancer, higher neonatal mortality, and a higher incidence of low infant birth weight (Shi 1994; Shi et al. 2003b). A greater use of specialty care is associated with detecting colorectal cancer at a later stage (Roetzheim et al. 1999), and with lower quality in general (Baicker and Chandra 2004). Other studies find that quality and outcomes of care are no better or are worse in areas with higher ratios of specialists to Medicare population (Fisher et al. 2003a, 2003b).

In an international context, countries with more primary care physicians have lower mortality rates, but the same does not apply to specialty physicians (Starfield et al. 2005). Forrest (2006) writes that "there is no evidence that more specialty care improves population health. Nations with a strong primary care infrastructure have better health outcomes than those such as the United States that emphasize specialty medicine" (1062). Starfield and colleagues concur: "Increasing the supply of specialists will not improve the United States' position in population health relative to other industrialized countries, and it is likely to lead to greater disparities in health status and outcomes" (Starfield et al. 2005, W5-97).

In summary, "there is considerable evidence for the benefits [on health outcomes] of an increase in supply of primary care physicians, and no evidence for a similar effect for specialists" (Starfield et al. 2005, W5-102). The differences in outcomes between primary and specialty care could be due to a number of factors, including the importance of primary care to vulnerable populations (Forrest 2006) or the adverse effects from inappropriate or unnecessary specialist care (Starfield et al. 2005). Primary care physicians tend to see problems in their early stages, have a more holistic approach to care, and have long-term relationships with patients, while specialists see patients with more advanced stages of illness, do not deal with anything other than the particular illness, and do not maintain long-term relationships with patients (Rosser 1996).

With RNs, most studies show that higher nurse staffing in hospitals and nursing homes is associated with lower rates of patient mortality and adverse events (Kane et al. 2007; Harrington et al. 2000). In hospitals, higher RN or licensed nurse (RNs and LPNs) staffing is related to lower rates of

- falls (Dunton et al. 2004; Krauss et al. 2005; Unruh 2003; Whitman et al. 2002),
- failure to rescue (death of a patient following a life-threatening complication) (Aiken et al. 2002, 2003; Needleman et al. 2002),
- upper gastrointestinal bleed (Needleman et al. 2002),
- medication errors (Whitman et al. 2002),
- mortality (Aiken et al. 2003; Elting et al. 2005; Mark et al. 2004; Person et al. 2004; Rothberg et al. 2005),
- pneumonia (Cho 2003; Kovner et al. 2002; Needleman et al. 2002; Unruh 2003),
- pulmonary compromise (Unruh 2003),
- shock (Needleman et al. 2002),

- skin breakdown (Unruh 2003),
- surgical or treatment complications (Dang 2002), and
- urinary tract infections (Needleman et al. 2002; Unruh 2003).

Higher RN staffing in nursing homes is related to lower resident mortality (Cohen and Spector 1996), fewer deficiencies (Harrington et al. 2000), and better scores on quality indicators (Rantz et al. 1997; Unruh, Zhang, and Wan 2006; Wan, Zhang, and Unruh 2006).

The positive effect of nurse staffing on patient outcomes is believed to be due to the need for adequate numbers and skill levels of nursing personnel to properly care for patients. In hospitals and nursing homes where staffing levels are low, patient safety and quality of care may be compromised. On the other hand, the relationship between nurse staffing and patient outcomes may not be positive at higher levels of staffing. If staffing continues to increase past an optimum point, the gains in quality could end or become negative (Hendrix and Foreman 2001; Zhang et al. 2006).

Effects of Workforce Shortages or Surpluses on Expenditures

There is some evidence that healthcare costs are higher in regions with more physicians in general (Fisher et al. 2003a, 2003b; Goodman and Fisher 2008).[14] As with access and quality, however, higher regional expenses may be more closely associated with the number of specialists in a region than with primary care physicians. In two papers, Fisher and colleagues report that a higher ratio of specialists to Medicare population is related to higher surgical rates and expenditures; higher-spending areas are related to higher utilization of specialists; and quality and outcomes of care are no better or are worse in high-spending areas (Fisher et al. 2003a, 2003b). Baicker and Chandra (2004) find lower costs in states with a greater use of primary care physicians, and the opposite in states with a greater use of specialists. Friedman (2008) observes that a shortage of primary care physicians is related to a higher use of the emergency room. Finally, when patients are treated for pneumonia by specialists rather than generalists, their treatment costs are higher with no difference in outcomes (Whittle et al. 1998). This occurs even when pneumonia etiology and comorbidities are taken into account.

With RNs, the main issue is whether it is cost effective to use a greater proportion of RNs to other nursing staff (skill mix), a higher RN-to-patient ratio, or both. While higher RN skill mix or RN-to-patient ratios could increase total labor costs, these higher levels of staffing may be more productive and could result in lower average costs per patient. Studies of the productivity effect, however, have mixed results (Glandon, Colbert, and Thomasma 1989; Bloom, Alexander, and Nuchols 1997). Another way in which higher RN staffing could be cost effective is by contributing to nurse satisfaction, which may reduce job turnover, which is estimated to cost around $82,000 per turnover (Jones 2008). While the cost savings of lower RN turnover may not be greater than the costs of hiring additional RNs, it offsets those costs to some degree (Needleman 2008).

Higher RN-to-patient ratios or higher RN proportions are also thought to be cost effective because they are related to shorter patient lengths of stay (Brown, Sturman, and Simmering 2002) and fewer adverse events, thus saving the hospital added patient days and resources. Based on the cost savings from reduced patient adverse events, Needleman and colleagues (2006) find that raising the proportion of RNs without increasing the licensed nurse hours of care is the only staffing strategy that would result in a net financial benefit. Needleman and colleagues and Rothberg and colleagues (2005) find that increasing the RN-to-patient ratio decreases costs by lowering patient mortality and adverse events. However, the cost savings from the lower patient mortality and adverse events never completely offset the higher labor costs from increasing the RN-to-patient ratio. Additionally, as the RN-to-patient ratio increases, the cost effectiveness declines. This is because there is an incrementally less positive effect on patient outcomes (and therefore costs) with each additional increase in the RN-to-patient ratio.

8.7 Public and Private Policies to Optimize the Healthcare Workforce

The research we reviewed in this chapter has shown that healthcare labor markets are complicated and do not operate like perfectly competitive markets. Prospective payment and fixed prices of public programs like Medicare and Medicaid influence healthcare institutions' demand for healthcare labor. Substantial educational requirements and professional regulation impose barriers to supply entry. Local markets may have elements of monopsononistic power. Wages and salary tend to be "sticky." When wages do change, demand and supply may not readily respond. Consequently, it is common for healthcare labor markets to experience imbalances.

As a result, it is unlikely that the healthcare labor markets alone can solve the issues of workforce adequacy, access, quality, and costs without governmental intervention. However, public policies attempting to realign these markets must take care not to make things worse. For example, increasing the total numbers of physicians won't necessarily improve the primary–specialty or urban–rural imbalances. The policies could even exacerbate existing maldistributions. For example, increased funding for graduate medical education (GME), if distributed unevenly (e.g., fewer dollars to public hospitals), could *reduce* the number of physicians trained to work with underserved populations (Shipman, Lurie, and Goodman 2004). This is why estimates and projections of healthcare needs, demand, and supply in the individual markets (including the workforce distribution within the markets) and knowledge of the interactions of those markets are important, and why those analyses must be the basis of healthcare workforce planning.

With careful analyses and planning, policy changes could improve the functioning of the healthcare labor markets. In the following subsections we suggest some of the possibilities that emerge from the research literature.

Optimizing Demand for the Healthcare Workforce

Usually healthcare workforce planning focuses on finding ways to match supply to demand expectations. Methods of stabilizing or reducing per capita healthcare utilization, which could then reduce demand for the healthcare workforce, are often bypassed. This is especially important as the United States considers providing universal coverage, which would increase the number of people demanding healthcare. Several authors recommend a more coordinated prevention approach (Goodman and Fisher 2008; Goodman and Grumbach 2008; Forrest 2006). Friedman (2008) lists specific polices, which include coordination of care to reduce duplicate services and waste; disease management to help patients cope with their conditions and achieve a high quality of life; prevention of avoidable problems through immunization, screening, and counseling; and early detection of disease.

Optimizing Physician Supply

Both the Association of American Medical Colleges (AAMC) and COGME recommend increases in the physician workforce. COGME recommends expanding the workforce by 3 percent by 2020 (COGME 2005). AAMC would like to see a 30-percent expansion of medical schools and a lifting of the cap on Medicare funding for graduate medical education (Association of American Medical Colleges 2006; Goodman and Fisher 2008). Yet there is enough controversy over the estimates of current and future physician supply and enough uncertainty about the future direction of healthcare demand to recommend caution about making such general increases.

Goodman and Fisher (2008) discuss several additional reasons to be cautious about a general increase in physician supply.

1. Physicians do not choose to go to areas where the need is greatest. Between 1979 and 1999, four out of five new physicians settled in regions where the supply was already high.
2. Given reimbursement systems that favor procedure-oriented specialties, unrestricted expansion of graduate medical education would probably make the primary care–specialty imbalances worse.
3. Expansion of physician supply will be expensive. If supply were expanded by 30 percent, authors estimate that the costs would be $5 billion to $10 billion per year, depending on the number of specialists

trained. Plans to increase physician supply "should be crafted to reduce, not exacerbate, regional disparities" (Goodman and Fisher 2008, 1660).

Whether overall physician supply is increased or not, policies that encourage a better distribution of physicians across practice and geographical settings are needed. The box on page 283 lists several policies that could improve these areas. We briefly discuss the first two from this list: revising medical school curricula and offering loan repayments that use incentives to practice in areas of need upon graduation.

Changing medical school curricula to emphasize primary care and rural practice has a positive effect on the student selection of those practices. Curriculum change should include class time and clinical time in the area. The Minnesota Rural Physician Associate Program, which puts medical students through an intensive curriculum of community-based healthcare, was found to have a 59 percent participant recruitment rate to rural areas (Brooks et al. 2002). Voluntary rotation of medical students through a rural preceptorship in Colorado made those students more likely to practice in a rural area (Brooks et al. 2002). Other studies show similar effects.

Reducing a physician's medical school debt by offering loan repayment programs linked to practicing in areas of need could also increase primary care physicians and practice in underserved areas. These programs, offered by federal, state, and local governments and private organizations, repay medical school loans in exchange for recipient practice in a medically underserved area such as community health centers, public hospitals, and public health settings (Friedman 2008). Most contracts require a two- to four-year service commitment upon graduation.

Optimizing RN Supply

Policies regarding the RN workforce must address inadequate recruitment of new RNs into the workforce, problems retaining RNs, and immigration issues. To increase the number of individuals going into nursing, the most important policy is to increase the capacity of the educational system. Due to a severe shortage of nurse educators, one of the most important policies for improving educational capacity is to increase the number of RN faculty. Schools of nursing also need more classroom space and practicum opportunities in hospitals and other clinical sites.

Increasing the number of RN educators has a demand and a supply component. On the demand side, the number of faculty positions in nursing schools could be augmented through private, state, or federal grants. In January 2007 the Nurse Education, Expansion, and Development Act (NEED Act) was introduced in the U.S. House of Representatives and a companion bill was introduced in the Senate that would amend Title VIII of the Public Health Service Act to authorize capitation grants for schools of nursing to

Policies for Improving the Distribution of Physicians

Experts have suggested the following policies to reduce imbalances in physician primary and specialty care and in physician geographical location. Although the list is not all inclusive, it suggests that there are many ways to approach distribution issues. It should be noted that the placement in the list does not indicate priority or relative effectiveness, as it is not known which of the policies are more effective than others. Some of the suggestions may be rather controversial, such as preadmission assessment of student attitudes toward primary care.

- Revise medical school curricula to increase the focus on primary and rural care (Brooks et al. 2002).
- Offer more loan repayment programs that use incentives to practice in areas of need upon graduation (Weiner 2007).
- Expand Title VII funding. Title VII funding, which reduces medical student debt, has been found to increase the number of medical school graduates who become family physicians in rural and low-income areas. The thinking is that if students have less debt upon graduation, they are more likely to choose primary care in underserved areas (Friedman 2008).
- Keep a funding cap for GME education to prevent unrestricted expansion of GME while targeting funding for primary care residencies and geriatric and palliative care fellowships (Goodman and Fisher 2008).
- Increase GME payments to programs with more primary care residents (Berkowitz 2004). This program, similar to the previous policy, would encourage growth in the capacity of primary care curricula, facilities, and educators in medical schools.
- Change medical school entry practices to select students who are more likely to practice in rural areas. This would be done through preadmission assessment of students' attitudes and interests (Brooks et al. 2002; Freeman, Ferrer, and Greiner 2007).
- Change reimbursement systems to better reward primary care and to reduce the relative income disparity between primary care and specialty physicians (Dovey et al. 2002; Goodman and Fisher 2008). The Medicare Payment Advisory Committee, an independent congressional agency that advises the government on healthcare payment issues, has recommended that Medicare pay primary care physicians more, but an issue that arises is where to obtain the money (Friedman 2008).
- Promote systems that rely on primary care providers, such as prepaid group practices, integrated delivery systems, and reform of Medicare payment (Goodman and Grumbach 2008).

increase the number of faculty and students (American Association of Colleges of Nursing 2008). Capitation grant programs have been used effectively to address past nursing shortages. State governments, private endowments and foundations, and individual hospitals are additional sources of funding for increased faculty positions (Yordy 2006).

A problem on the supply side of the RN faculty shortage is that not enough RNs go on to get advanced degrees and become educators. For the RNs who do get advanced degrees, education does not pay as well as other employment opportunities. Nursing school faculty are paid much less than advance practice nurses in nonacademic jobs (around $50,000 per year for faculty compared to $80,000 for nonacademic advance practice jobs) (Maryland Statewide Commission on the Crisis in Nursing 2005). Federal and state governments and private foundations could increase the supply of RN educators by increasing funding for graduate school scholarships and loans and by providing funding to increase RN faculty pay and benefits. For example, in 2007, Virginia increased state university nursing faculty salaries by 10 percent (UVaToday 2007). Other states, such as Idaho, are looking into similar salary increases (Russell 2007). An example of private support for graduate school scholarships is the Robert Wood Johnson Foundation's career development award, administered by its Nurse Faculty Scholars Program (Robert Wood Johnson Foundation 2008).

As the educational system's capacity enlarges, policies that increase the matriculation of nursing students can be implemented. Private, state, or federal grants can be awarded to schools or individuals to increase the number of students entering nursing. The NEED Act of 2007 calls for an increase in funding to nursing students. In addition to financial inducements, attracting individuals into the profession of nursing is important. Media campaigns on the importance of nursing have been common, but perhaps the most important inducement will be to improve the work environment so that the work of nursing is attractive compared with other professions.

Retention of RNs is as important as improving the inflow of nurses. Improving the work environment is paramount in retention. Section 8.4 listed work environment factors that have been shown to affect the satisfaction and job retention of nurses. Although improvements in these areas require changes at the institutional level, public policy can influence or even regulate these changes. For example, mandatory staffing ratios (as enacted in California) require certain levels of nurse staffing at the institutional level. Such regulations, however, are heavy-handed and controversial.[15] A less authoritarian approach is a national recognition program that encourages hospitals to create positive work environments. Two programs that have been associated with positive hospital work environments are the Magnet Recognition Program and Transforming Care at the Bedside (TCAB). Magnet Recognition is awarded by the American Nurses Credentialing Center to hospitals that meet a number of standards indicating excellence in nursing services (American Nurses Credentialing Center 2008). TCAB has multiple goals, among which are creating a satisfying and supportive workplace and increasing the time nurses spend at the bedside (Robert Wood Johnson Foundation 2008).

Some aspects of RN attrition, such as the retirement of older RNs, cannot be helped. However, policies can be adopted that keep older individuals in the workforce longer, such as reducing workloads, improving the ergonomics of the workplace, and offering non–patient care roles for the older RN workforce (Norman et al. 2005).

RN immigration policies must also be considered. On the positive side, immigration helps boost RN supply and ease the current shortage, although so far it has not been enough to close the gap completely. Immigration also contributes to enhancing ethnic and racial diversity in the nursing profession, although the increase so far has been mostly in Asian nurses, not in Latino or black nurses, who are underrepresented in the profession.

On the negative side, a reliance on immigration can postpone the domestic demand or supply changes needed to reduce the gap. In other words, boosting the supply of U.S. RNs through the importation of foreign graduates reduces the incentive to expand educational capacity, increase matriculates, raise wages, or improve working conditions in the United States. As a consequence, future shortages could be exacerbated, especially if the flow of foreign graduates slows down in the future, or if foreign-educated nurses react as do U.S.-educated nurses to poor work environments by becoming dissatisfied and leaving the profession.[16]

An additional consideration is the effect of immigration on the emigrating countries. Working as an RN in the United States is an attractive opportunity for individuals in other countries because of the higher salaries and other professional opportunities. It is so attractive that non-RN healthcare professionals, such as physicians, are retraining to become RNs (Aiken 2007). However, it may create or exacerbate healthcare workforce shortages in the emigrating countries.

With these points in mind, a prudent immigration policy would be—as suggested by Aiken (2007)—to "manage" nurse migration internationally. This policy would "include provisions to balance the rights of individual nurse migrants and their families, the interests of their countries of origin, patient concerns about quality and communication, and employers' needs" (Aiken 2007, 1315).

At the same time, immigration should not be considered a long-term solution to the nursing shortage in the United States. Improvements in the matriculation and retention of RNs must continue even if immigration eases the current shortage somewhat. Furthermore, developing policies to level the playing field internationally would slow the flow of emigration from countries with much lower wages and less rewarding professional nurse roles. Since research indicates that large wage increases would be needed to affect migration, policies that focus on nonwage changes such as improving the professional role of nurses in emigrating countries have been suggested (Aiken 2007).

8.8 Chapter Summary

This chapter introduced the U.S. healthcare workforce as a set of interconnected labor markets that are substitutes for and complements of each other. Economic theory of labor markets predicts that they have typical demand and supply responses to wages and other economic changes. But these markets also have characteristics that cause them to respond differently than perfectly competitive markets would. For example, professional barriers such as licensing and long educational periods limit supply and slow supply responses to shortages. Market power in the form of monopsony or oligopsony can keep wages and employment below equilibrium levels.

Healthcare labor markets, therefore, do not meet many of the assumptions of perfectly competitive markets. Because these markets are imperfectly competitive, if left to themselves, they will have recurrent or persistent imbalances. The physician market is noted for its significant geographical and specialty imbalances. Nursing is noted for chronic shortages, especially in direct care settings.

Policies that intervene in the markets to improve their functioning can be developed, but policymakers must be careful that interventions are based on accurate information about current and future demand and supply so that the policies will not have unintended consequences. The accuracy of forecasts of future demand and supply depends upon the assumptions and type of model used.

According to several forecasts, unless the physician workforce is expanded there will be a future physician shortage. Some experts caution that more physicians overall may not improve the existing primary care–specialty and urban–rural maldistributions of physicians. Rather than an expansion of the physician workforce, they say, redistribution is needed. With the nursing workforce, there is no disagreement that the workforce must be expanded and more nurses must be retained in order to avoid a severe shortage in the future.

The chapter closed with several policies to optimize the physician and nursing workforces. A demand-side policy was suggested to reduce demand for the healthcare workforce by reducing healthcare utilization. This could be accomplished through a greater emphasis on coordination of healthcare, disease management, and prevention. To improve physician distribution, policy recommendations included changing medical school curricula and providing loans to medical students in exchange for service in underserved areas. RN supply could be increased by expanding the educational system, increasing new graduates, and retaining more RNs in the profession by improving working conditions.

Notes

1. One other issue of importance to economists and policymakers—the extent to which physicians induce demand for their services—was covered in Section 6.1.
2. This table, compiled from 2007 and 2008 data from the Bureau of Labor Statistics (BLS), does not include all occupations in the healthcare workforce. In

particular, it omits many of the assistant and technician roles listed in the BLS *Occupational Outlook Handbook*, and it does not list providers involved with alternative forms of healthcare such as acupuncture and homeopathy.

3. MDs and DOs are similar. They have a similar education, and both can practice in all of the various primary care and specialty areas. The main difference between the two is that MDs focus on treating specific illnesses or conditions, while DOs have a more holistic approach and may include musculoskeletal manipulation in their practices.

4. For example, hospitals may extend the usual nursing assistant duties beyond personal care (bathing, feeding, position, and assisting with getting out of bed), to include tasks normally assigned to RNs such as taking vital signs, changing dressings, or inserting urinary catheters.

5. Higher wages may at some point lead to fewer hours of work and a backward-bending labor supply curve, as illustrated in Figure 6.2.

6. The discussion in the remainder of Section 8.2 is most relevant to the demand and supply of healthcare workers who are employees of a healthcare organization, including professionals such as physicians. However, it also applies to independently practicing professionals, such as a significant sector of the physician workforce.

7. Section 2.2 discusses diminishing marginal productivity and provides examples.

8. This is a simplification, because elasticity actually changes along demand or supply curves, with the upper half becoming progressively more elastic going up the curve, and the lower half becoming progressively more inelastic going down the curve.

9. Present value analysis involves transforming future values into present values through the use of an interest rate that "discounts" the future value to what it would be worth in the present. This is a major component of cost-benefit analysis and cost-effectiveness analysis, but it is not explored in this book.

10. For more about calculating ROI and examples of ROI in healthcare, see the article by Weeks and Wallace (2002).

11. The hours-adjusted internal rate of return is the interest rate that equalizes the present value of future incomes minus the costs, adjusted for the number of hours a person works in a lifetime.

12. It is beyond the scope of this book to discuss these factors in detail. For more information, readers may consult the authors cited in the list.

13. The last BHPr forecast was done in 2002 and was based on 1996 and 2000 demand and supply data from the quadrennial National Sample Survey of RNs, Area Resource Files, Bureau of Labor Statistics, Occupational Employment Statistics, American Hospital Association Annual Survey, National Home and Hospice Care Survey, and other sources (Biviano et al. 2004).

14. The impact of physician-to-population ratios on expenditures was reviewed briefly in the discussion of physician-induced demand in Chapter 6.

15. The controversy over and experience with mandated nurse staffing ratios is beyond the scope of this book. For readers wishing to study this issue more, see Keepnews (2007).

16. Flynn and Aiken (2002) have discovered that foreign-educated nurses react like U.S.-educated nurses to poor work environments: They develop job dissatisfaction, burn out, and leave their jobs.

THE ROLE OF GOVERNMENT

Up to this point, we have argued that market competition in healthcare will not necessarily lead to efficient outcomes—that is, maximum output (health itself, utilization, or satisfaction) at minimum costs. Not only does government involvement have the potential to enhance efficiency, but it is also essential to achieving equitable outcomes. We explore equity and redistribution in Chapter 9, which critiques the central philosophical tenet underlying the presumed advantage of markets—utilitarianism—and presents alternative conceptions of social welfare.

Chapter 10 brings together issues discussed earlier involving demand, supply, and equity by examining the experiences of a number of developed countries. It begins with a discussion of 15 decisions that countries make in organizing their healthcare systems. We then examine these countries' health outcomes and resource expenditures. The chapter ends with ten lessons on the role of government in healthcare systems.

Chapter 11 is a brief conclusion to the book, summarizing the argument that market forces should not be presumed superior to government involvement. Evidence, not theory, must drive the evaluation of alternative systems.

EQUITY AND REDISTRIBUTION

Although economists often focus on efficiency, most people are more concerned about fairness. Daniel Hausman and Michael McPherson (1993, 676) write, "Notions of fairness, opportunity, freedom, and rights are arguably of more importance in policy making than are concerns about moving individuals up their given preference rankings." Issues of equity and redistribution, despite their importance, have not received sufficient attention from health economists.

Section 9.1 summarizes traditional economic theory's treatment of the redistribution of wealth. Section 9.2 critiques this theory, focusing on problems with "ordinal utilitarianism," the philosophy on which most policy conclusions are based. Section 9.3 considers how issues of equity and redistribution relate to health.

9.1 The Traditional Economic Model

Issues of equity and the redistribution of wealth play little part in the traditional microeconomic model. Rather than concerning itself with how people come into possession of their initial stock of wealth, the traditional model devotes nearly all its attention to how they allocate the resources over which they have already been assigned property rights (Young 1994).

Figure 9.1 is a modification of the Edgeworth Box shown in Figure 2.24. For simplicity, we assume that society produces only two goods (X and Y) and that only two people, Paul and Jane, consume these goods. We saw in Chapter 2 that any allocation of the two goods that falls along the contract curve 0–A is economically efficient because no reallocation will make one of the consumers better off without making the other worse off. (Unlike in Chapter 5, we will ignore the issue of envy here.)

With the Edgeworth Box, we can see how any initial allocation of resources will be transformed, through trading, to a final equilibrium. Suppose that Paul is initially endowed with about three-quarters of good X and just less than half of good Y (with Jane getting the remainder of each), as depicted at point D. This is not a Pareto-optimal point, because it is possible to make one or both of the consumers better off. Paul and Jane will therefore engage in trading, and afterward, the final allocation will fall along the contract curve somewhere between points A and B. The exact point depends on the relative bargaining skills of the two people.

FIGURE 9.1: Edgeworth Box

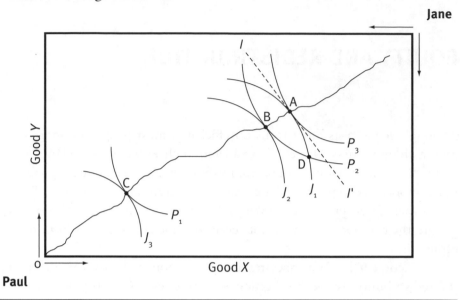

However, only one point on the contract curve will also maximize *social* welfare. (See Section 2.5 for a discussion of social welfare functions.) To reach that point, the economic model assumes that society will engage in redistribution of the initial endowments of wealth until the market reaches equilibrium through trading.

Thus, under the traditional model, competition ensures the efficient use of resources. Wealth is redistributed through the transfer of money (since in the real world there are numerous goods, not just two) to ensure a distribution of resources that is in accordance with society's desires. (The issue of how to carry out such redistribution through taxation, without marring the efficiency brought about by competition, was already addressed in Section 5.1.)

9.2 Problems with the Traditional Model

The traditional model has been criticized for the way it deals (or, perhaps more accurately, does not deal) with equity and fairness and with the distribution of resources. These objections share a common element: They dispute the notion of ordinal utilitarianism, on which the traditional model is based.

This section critiques two of the assumptions listed in Table 3.1:

Assumption 5: Social welfare is solely the sum of individual utilities.
Assumption 14: The distribution of wealth is approved of by society.

Overview of Utilitarianism

Utilitarianism is the philosophy that assumes that social welfare is simply the sum or aggregate of all individuals' welfare. Under this philosophy, utility is a personal psychological perception, and, to the economist, it is based on the goods a person possesses.

As we discussed in Section 2.1, classical utilitarians such as Jeremy Bentham believed that these utilities could be not only quantified, but also added across individuals. Modern economics rebelled against this concept, stressing *ordinal* rather than *cardinal* utility. Under ordinal utility, individuals choose the bundle of goods they prefer over any other instead of quantifying the utility derived from one bundle versus another.[1]

The term "utilitarianism" encompasses a number of seemingly distinct beliefs.[2] As we noted, under classical utilitarianism, individual utilities can be quantified using a metric that is consistent across individuals. Ordinal utilitarianism requires only that individuals be able to rank alternative bundles of goods (which allows economists to employ indifference curves). Under incremental utilitarianism, goods should be put in the hands of those who accrue the most gain from them. One hybrid form of utilitarianism brings intensity of preference into play (e.g., one good brings three times as much utility as another to a person), but does not permit utilities to be added across individuals.[3]

Problems with Ordinal Utilitarianism

This section explores three problems with the modern concept of utilitarianism, each of which has important implications concerning equity and the distribution of wealth. The first problem concerns lack of breadth: Utilitarianism ignores issues of social justice and fairness. Much of the present chapter is devoted to this. The second problem concerns lack of depth: Utilitarianism is defined solely in terms of a single, goods-based, psychological metric, ignoring other potentially important conceptions of what drives individual and social welfare. We touch on this in our description of "extra-welfarism." The third problem is perhaps more practical: Utilitarianism mistakenly assumes that the socially optimal redistribution of wealth should take the form of cash grants rather than transfers of the goods and services themselves. This problem is explored in Section 9.3.

Social Justice and Fairness

Modern economics in general, and utilitarianism in particular, does not concern itself with what is right or fair. Rather, it assumes that the possession of goods brings utility to individuals and therefore to society, which is simply the aggregate of all individuals.

No concern is given to whether the overall distribution of wealth is *justified*. This is not to say that issues of income distribution are ignored. In fact, the people in a society may indeed be concerned about distributional issues and may choose to tax the rich to provide for the poor. But in such a situation, the distribution is the result of *social choice* (as exemplified by the social welfare function) and not necessarily based on *social justice*.

To understand this crucial distinction, consider the difference between altruism and equity. The former is based on preferences. For example, I want the poor to have more, so I provide donations or vote to increase taxes. Providing for the poor makes *me* better off because their welfare enters my utility function. In contrast, according to Adam Wagstaff and Eddy van Doorslaer (1993, 8),

> Social justice (or equity), on the other hand, is not a matter of preference. As [Anthony] Culyer puts it: "the source of value for making judgments about equity lies outside, or is extrinsic to, preferences. . . . The whole point of making a judgment about justice is so to frame it . . . independently of interests of the individual making it." Social justice thus derives from a set of principles concerning what a person ought to have *as a right*.

The best-known modern exposition of social justice and rights is John Rawls's (1971) book *A Theory of Justice*. The next two subsections describe and critique Rawls's viewpoint.

Rawls's Theory   Rawls's theory, which he calls "justice as fairness," provides an alternative to utilitarian philosophy. To determine what is fair, he invokes the "original position," in which people choose the principles of a just society from a position where "no one knows his place in society, his class position or social status, nor does anyone know his fortune in the distribution of natural assets and abilities, his intelligence, strength, and the like" (Rawls 1971, 12). Neither does one know the sort of society in which he or she will be placed. It may be a democracy, or it may be a dictatorship in which there is a small ruling class and the rest of the population is assigned to slavery. Rawls's goal is to determine the system of justice that rational, self-oriented people would choose when placed in the original position.

Rawls (1971, 62) posits that people in the original position would accept the proposition that primary goods, defined as "rights and liberties, powers and opportunities, income and wealth," should "be distributed equally unless an unequal distribution of any, or all, of these values is to everyone's advantage. Injustice, then, is simply inequalities that are not to the benefit of everyone."

The upshot—the system of justice that Rawls believes would be adopted by a society whose members have considered these issues in the original position—is what he calls the "difference principle." Under the difference principle, society is best off only when it makes its worst-off people better off. In other words, society's resources should be devoted to increasing the

FIGURE 9.2: Social Welfare Under Rawls's Theory

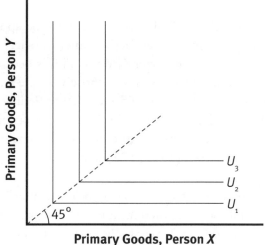

SOURCE: Reprinted by permission of the publisher from *A Theory of Justice* by John Rawls, p. 76, Cambridge, Mass: The Belknap Press of Harvard University Press, Copyright 1971, 1999, by the President and Fellows of Harvard College.

primary goods the most disadvantaged people possess. The only time that resources will go to those who do not occupy the bottom rung is when the benefits of doing so will trickle down to the most disadvantaged group.

This result—that in the original position, people will adopt this method of allocating primary goods—is called "maximin."[4] In essence, people will choose to maximize the lot of those who have the minimum. The unusual nature (at least to an economist) of this philosophy can be seen in Figure 9.2, which shows a set of L-shaped social indifference curves derived under the theory. Let the x-axis be the primary goods enjoyed by person X and the y-axis those enjoyed by person Y. Each curve shows distributions that are equally desirable from society's viewpoint. Higher curves (i.e., those farther from the origin) represent higher levels of social welfare. The 45-degree line shows equal distributions of primary goods.

The indifference curves are L shaped, indicating that society is no better off when Y has more primary goods if those X possesses do not increase. The only way to increase social welfare—that is, to get on a higher indifference curve—is to provide more to the person who has the least.

Why would people, placed in the original position, come up with such a conception of justice? Rawls (1971, 150–51) has a simple answer:

Since it is not reasonable for [a person] to expect more than an equal share in the division of social goods, and since it is not rational for him to agree to less, the sensible thing for him to do is to acknowledge as the first principle of justice one requiring an equal distribution. Indeed, this principle is so obvious that we would expect it to occur to anyone immediately.

Although Rawls's theory is abstract and cannot be applied directly to many problems,[5] one implication overrides all others: Society should engage in far more redistribution than it currently does. This is because many redistributive programs are not targeted solely at those who are worst off in society. Examples in the United States would include the deductibility of home mortgage payments and charitable contributions in the taxation of income. In fact, one could argue that relatively little goes to those who are worst off. In this regard, Gordon Tullock (1979, 172) writes,

> So far as I know there is absolutely no reason to believe that majority voting or any of the variants of democratic government transfer an "optimal" amount. Indeed, I would argue that they do very badly, since the bulk of the transfers they generate are transferred back and forth within the middle class; and, so far as I know, there are no arguments that would indicate that these transfers are desirable.

Although Rawls did not list health as one of the primary goods, some analysts have disagreed with his omission. According to Ronald Green (1976), "Access to health care is not only a social primary good, but possibly one of the most important such goods [because] disease and ill health interfere with our happiness and undermine our self-confidence and self-respect" (120). A universal health plan would offer "basic preventive and therapeutic services" (Green 1976, 120).[6]

Norman Daniels (1985, 2001) has explored the extension of Rawls's theory to health. He notes that

> by keeping people close to normal functioning, healthcare preserves for people the ability to participate in the political, social, and economic life of their society. It sustains them as fully participating citizens . . . in all spheres of social life. . . . By maintaining normal functioning healthcare protects an individual's fair share of the normal range of opportunities (or plans of life) reasonable people would choose in a given society. (Daniels 2001, 3)

Daniels goes on to assert that a universal health insurance program is consistent with a Rawlsian view of a just society. The topic of universal insurance coverage is further explored later in this chapter.

Critique of Rawls's Theory   Although Rawls's theory is usually praised even by its critics, a number of objections have been leveled against it, which are discussed below.

Rawls assumes that rational people would choose the maximin principle to distribute primary goods. Many analysts, particularly economists, disagree, claiming that to reach this conclusion, one must assume a huge amount of risk aversion among the population. Suppose that people were asked to choose between two alternative societies, one in which 95 percent of the people were endowed with $10,000 in resources and the other 5 percent with $1,000, and another society in which everyone was endowed with $1,500. It seems unlikely that most people would choose the latter, but that is what Rawls predicts. Indeed, survey research on how people claim they would behave under the original position indicates that they would prefer the first scenario, so long as they did not view the $1,000 as too low for subsistence. In general, people prefer maximizing average income subject to some minimum constraint or floor to the maximin solution (Miller 1992).

People Would Not Choose Maximin

In fairness to Rawls, however, there are two responses to the above argument. First, Rawls makes it clear that under the original position, one does not know in what kind of society one will be placed. Given that uncertainty, one might choose maximin rather than risk being a member of the (subjugated) masses, so why not choose a system in which resources are equally distributed? In surveys such as those Miller (1992) discusses, people likely imagined themselves in a democratic society like the one they were used to.

Second, although one could argue that Rawls's theory will result in unreasonable choices "on paper," he admits that such odd results might be unlikely under real-world circumstances. In the example, the implication is that, somehow, the subjugation of 5 percent of the population will allow the other 95 percent to accrue far more wealth. In this regard, Rawls (1971, 157) states, "it seems extraordinary that the justice of increasing the expectations of the better placed by a billion dollars, say, should turn on whether the prospects of the least favored increase or decrease by a penny." This is indeed unlikely; testing the validity of the theory using numbers like these might in itself be unfair. Nevertheless, Rawls's theory might sacrifice too much efficiency in return for little equity.

Under Rawls's theory, the group that is worst off receives a greater portion of primary goods. This is not necessarily desirable. Why not help the nearly worst off at the same time you are helping the worst off; might not that be what people would choose in the original position (Sen 1982)?

More Groups Should Receive Favorable Treatment

This raises a related issue: How do we know who is worst off? In the theory, Rawls uses a "representative person" within each subgroup of society. The problem is that some of these representative people may be better off in some characteristics (such as health) and worse off in another (e.g., income). If that is the case, to whom would the first primary goods be assigned? Furthermore, the way society makes decisions clearly demonstrates that not all aspects of a person's background are considered when distributing scarce resources. To give one example from the literature, the fact that you do not get a kidney for transplantation (and therefore must remain on dialysis) will not typically increase your chances of being admitted to a university over other qualified candidates (Young 1994). Societal decision making is typically done on a local rather than a global basis (Elster 1992; Young 1994). Those who decide on college admissions do not decide on kidney allocation, nor do they usually consider such factors.

Other Factors Should Form the Basis of Reallocation

Subsequent material examines other views of welfare (besides utilitarianism), so we will mention this argument only briefly. Just as utilitarianism is limited in its conception of resource distribution, so, it can be argued, is Rawls's theory.

In the theory, the only basis for redistribution is a person's position in society with respect to his possession of primary goods. This viewpoint is limited for the following two reasons:

1. Under the theory, people are entitled to an equal share of resources irrespective of their work effort, motivation, or any other factor. This is because the characteristics a person is born with are according to Rawls, really just the result of a "natural lottery," which "is arbitrary from a moral perspective." As a result, he believes that "[e]ven the willingness to make an effort, to try, and so to be deserving in the ordinary sense is itself dependent on happy family and social circumstances" (Rawls 1971, 74). Thus, if people exhibit a lack of motivation, it is not clear that they should be endowed with a smaller share of primary goods because, in essence, the lack of motivation is not their fault. Needless to say, relying on such criteria to carry out policy could result in a large sacrifice of efficiency.

2. Equalizing resources does not necessarily solve people's problems, because they might not be able to use the resources in a manner that will be of benefit to them. In fact, some people (e.g., the disabled) might need more resources than others.

Nozick's Libertarian Critique of Rawls

As one might imagine, philosophers (and economists) have reached different conclusions about what things people should have as a right. Perhaps Rawls's chief critic was his Harvard colleague Robert Nozick (1974), who proposed an "entitlement theory"—a libertarian philosophy in which the distribution of wealth is just, if (1) the original assignment of wealth was arrived at fairly and (2) the current distribution was arrived at through voluntary exchange.

Nozick develops a conception of a *just* role of government, concluding that this would be a "minimalist state" in which government's role is limited to such things as mutual protection and enforcement of contracts; "any state more extensive violates people's rights" (Nozick 1974, 149). He concludes,

The minimalist state treats us as inviolate individuals, who may not be used in certain ways by others as means of tools or instruments or resources; it treats us as persons having individual rights with the dignity this constitutes. Treating us with respect by respecting our rights, it allows us . . . to choose our life and to realize our ends and our conception of ourselves, insofar as we can, aided by the voluntary cooperation of other individuals possessing the same dignity. How *dare* any state or group of individuals do more. Or less (Nozick 1974, 334–35).

Two aspects of Nozick's entitlement theory pertain to justice. The first is the "principle of justice in acquisition of holdings," which pertains to how a person originally obtains a resource, and the second is the "principle of justice in transfer of holdings," which concerns resources obtained from others. Essentially, Nozick says that if a person originally obtained a resource without violating anyone else's rights, or from another person voluntarily, then he or she is entitled to it.

Unlike Rawls, Nozick believes that people should be able to enjoy the full fruits of any natural advantage they possess. If, say, a person is born smart, and becomes rich as a result, that individual should keep all of her wealth if she did not violate anyone else's rights in obtaining it. Rawls, however, would likely contend that being born smart is a lucky advantage that does not make the person deserving of additional primary resources. Nozick interprets Rawls's view as saying that "everyone has some entitlement or claim on the totality of natural assets . . . with no one having differential claims. The distribution of natural abilities is viewed as a 'collective asset'" (Nozick 1974, 228).

At one point in his book, Nozick uses health as an example. He presents and then refutes an argument made by Bernard Williams (1962), who claimed that societal resources should be redistributed to those in poor health who cannot afford necessary medical care. Nozick (1974, 235) counters that Williams

ignores the question of where the things or actions to be allocated and distributed come from. Consequently, he does not consider whether they come already tied to people who have entitlements over them (surely the case for service activities, which are people's *actions*), people who therefore may decide for themselves to whom they will give the thing and on what grounds.

Many objections can be raised about Nozick's conception of justice. Where does one draw the line on whether a wealthy person acquired his or her resources fairly? What if a person inherited it from a relative who obtained it by questionable means? Perhaps the major objection from a philosophical standpoint is that people who start at a disadvantage are likely to remain at one. Nozick says that holdings that were acquired fairly must not be taken involuntarily from an individual. Who is to say what is a fair way of acquiring resources? And how can it be called fair if some people are born in such a disadvantaged position that they effectively have no way to overcome it? Even Nozick (1974) admits that he is "as well aware as anyone of how sketchy [his] discussion of the entitlement conception of justice in holdings has been" (230). A less charitable view is that it is a philosophy espousing the rule of "finders keepers" (Elster 1992; Stone 2001).

Other Conceptions of Social Welfare

A Theory of Justice was an important book because it provided a base for other alternative conceptions of social welfare. Rawls poked a number of holes in the utilitarian philosophy; since then, others have enlarged them. A few key ideas will be presented here. Those interested in pursuing the topic may wish to consult the references for additional reading.[7]

The Role of Equality

Readers often have difficulty understanding why philosophers might not believe that people should be granted full property rights over the resources that they have inherited or earned. Rawls (1971, 102) states that "[n]o one deserves his greater natural capacity nor merits a more favorable starting place in society," and interestingly, most philosophers and many economists agree. Kenneth Arrow (1983, 98–99), the consummate "economist's economist," notes that under Rawls's theory,

> Even natural advantages, superiorities of intelligence or strength, do not in themselves create any claims to greater rewards. . . . Personally, I share fully with this value judgment. . . . But a contradictory position—that an individual is entitled to what he creates—is widely and unreflectively held; when teaching elementary economics, I have had considerable difficulty in persuading the students that this *productivity principle* is not completely self-evident.

The literature on moral philosophy clearly states that in creating a fair society, something must be equalized. Amartya Sen (1992, 17) provides a reason:

> It may be useful to ask *why* it is that so many altogether different substantive theories of the ethics of social arrangements have the common feature of demanding equality of *something*—something important. It is, I believe, arguable that to have any kind of plausibility, ethical reasoning on social matters must involve elementary equal consideration for all at *some* level that is seen as critical. The absence of such equality would make a theory arbitrarily discriminating and hard to defend. A theory must accept—indeed demand—inequality in terms of many variables, but in defending those inequalities it would be hard to duck the need to relate them, ultimately, to equal consideration for all in some adequately substantial way.

Sen notes that even Nozick's (1974) libertarian philosophy calls for the equalization of something—libertarian rights.

Unfortunately, the decision that something ought to be equalized raises more questions than it answers. The main problem, of course, is that such a decision does not tell us *what* should be equalized. Before confronting this, we must distinguish between two similar-sounding but quite different concepts: "equality" and "equity." The former implies equal shares of something, the latter, a "fair" or "just" distribution, which may or may not result in equal shares.

The difference between the two terms is illustrated by the two common forms of equity: horizontal and vertical. Horizontal equity implies that similar people are treated the same with respect to some characteristic (the choice of which is a major issue in itself)—this is equality. But vertical equity is different. According to Gavin Mooney (1996a, 99), it is "the unequal but equitable treatment of unequals." For example, we might, in the name of equity, establish a lower tax rate for the poor than for the rich.

Deborah Stone (2001) illustrates the distinction among all of these terms by discussing how to divide up and distribute "a delicious bittersweet chocolate cake" among students in her public policy class. One way, of course, is to give equal slices to all, but that seemingly fair method may lead to protests that "equality" does not result in an "equitable" distribution. Some possible objections to equal slices, each of which results in a different distribution of cake, include the following:

- Everyone in the university should get a slice, not just class members.
- Higher-ranked persons deserve bigger slices (or more frosting).
- Because males traditionally have had less access to homemade cake, each sex should get half the cake to divide among their members.
- Those who were given smaller main courses should get more cake.
- People who can't appreciate the cake should get less (or none).
- *Access* to the cake, not the cake itself, should be equalized by giving everyone a fork; competition for the cake would then ensue.
- The cake should be distributed by lottery.
- The allocation should be decided on by voting.

It is not hard to come up with close analogies to each of these arguments when allocating scarce medical goods and services.

As noted above, resource allocation theories require the equalization of something. What is being equalized under utilitarianism? The answer is not as straightforward as it might seem, because the concept embraces several different formulations. In general, though, utilitarianism is less about equalizing something as about maximizing something else (Sen 1992). Under classical utilitarianism, the sum of all individuals' utility is being maximized.

Under ordinal utilitarianism, society is best off when each individual succeeds in maximizing his own utility. As discussed in Section 2.5, however, some income redistribution is necessary to maximize the social welfare function.

We are most concerned with ordinal utilitarianism because it forms the basis of modern economics. What is being equalized under ordinal utilitarianism? One possibility is that each individual's interests are being treated equally; my utility counts as much as yours. Another possibility is that people have equal rights to produce and trade to maximize their utility. This is not to say that their ability or opportunity to do so is equal, but that no explicit restrictions prevent participation in a competitive market. It is not hard to see why moral philosophers, in considering the vagaries of social advantage in the real world, would find this concept wanting.

What, then, should be equalized?[8] One line of thought, advocated by Ronald Dworkin (1981), is that people's "resources" should be equalized—a philosophy that is similar to Rawls's equalization of primary goods.[9]

Another line of thought, put forth by John Roemer (1995), is that people's "opportunity" should be equalized. The idea is that people should be responsible for their own actions once a "level playing field" is established. Roemer distinguishes between factors that are beyond one's control and factors that are within one's control. He gives the following example: Suppose we want to compensate people who contract lung cancer (to help them afford medical care). We first come up with a list of factors over which people have little control; Roemer uses age, ethnicity, gender, and occupation. We then look at smoking behavior within these subgroups. Suppose that the average 60-year-old, male, African American steelworker has smoked for 30 years, and the average 60-year-old, female, white college professor has smoked for eight years. These figures provide a gauge for the behaviors of others who fall into these subgroups. If an African American steelworker and a white professor then contract lung cancer after smoking for 20 years and 15 years, respectively, the steelworker would receive more compensation, because his behavior was more responsible *given the circumstances over which he had little or no control.*

Equalizing Capabilities

Sen (1992) advocates another candidate for equalization: "capabilities." These "reflect a person's freedom to choose between alternative lives" (Sen 1992, 83). The idea here is to give people the ability to achieve the things they want. Capabilities relate not to resources themselves, but to what resources can do for a person. As Cookson (2005, 819) summarized, "people differ radically in their ability to convert resources into valuable activities and states of being, due to diversity in people's internal characteristics (e.g., health, strength, stamina, charisma) and external circumstances (e.g., location, social position, employment, family characteristics)." Equality of capabilities might mean that more resources are given to a disabled person because that person might need more to be capable of achieving his goals. Or it might mean giving unskilled laborers the skills to achieve more, rather than simply plying them with cash grants.

Equalizing capabilities differs from Rawls's theory and from equalizing resources. Under those systems people are given physical resources but not necessarily the ability to use them to achieve what they want. And it differs from equality of opportunity because giving people an opportunity does not necessarily mean that they will be able to use that opportunity to their own advantage.

The notion of capabilities has received attention in recent years, particularly in the field of economic development (Cookson 2005; Robeyns 2006). In some of his later writings, Sen (2002, 660) concluded that health is a key capability, stating that

> health is among the most important conditions of human life and a critically significant constituent of human capabilities which we have reason to value. Any conception of social justice that accepts the need for a fair distribution as well as efficient formation of human capabilities cannot ignore the role of health in human life and the opportunities that persons . . . have to achieve good health— free from escapable illness, avoidable afflictions and premature mortality.

Health economists have also found the concept of capabilities attractive (Coast, Smith, and Lorgelly 2008), although applying it to the healthcare area has been challenging due to the difficulty of reaching agreement on what particular capabilities to focus on and how to weight them to come up with a single index (Richardson and McKie 2005). One observer from the field of feminist economics offers a list of ten "central human capabilities," among which is "bodily health," which she defines as "being able to have good health, including reproductive health; to be adequately nourished; to have adequate shelter" (Nussbaum 2003, 41).[10]

Richardson and McKie (2005) demonstrate how the standard economic view of maximizing utility does not do a good job capturing the population's view of how resources should be allocated. Equalizing capabilities, as Sen called for, appears to be a much better match. We consider two of their examples here.

The first concerns the treatment of illnesses. A utility maximization model would conclude that, for a given amount of expenditures, we should focus public health investments on the program that improves aggregate health the most, irrespective of the initial health state of participants in alternative programs. A common measurement of health benefits is quality adjusted life years, which is the expected number of healthy years of life that a person has left. (A year of non-optimal health is given a value of less than 1.0.) Interestingly, survey results from a number of countries (including the United States) show that such an allocation formula does not reflect people's values. Most people prefer giving priority to those who begin in poorer health. It would appear that some notion of fairness trumps economic efficiency.

Richardson and McKie (2005, 229) note that severity of illness is the main criterion by which scarce hearts and livers are allocated for transplants in the United States. How social priorities differ from the utility maximization paradigm comes across quite clearly.

> Those with the best prognosis after receipt of an organ are those with the least severe illness, and maximum health gain would be achieved by giving this group priority. The actual policy is to give the highest priority to those with the most severe problem. This results in the "perverse" situation where the relatively healthy must wait until their health state has deteriorated sufficiently for them to satisfy the severity criterion . . . This policy can only be described as "perverse," however, if health gain is the overriding social objective. In the present case, health gain is explicitly of secondary importance to severity.

The second example relates to a concept called "The Rule of Rescue." The idea is that while focusing resources on health interventions may do the most good in the aggregate, in reality people tend to prefer spending on rescuing identifiable people who are in peril. While this may seem to be bad social policy, McKie and Richardson (2003) demonstrate that the issue is far more complex than it first appears.

News stories commonly report expensive, against-all-odds searches for miners stuck underground. The searches often persist even when there is little chance of successful rescue. Applying this to health, McKie and Richardson (2003, 2407–08, emphasis added) write,

> Surely these policies divert resources from other activities where the benefits would be greater? Why do some patients receive a second or third heart or liver transplant, when the first-time recipients have a higher 1-year survival rate? When organs are in short supply why not give priority to first-time transplants if they have a better chance of survival?

They go on to answer their own question:

> These practices manifest a psychological imperative that is hard to resist: namely, the imperative to rescue *identifiable* individuals facing avoiding death, without giving too much thought to the opportunity cost of doing so. . . . people cannot stand idly by when an identified person's life is visibly threatened if rescue measures are available.

There are two problems with this ethic. First, it provides advantage to those who happen to be identifiable in some way (as opposed to what Richardson and McKie refer to as a "statistical life") and second, it does seem like a poor allocation of resources.

How, then, can it be justified, given that "being identified does not seem to be a morally relevant criterion for discrimination," since "those anonymous individuals who quietly die from preventable cancers in hospital wards are no less real than the trapped miner" (McKie and Richardson 2003, 2415)? The authors provide two provocative justifications: (1) Observers of the rescue receive utility from knowing that an attempt to help the victim is being made, and (2) people receive utility from the affirmation that they live in a "humane" society whose members don't stand idly by in the face of calamities—which, incidentally, could also befall them.

This is not to say that we should favor the identifiable over the statistical life, but rather, as McKie and Richardson (2003, 2417) conclude, that

> there is probably no unambiguous advice that may be offered to health econo-
> mists, health service researchers or policy makers except to remember that the
> evaluation of health services is not simply a technical matter but a quintessentially
> ethical endeavour, and that in complex societies with divergent values there may
> be a range of considerations that may "trump" the utilitarian rationality.

9.3 Equity, Distribution, and Health

Thus far, the focus of this chapter has been on problems with the concept of ordinal utilitarianism, the key tool in the economics of social welfare. By relying on it, the economics field has been able to sidestep such important issues as determining a fair and equitable allocation of resources. Most of the literature cited, however, comes from the philosophy and distributive justice fields. In this section we raise four related applications: (1) the need to focus not just on the perceived utility of members of society, but also on their health; (2) whether factors other than their own utility—specifically, commitment to a cause—might drive individuals to improve the welfare of others, including health; (3) whether it is more desirable for society to redistribute resources in cash or in services such as healthcare; and (4) national health insurance.

Focusing on People's Health as Well as on Their Utility

Under the conventional economic model, society strives to allow people to maximize their utility. This is because, under utilitarianism, social welfare is simply the aggregate of individual utilities. Because utility is purely subjective, not directly measurable, and not comparable among different people, public intervention is typically not advised. Instead, people should spend their resources in whatever manner they think will maximize their welfare.

But as we argued above, one of utilitarianism's shortcomings is its silence on whether people should be penalized for things over which they have little or no control. For a theory to have any moral sway, something important needs to be equalized. This "something" has to do with people's opportunities, or alternatively, their capabilities to achieve their goals.

For decades, health economists have debated whether health is "different."[11] Much of this literature has focused on informational problems—certainly an important issue, but other sectors of the economy have major (although perhaps not quite as severe) information problems. Other literature has focused on the possibility that health is associated with stronger positive externalities. Arrow (1963b, 954), for example, states, "The taste for improving the health of others appears to be stronger than for improving other aspects of their welfare." This provides a somewhat stronger case that health is special, but one can imagine other needs—food, education, housing—that are equally compelling.

Health's true difference concerns opportunities and capabilities: Good health provides people with the opportunity and/or capability to achieve other desired things. As A. J. Culyer (1993, 300) writes, "One reason for such beliefs may do with the important role [things like health] have in enabling people to fulfill their potential as persons." He also states that,

> If it is felt that all residents of a political jurisdiction ought to have equal opportunities for their lives to flourish, then it follows that *health care* is one of the goods and services whose right distribution must be ensured. (Culyer 2001, 276)

Such a viewpoint is consistent with the reason Lester Thurow (1977, 93) gives: "[S]ociety's interest in the distribution of medical care springs, not from unspecified externalities that affect private-personal utility, but from our individual-societal preferences that 'human rights' include an *equal* 'right' to health care."

The idea that society should consider other, nonutility aspects of welfare has been coined the "extra-welfarist" approach (Brouwer et al. 2008).[12] Under a welfarist approach, only individual levels of utility matter to society. In health, these nonutility aspects relate to access to health services, good health, or both.[13] Some researchers, such as Lu Ann Aday, Ronald Andersen, and Gretchen Fleming (1980, 26), have advocated access to health services as the key dimension of equity, whereby "[t]he greatest 'equity' of access is said to exist when need, rather than structural or individual factors, determine[s] who gains entry to the health care system." Work by Mooney et al. (1991, 479) appears consistent with this viewpoint. They advocate "equal access for equal need," because this "provides individuals with the *opportunity* to use needed health services."

Other analysts, notably Culyer (1989), have advocated health status rather than access to care as the key outcome[14] and the determinants of health as the key research issue.[15] If one considers health rather than utility as the outcome, the meaning of economic efficiency is different from the one economics typically uses. Culyer (1993, 312) states that efficiency is achieved "by prioritizing the more 'urgent' and so distributing health between A and B [such] that, at the margin, the cost of A's and B's additional health is equal to the social value attached to the health of each." Recall that from a utilitarian standpoint, in contrast, whoever can pay the most will receive priority.[16, 17]

Under this allocation rule, society is interested less in what people demand as evidenced by their willingness to pay than in how far a given amount of money can go toward improving health—a nonwelfarist viewpoint. This view and the one centered on access to care dictate health policy worldwide much more than the conventional economic model does. The access-centered view is consistent with government-sponsored programs that seek to equalize people's ability to obtain needed medical care. The health-centered view has influenced the growing reliance on cost-effectiveness analyses in health-related studies and the relatively new focus on clinical outcomes and effectiveness in health services research.

In contrast, a renewed interest in the United States and other countries in rationing the use of services by higher out-of-pocket price—a topic explored in Section 4.5—is becoming a source of worry. Such policies may quell the use of services: According to conventional theory, more efficient economic outcomes will result if people forgo services that they do not find very useful. But if one views access to health services, or health itself, as the outcome society is trying to maximize, the results could be different. Policies aimed at reducing demand may reduce access, health status, or both more than society deems optimal. These issues are taken up again in Chapter 10, where the experiences of a number of developed countries' healthcare systems are explored.

Commitment: Another Factor Driving Individual Behavior

Economists typically do not question why people derive utility from particular goods. Modern theory is interested simply in which bundle of goods a person prefers; the preference need not be justified. An economic system that is able to satisfy such preferences is desirable, because the preferences themselves are beyond questioning.

Objections to this viewpoint include the following:

- It essentially sanctions preferences that we might view as immoral; for example, equal favor is given to preferences that may cause harm and those that are loftier. In this regard, Mark Sagoff (1986, 302) writes, "It cannot be argued that the satisfaction of preferences is a good thing in itself, for many preferences are sadistic, envious, racist, or unjust."
- It sanctions preferences that might be, in some sense, faulty (e.g., behaviors that are self-destructive). One example is shortsightedness. Sagoff

(1986, 304) writes, "Literary and empirical studies amply confirm what every mature adult discovers: happiness and well-being come from overcoming or outgrowing many of our desires more than from satisfying them."

• It focuses on goods rather than on values such as freedom. This leads to the prediction that people will be equally happy with a particular bundle of goods whether it is assigned to them or freely chosen (Hahnel and Albert 1990).

This conception of utility also does a poor job in predicting other aspects of people's behavior, such as why people bother to vote. Given the infinitesimally small chance that your vote would decide an election, why go to all the effort? Another example is income taxes. Why be honest when it is so easy to cheat and so unlikely that you will be caught (Aaron 1994)? As a final illustration, consider the following summarization of Howard Margolis's (1982) discussion of people's contributions to charity:

Suppose that a public radio station embarks on a fundraising campaign, and you decide to contribute $10 (but not $11); that is, you maximize your utility by spending $10 for this charity instead of other goods and services. But just as you are about to call in your pledge, the station announces that someone else has just given $10. Under the conventional model, this new information will make you will forgo your contribution—the station is already $10 richer; you can now keep the $10 and be that much better off than before. Not contributing allows you to have your cake and eat it too.

If people really behaved this way, public radio (or for that matter, almost any charity) could not exist. Once a single, large donor announced his or her intention to contribute, getting anyone else to contribute would be nearly impossible. The outcome would be economically inefficient, because charities would receive far less in donations than the public desires.

Fortunately, something still drives people to contribute to charities. A broader definition of utility is necessary to explain such paradoxes. Amartya Sen (1982) distinguishes between two concepts, sympathy and commitment. A person who acts on feelings of sympathy is indeed showing his personal preferences through his actions. Commitment, however, is different. You would rather do something else, but you do not because you are committed to a particular cause. Sen uses recycling as an example. He argues that people recycle not because they enjoy it or because they believe that they will make a marked difference in the cleanliness of the environment, nor do they think others will follow suit. Rather, they do it because of their commitment to a cleaner environment. He states, "one way of defining commitment is in terms of a person choosing an act that he believes will yield a lower level of personal welfare to him than an alternative that is also available to him" (Sen 1982, 92).

Margolis (1982) explains people's behavior by positing that they have two distinct altruistic motivations. One, which he calls *goods altruism*, is the one of which we normally conceive: People receive utility when other less-well-off people have more goods to consume. The other is *participation altruism*, under which people receive utility from giving resources (including their time) away because it makes them feel good about themselves. This dual form of altruism, according to Margolis, can explain the paradoxes of why a person would vote, give to charity, or not cheat on taxes.

More recently, Henry Aaron (1994, 15–16) provided a critique of utility theory, calling for "a new economics of human behavior." Although spelling out the details is beyond the scope of his work, he believes that

> each person [has] more than one, possibly many, utility functions. In one or more of these sub-functions the arguments, as in standard theory, are particular goods and services. In others the arguments are intangible objectives such as adherence to duty, altruism, or spite, characteristics necessary for reputation or self-respect. Particular economic commodities may enter more than one function. In contrast to standard theory, however, the marginal utility of a given object may vary widely in different utility functions and may even have different signs.

Thus, there are a number of reasons to believe that people benefit from knowing that others have the resources necessary to provide for their own and their family's healthcare. But whether these resources should be provided in the form of cash or as services remains a question.

Providing Health Services Rather Than Cash

A common application of ordinal utility theory is the supposed superiority of cash over in-kind transfers. The argument is as follows: Suppose that society wishes to transfer resources from wealthier to poorer individuals and has two choices for doing so: giving people money or giving them goods or services directly. The former would always be superior, because letting people choose exactly how to spend their money allows them to maximize their utility (i.e., reach their highest affordable indifference curve). In contrast, if goods or services are provided, maximizing utility would be almost impossible. We could never do more to maximize utility than by transferring cash, and we could only do as much if the goods transferred were *exactly* what would have been purchased had the grant been in the form of cash.

The issue, to most economists, is one of consumer sovereignty. Should people be allowed to make their own choices, or should society tell people how to spend their resources? Ordinal utilitarianism shows a clear preference for cash transfers because it assumes that people will make choices that are in their best interest. The question of whether people will really spend money in the way that is best for them is discussed at some length in chapters 4 and

5. In this section we assume that however the person spends the money will indeed maximize his or her utility.

There are three other reasons to believe that providing goods and services is superior to providing cash; each will be addressed briefly in the following subsections.

The Desires of Donors

The most important reasons to provide goods over cash are that

- we do care about the utility of the people who make the donations (or pay the taxes), and
- these donors or taxpayers do care about how their money is spent.

Because these two issues are related, we will deal with them together.

Why would we ignore the wishes of the donors? One possibility is the supposition that how the recipients spend the money is none of the donors' business. But this belief contradicts a tenet of economic theory—that preferences do not have to be justified. If donors care about how the money is being spent, this must be taken into account in determining what is in society's best interest. And if total welfare is simply the sum of all individuals' welfare, it is incumbent on the analyst to consider everyone's preferences, including those of the donors.

What, then, do donors care about? George Daly and Fred Giertz (1972) posit that two kinds of (positive consumptive) externalities should be considered in providing transfer payments to those who are less well off. One, which they call a "goods externality," exists when the donor obtains utility from a recipient having specific goods such as housing, food, education, or health services. The other, labeled a "utility externality," exists when the donor cares only about the recipient's utility, regardless of the goods through which it is obtained.

The question Daly and Giertz (1972, 135) pose is, "Do people, individually or collectively, extend aid to others in hopes of improving the real welfare of the recipients or in order to alter their consumption pattern?" To answer it, they observe people's preferences in private charity, where donations are purely voluntary, and they find that private charities "almost invariably redistribute it in the form of particular commodities." Furthermore, the justification for public redistribution programs (e.g., housing support), is often explicitly to alter recipients' consumption patterns. In this regard, the authors add,

> [A] majority of voters might approve of public housing for slum areas but be strongly opposed to the transfer of money to people living in those slums. . . . For donors the crucial issue may be not the level of well-being achieved by the recipient but rather *how* he achieves it (Daly and Giertz 1972, 136).

Although some people may claim that they are only interested in the utility of the recipient, this attitude seems a bit far-fetched, as the following quotation by David Collard (1978, 122) suggests:

> The overwhelming weight of impressionistic evidence is that people are concerned less with other people's incomes or utilities than with their consumption of specific commodities. Any reader who believes himself to be entirely non-paternalistic in his concern is asked to perform the following mental experiment. I notice that my neighbour is badly fed and badly clothed so I give him some money which he then spends on beer and tobacco. Do I feel entirely happy about this or do I somehow feel that my intentions have been thwarted?

As Section 2.2 showed, the presence of positive externalities of consumption necessitates a transfer of income to ensure an economically efficient, Pareto-optimal outcome. But suppose that donors, fearing that recipients will squander their donations, decide not to give (or vote to reduce taxes). This reduces donations to a level that is less than economically efficient. By allowing for in-kind rather than cash subsidies (and illiquid ones at that), more money is likely to be donated, resulting in a more efficient outcome (Daly and Giertz 1972).

Ensuring Sufficient Donations

Another topic raised in Chapter 2 is the fact that few, if any, "neutral" transfer payments exist. In general, taxes and subsidies result in a work disincentive that leads to a suboptimal amount of production. Welfare payments may reduce the incentive to work; as earned income rises, welfare payments decline.

Improving Productivity

A. C. Pigou (1932, 725–26), in his classic book *The Economics of Welfare*, raises an important reason in-kind transfers might be superior to cash:

> [T]ransference of objects not capable of being sold or pawned, and designed to satisfy needs, which, apart from the transference, a recipient would have left unsatisfied, have a different effect. The last unit of money which a man earns for himself in industry will be required to satisfy the same needs, and will, therefore, be desired with the same intensity as it would have been if no transference had been made. Hence no contraction will occur in the contribution which, by work and waiting, he makes to the national dividend.

This point has apparently been overlooked by most analysts: Provision of a good or service that the recipient would not otherwise have purchased provides no work disincentive. (An example would be medical care services that a poor person could not otherwise have afforded.)

The previous discussion showed several reasons it is better to provide services than cash in redistribution. Of course, this contrasts sharply with the predictions of the conventional economic model, which posits that cash contributions will always be superior. Needless to say, most health policymakers have eschewed the conventional model. What they have tended to do instead is promote insurance coverage or reimbursement for services. No country relies on giving low-income people money and leaving them to choose whether to purchase health coverage.

An examination of how the one industrialized country that has not adopted national health insurance—the United States—carries out redistribution provides further evidence. In 2002, $522 billion in cash and noncash benefits were provided to persons with low income in the United States. Of this amount, only 20 percent was cash aid. The remaining 80 percent was for the direct provision of goods and services such as medical care, food, and housing. In fact, nearly three times as much was spent on providing just one in-kind service—medical care—than was spent on cash subsidies (U.S. Census Bureau 2006, 361).

Providing health insurance coverage is not the same as providing services directly, however. Unlike the latter, where the recipient is given no choice, a person who has health insurance can choose from the services the insurance program covers. In that respect, insurance coverage bears some resemblance to cash. But choices are limited to a specified set of health-related goods. Donors (private charity) and taxpayers (public programs) would be unlikely to tolerate recipients spending these resources on non–health related items.

Thus, we see that social policy worldwide is not consistent with what the conventional economic model predicts. And developed countries (excluding the United States) have gone the extra step of providing guaranteed health insurance coverage for the entire population.

National Health Insurance

If societies believe that either equal access to health services or equal access to good health is necessary in the name of social justice, national health insurance is clearly justified. Wagstaff and van Doorslaer (1993) researched views on equity in several developed countries and concluded that such programs are consistent with the prevailing ethical viewpoints of nearly all developed countries.[18]

The United States is the one developed country without a national health insurance program; the reason for this has been debated for decades. One possible explanation is that the United States holds a different ethic than other countries. Robert Blendon and colleagues (1995) report on a survey that found that only 23 percent of Americans agreed with the statement, "It is the responsibility of the government to take care of the very poor people who can't take care of themselves." The numbers for other countries were considerably higher: 50 percent of Germans, 56 percent of Poles, 62 percent of British and French, 66 percent of Italians, and 71 percent of Spaniards agreed with the statement (Blendon et al. 1995).

Of course, the way questions are worded affects the results of such studies. This one focused on the poor and did not specifically mention health. A recent survey asked Americans, "Do you think it is the responsibility of the federal government to make sure all Americans have healthcare coverage, or is that not the responsibility of the federal government?" Sixty-nine percent said that they thought it was government's responsibility (Center for American Progress 2007). Of course, the percentages might have been much higher for other countries if they had been included in the study.

The views of Americans relative to others correspond with international findings on the actual amount of equity in different countries. The United States and Switzerland, both of which have large private insurance markets, were the least equitable of 13 countries studied (Wagstaff et al. 1999). The results with regard to the equity of service delivery are harder to generalize (van Doorslaer et al. 2000).

National health insurance makes sense when one considers the alternative conceptions of social welfare that we discussed earlier in this chapter. If, as Margolis (1982) and Aaron (1994) argue, people have more than one element in their utility functions—if, in addition to goods-based utility, they also derive satisfaction from helping others—then they may derive utility from being part of a society that helps those who do not have access to health services or good health.

In this regard, Mooney (1996a, 100) writes,

Individuals recognise that they are members of a society and that they get some form of utility or increased well-being from being in a society, being able to make a contribution to that society, and being an active participant in that society. The source of this form of utility seems much more to be non-individualistic or at least stemming from a recognition on the part of the individual that he or she is a member of a society and that such membership does convey certain benefits but also perhaps certain responsibilities.

This attitude has been termed "communitarianism," where, as applied to health, there is a "desire on part of the members of that society to create a just health care service as part of a wider just society" (Mooney 1996a, 101).[19] A key element in enacting the appropriate health system is determining the extent to which the country's population holds such an ethic—a fruitful area for future research.[20]

Researchers worldwide have investigated these issues, often from a "social capital" perspective. Although many definitions of social capital exist,[21] most involve the empowerment of individuals through membership in a group with which they share characteristics. Similarly, many different pathways between social capital and health have been hypothesized. One is social cohesion, the idea that a society with large gulfs between the well and poorly off or between races results in numerous adverse consequences for the individual (e.g., additional psychological stress), and for the group (e.g., unresponsive government) (Kawachi and Kennedy 1999). Another pathway is social relationships: Some researchers have found that the quantity and quality of human interactions affect health status (House, Landis, and Umberson 1999).

Not all researchers agree. Some believe that social capital is a void concept or even a nefarious one. According to Pearce and Smith (2003, 122), "Intervening in communities to increase their levels of social capital may be ineffective, create resentment, and overload community resources, and to take such an approach may be to 'blame the victim' at the community level while ignoring the health effects of macrolevel social and economic policies."

In summary, the case for a national health insurance program is strong. Universal coverage is consistent with prevailing notions of fairness; people should not be penalized for circumstances—such as their sociodemographic background or their current health—over which they have little control. The case for providing coverage to all children is especially compelling, since they are clearly not responsible for their circumstances. Unlike other characteristics, good health is instrumental in people's capabilities to achieve their personal goals. Financial barriers to obtaining care are doubly unfair: They not only result in poorer health, but they also frustrate people's ability to attain the other things that they value. Furthermore, most people draw pride from being part of a society in which the well-being of others is an important part of the welfare of all members. That nearly every developed nation is committed to providing health insurance to its population, regardless of the individual's ability to pay, is not surprising.[22]

9.4 Chapter Summary

The field of economics has given short shrift to issues surrounding equity and redistribution. Moreover, the traditional model of ordinal utilitarianism does not adequately capture societal views of social justice. Markets by themselves—or markets accompanied by cash redistributions—do not reflect societal preferences for providing those in need with access to healthcare services. Other countries have enacted national health insurance programs to ensure that all members of society are treated fairly with regard to healthcare, a commodity that is instrumental in allowing them to achieve their personal goals.

Notes

1. Some critics, however, believe that modern economists have gone too far in eschewing interpersonal comparisons of utility. Little (1957), for example,

claims that most people are able to make valid judgments about whether one person is happier than another or gets a greater amount of utility than another person from a particular good.

2. For a discussion of the different types of utilitarianism, see Elster (1992).

3. Elster (1992) has coined this "Neumann-Morgenstern utility" after the founders of game theory.

4. This stands for *maximum minimorum*.

5. See Elster (1992) for a more thorough discussion of this criticism.

6. For more views on this topic, see Daniels (1985).

7. Some especially useful books about this topic have been written by Amartya Sen (1987, 1992).

8. We make no attempt to review the literature on this topic; those seeking additional information may wish to consult Sen (1992) and Hausman and McPherson (1993).

9. Dworkin (1981) devotes several pages to explaining the difference between his theory and Rawls's theory. One difference is that Dworkin claims that his theory is tailored to the individual, whereas Rawls focuses on a representative person in a social class. Individuals are more responsible for their actions (how they spend their resources) under Dworkin than under Rawls.

10. The other nine capabilities Nussbaum (2003) lists are life; bodily integrity; senses, imagination, and thought; emotions; practical reason; affiliation; relation to other species and nature; play; and control over one's environment.

11. See, for example, Pauly (1978) and Reinhardt (1978).

12. Brouwer and colleagues (2008) provide a thorough discussion on what distinguishes welfarism from extra-welfarism. They postulate that there are four differences: (1) the outcomes being considered—extra-welfarism includes aspects besides personal utility, including perhaps health; (2) who evaluates the outcomes—it is the individual in a welfarist approach, but it could be others, such as expert decision makers, under extra-welfarism; (3) the weighting of outcomes—under welfarism, the Pareto principle tends to prevail (see Section 2.1), whereas in extra-welfarism, researchers or policy makers can provide different weights or emphases to different groups of people (e.g., the poor); and (4) the role of interpersonal comparisons (allowed under most extra-welfarist viewpoints but not generally under welfarism).

13. For a discussion of the pros and cons of equalizing health, utilization, or access, see Chapter 5 of Mooney (1994).

14. Some of Culyer's later writings move away from this position. In Culyer (1993, 318), he writes: "I now think that it is more helpful in studies of distribution to focus on the need for health care than on the need for health. . . . [Adam] Wagstaff and I have also come to a stipulative definition of need as 'the minimum resources required to exhaust an individual's capacity to benefit from health care.'"

15. For a thorough model of the determinants of health, see Evans and Stoddart (1990).

16. Alan Williams (1997, 199) advocates a similar view, called the "fair innings" argument. He writes that it "reflects the feeling that everyone is entitled to some 'normal' span of health. . . . The implication is that anyone failing to achieve this has in some sense been cheated, whilst anyone getting more than this is 'living on borrowed time.'" One implication of this view is that more medical resources should be devoted to the young, who have not yet had their fair innings, with correspondingly less spent on the elderly.

17. Note, however, that Culyer's statement is inconsistent with "The Rule of Rescue" discussed earlier—no surprise, since most economists, even the extra-welfarists, are uncomfortable about following a rule that, at least on the surface, appears to squander resources and be unfair.

18. For a summary of research on this topic, see van Doorslaer, Wagstaff, and Rutten (1993).

19. A related area of inquiry is how people's sense of community affects their attitudes. In a study conducted among 1,200 Florida residents, Ahern, Hendryx, and Siddharthan (1996) found that a person's positive or negative feelings about his or her community was the best predictor of that person's perceived experiences with the health system.

20. For an extensive discussion of these issues, see Mooney (1996b).

21. See Macinko and Starfield (2001) for a summary.

22. The Appendix contains brief descriptions of the health insurance systems in ten developed countries.

HEALTHCARE SYSTEMS IN DEVELOPED COUNTRIES: ORGANIZATION, OUTCOMES, COSTS, AND LESSONS

So far, we have focused on health economic issues—demand, supply, and distribution—highlighting concerns about the application of traditional economic theory in the healthcare arena. While we have discussed real-world experiences throughout, we have not paid much attention to the successes and failures of different countries, each of which has its own healthcare system organization.

This chapter examines the ways different countries organize their healthcare systems and how this influences outcomes. Section 10.1 presents varying organizational approaches to the structure of the healthcare system, service coverage and delivery, regulation of prices, expenditures, volume, and control of the supply of inputs. Section 10.2 focuses on actual performance: the successes and failures of ten developed countries in achieving access to high quality care in the context of how much they spend. Finally, Section 10.3 uses these experiences to provide ten lessons concerning the role of government in healthcare systems.

10.1 Different Approaches to the Role of Government in the Healthcare Sector

Every country has its own way of involving government in the financing and delivery of health services. These methods, of course, are not set in stone. Most nations continually tinker with their systems. Maynard (2005, S255) notes that "The Netherlands and the UK . . . are caught up in a frenzy of repetitive change" and these countries are not alone. Altenstetter and Busse (2005, 122) refer to "frenzied reforms" in Germany. Occasionally, countries enact major changes—for example, the movement toward more competition through "internal markets" in the United Kingdom (described in more detail in the Appendix), which began during the Thatcher administration but has morphed into Primary Care Trusts since the Labour Party came into power in 1997.

Views differ on the proper role of government in the healthcare sector. Nevertheless, there is some agreement on where government should have a strong role and where it should have little. One area that is widely considered government's responsibility is monitoring the health services sector and making policy. Most would also agree that the production of medical supplies such as latex gloves should be left to markets. For example, Robert Evans (1983, 37), a critic of market-based systems, has written,

> Where commodities are concerned—pharmaceuticals, optometric goods, and health appliances—there is both analysis and empirical experience to suggest that an open, competitive market combined with product inspection and certification (but not licensure of providers) might significantly enhance efficiency and lower costs.

In such cases, the potential for a great deal of competition among producers exists, and information is not much of a problem because measurement of outputs is reasonably straightforward (Preker and Harding 2007).

Most societal choices in healthcare, however, fall between these two extreme cases. Consequently, the optimal degree of government involvement is not obvious. This section explores the different ways government is involved in the health services sector, illustrating the choices with examples from selected developed countries.

Tuohy, Flood, and Stabile (2004, 361) provide four different (but not mutually exclusive) models for how the interaction between the public and private sectors can take place:

1. Parallel public and private systems: For a given range of services, a separate privately financed system exists as an alternative to the public sector.
2. Copayment: Financing for a broad range of services is partially subsidized through public payment, with the remainder financed through out-of-pocket payments and/or private insurance. The degree of copayment may be scaled according to the patient's income.
3. Group-based: Certain population groups are eligible for public coverage; others rely on private insurance.
4. Sectoral: Certain healthcare sectors are entirely publicly financed; others rely much more heavily on private finance.

This is a useful way to categorize the alternative relationships between markets and government. Nevertheless, every country is presented with thousands of choices for how government should be involved in the organization, financing, delivery, and monitoring of health-related goods and services. Table 10.1 lists some of the major roles the government can play in four overall areas: the structure of the system, the nature of coverage and delivery, control of expenditures, and control of input supply. The remainder of this section elaborates on those roles.

TABLE 10.1: Alternative Roles for Government in the Healthcare Sector

---

- *Structure of the System*
  - Universality of coverage
  - Publicly vs. privately administered coverage
  - Coordination of payers
  - Site of administrative authority

- *Nature of Coverage and Delivery*
  - Role of private insurance
  - Benefits in publicly mandated systems
  - Cost-sharing requirements
  - How providers are paid
  - Choice of providers

- *Control of Expenditures*
  - Hospital fee schedules and global budgeting
  - Physician fee schedules
  - Direct regulation of volume

- *Control of Input Supply*
  - Hospital
  - Physician
  - Capital/medical technology

A basic understanding of the health systems in various developed countries will help the reader understand the remaining sections in this chapter. The Appendix includes short descriptions of the organization, financing, and delivery of services in ten selected countries: Australia, Canada, France, Germany, the Netherlands, Japan, Sweden, Switzerland, the United Kingdom, and the United States. These countries were chosen because of their size or because their healthcare systems are often discussed in policy circles.

The following discussion is, by necessity, fairly general. It is not possible to go into detail about how each of several countries has dealt with each of 15 societal decisions. Rather, we discuss each issue in general, give examples of selected countries that have approached it differently, and provide an overview of the advantages and disadvantages of alternative policy choices.

Structure of the System

Nearly all developed countries provide guaranteed healthcare coverage to almost all citizens. In most cases, such coverage is the cornerstone on which the

Universality of Coverage

system is based. Germany, for example, has a history of solidarity through a social code, *Sozialgesetzbuch*, which "holds that medical care should be provided solely according to an individual's needs, whereas the financing of care should be based solely on the individual's ability to pay" (Pfaff and Wassener 2000, 907). The federal government in Canada will contribute to provincial health plans only if care is provided to all citizens with minimal financial impediments. The United Kingdom's National Health Service was established more than 50 years ago to provide comprehensive universal coverage with no financial access barriers (Roemer 1991; Smee 2000). Sweden not only ensures equality of access to care, but strives for "a vision of equal health for all" (Anell 2005). Similar to Germany's ethic, Sweden's system is based on two sets of values: "*jamlikhet* (equality of all citizens) and *trygghet* (security)" (Saltman and Bergman 2005, 261). Solidarity has been a hallmark in France since 1945, through "the sharing of resources, equality of all in the face of illness, and free access to health care services" (Bellanger and Mosse 2005, S119). Similar social ethics are common among almost all European countries.

Coverage is not completely universal in several of these countries; some people do fall through the cracks. In some cases, individuals are required to sign up for coverage, and some do not. In other cases, some are allowed to opt out of public coverage but may fail to procure private insurance. Until their reforms in 2009 requiring universal coverage, Germany provided an example. About 10 percent of the population—generally those with the highest incomes—were not required to enroll in sickness funds (Worz and Busse 2005).[1] Most of this 10 percent instead chose private insurance, which tends to pay providers more and, as a result, may make these patients more financially attractive to providers. But some not eligible for government-mandated coverage, mainly those who are self-employed, do not enroll in private insurance. It is estimated that about 200,000 Germans—0.2 percent of the population—were uninsured in 2007 (Cheng and Reinhardt 2008).

The United States provides universal coverage only to a subgroup of the population—those aged 65 or older and those with disabilities—through the Medicare program. Although many low-income individuals also receive Medicaid coverage, it is hardly universal for this group. States have discretion in setting income thresholds, and individuals often must be "categorically eligible"—for example, a dependent child or the mother of dependent children. In 2006 just 46 percent of U.S. citizens below the poverty level had Medicaid, while 30 percent were uninsured (Office of the Assistant Secretary for Planning and Evaluation [ASPE] 2007, 402–05).

The advantages of universal coverage include the potential to

- improve the health and productivity of the population by making health services financially accessible to all;
- obviate the need for safety-net facilities for uninsured sick people who cannot afford care;

- decrease administrative costs, because processes such as verifying eligibility for the program will not be necessary;
- provide government with more power to keep provider payments in check (in cases where the coverage is from public entities);
- reduce problems of adverse selection in health insurance plans;[2] and
- enhance fairness in society (Rice 1998).

A possible argument against universal coverage is that it forces those who do not want coverage to pay for it, either through higher taxes or lower take-home wages. This situation was discussed in Chapter 4. As Mark Pauly (1968) argued, universal coverage, coupled with first-dollar coverage, could result in a reduction in social welfare if the costs of the extra utilization exceed the benefits. A possible counterargument is that providing coverage for preventive care could actually lower future expenditures for care, but the evidence for this is mixed.

Countries with near-universal coverage administer their healthcare systems in one of two ways (Saltman and Figueras 1998). The first system is sometimes referred to as "Beveridge style," after British academician William Beveridge, often credited with masterminding the post–World War II welfare state in the United Kingdom that included the National Health Service. Under such systems, which are also characteristic of Scandinavian countries such as Sweden, government is responsible for overseeing the provision of most services. Canada's system, although different in that it gives a larger role to private providers, is similar in that the government makes nearly all payments to providers for covered services—a system known as "single payer." These systems tend to obtain the bulk of their funding through tax revenues.

Publicly Versus Privately Administered Coverage

The other type is sometimes referred to as "Bismarck style," after nineteenth-century German Chancellor Otto von Bismarck, who (in part, as a way of staving off political support for socialism) enacted the modern world's first system of social welfare, which included health and old-age insurance. Under this kind of system, government does not oversee the provision of most health services directly. Rather, this is done by private nonprofit organizations such as sickness funds, which are often, although not exclusively, operated by occupational consortia. France and Germany use such a system. These systems rely more on contributions by employers and employees than on taxes (van Doorslaer et al. 1999).[3]

The Netherlands also financed its system this way until recently. The Dutch system has been evolving for 20 years, since the work of the Dekker Committee in the late 1980s, which advised coupling national health insurance with market reforms (Van de Ven and Schut 2008). Employers and employees still provide most of the contributions, but sickness funds are now hard to distinguish from private insurers, which compete for enrollees (Schut and Van de Ven 2005). This system is akin to the model of managed competition Alain Enthoven (2008) proposed in the late 1970s, which we mentioned in Chapter 1.

One of the main advantages of publicly administered coverage is its financing method. Tax systems usually do more to enhance equity than systems that rely on employer and employee contributions—although both are generally more equitable than systems that rely on private insurance. Tax systems may also be less disruptive to the economy. For example, mandatory payroll contributions may make it difficult for small employers to compete. In contrast, others tout privately administered systems as more removed from the political process (White 1995).

Coordination of Payers

In countries that rely on sickness funds or private insurers to administer healthcare coverage, an issue arises concerning the extent to which these entities coordinate provider payment. The United States has no statutory requirement for coordination or any formal system of coordinating payment. Each insurer establishes its own provider payment mechanism. Even when two insurers use similar systems (e.g., fee-for-service with withholds), the amount they pay usually differs.

In contrast, under an "all-payer" system, all insurers pay providers the same amount. Japan has what some consider the purest all-payer system. According to Ikegami and Campbell (2004), "[t]he fee schedule sets the price of all procedures, drugs, devices, and so on, and it applies uniformly to all plans for reimbursement to virtually all hospitals and physicians' offices" (27–28). In some cases (e.g., hospital payment in France), government regulators establish the budgets or fees (Bellanger and Mosse 2005). In Germany, government is less involved; a consortium of sickness funds negotiates joint rates with hospitals—in recent years, with rates increasingly based on diagnosis-related groups (DRGs) (Worz and Busse 2005). In such countries, all-payer rates are the norm for physician payment as well.

While all-payer rates are typical in many of these countries, some exceptions exist. Perhaps the most notable is Germany. Wealthier Germans (generally those in the top tenth income percentile) can purchase private insurance rather than going through sickness funds. In addition, rather than joining the sickness fund associated with their occupational category or region, Germans can instead enroll in a "substitute fund," which sometimes provides more benefits and which tends to pay providers more. Currently nearly anyone can join any sickness fund (Worz and Busse 2005).

All-payer rate setting has two main potential advantages. First, providers have less of an economic incentive to favor one type of patient over another. This contrasts with the situation in the United States, where, for example, some physicians avoid treating Medicaid patients because program payment rates have historically been lower than those paid by Medicare and by private insurers. The second advantage is the inability of providers to "cost shift"—to increase charges to one payer to compensate for lower payments from another. (Cost shifting was discussed in Section 6.3.) Cost shifting makes it difficult to control overall costs because providers can charge the patients of one payer more if another payer provides less.

The main potential disadvantage of all-payer rates is that all providers tend to receive the same payment, irrespective of their skills or the quality of care they deliver. Thus, a country needs to find other ways to reward providers. (Of course, where there is an abundance of physicians, better ones presumably will be rewarded with more business.) Some would also argue that individuals should be allowed to make themselves desirable to the best providers. This can occur in countries that allow people to opt out of the public system entirely, but is not possible under a pure all-payer system.

All countries administer their healthcare systems at the national and subnational levels. Some countries, however, rely more on one type than on the other. Most European countries administer at the regional level (Jonsson 1989). The United Kingdom was the main exception, but in recent years it also has moved toward regional involvement by having district health authorities carry out some budgeting (Le Grand 1999; Oliver 2005). Most significant health-related decision making in Sweden and Switzerland is done at the regional or municipal level, in part because regional government is vested with strong powers (Anell 2005; Zweifel 2000). In Canada, provinces have the vast majority of power over the operations of their systems.

Locus of Administrative Authority

In the United States, the Medicare program is administered at the federal level. Day-to-day administrative tasks, however, are carried out by regional intermediaries and carriers—usually insurers. Insurers also administer the prescription drug benefit that began in 2006. The Medicaid program receives considerable federal funding, but states run these programs—although they often must obtain federal "waivers" if they want to innovate.

Focusing government effort at the national rather than the regional level affords two main advantages. First, national government tends to have more resources available to ensure a sufficient level of expertise in conducting its activities. In the United States, Agency for Healthcare Research and Quality personnel tend to have more collective expertise in measuring quality of care than personnel in the Medicaid agency of a single state. Second, administration and enforcement at the national level leads to more uniformity and has the potential to ensure equity across different regions.

Nevertheless, there are advantages to carrying out most government activity at a subnational or regional level. The main one, of course, is that personnel at the regional level are more likely to understand the particular problems of their own populations and providers. Unlike central government, which often has a "one-size-fits-all" mentality, regional government may be able to craft solutions that meet local needs.

Nature of Coverage and Delivery

Role of Private Insurance   Generalizing about the role of private insurance across countries is difficult; each country has its own unique system. Among countries with universal coverage, two basic differences predominate. The first concerns the role of private insurers over and above what is provided under government-mandated coverage. The second is in whether insurers can compete against the government sector for enrollees.

Most countries allow private insurance to compete against government-mandated coverage. As noted earlier, about 10 percent of Germans have private health insurance. One of the attractions of private coverage is that it tends to pay providers more, although the German health minister recently noted that "because by far the largest part of the income of health care providers comes from the statutory [that is, government-mandated] system, [physicians] simply could not afford to reject patients from the statutory system" (Cheng and Reinhardt 2008, W209).

Canada is unusual in that it effectively prohibits private health insurers from selling coverage for services already included in a particular provincial health plan.[4] Although private insurance coverage for hospital and physician services is allowed in some Canadian provinces, hospitals and physicians seeing private patients cannot receive any payments from public sources—effectively eliminating a market for private insurance covering hospital and physician care. While private coverage is not prohibited in Sweden, only about 1 percent of Swedes have it (Saltman and Bergman 2005).

In countries with long waits for elective procedures, private insurance that pays more than the government-mandated system can be a very attractive feature. That is undoubtedly a major attraction of private insurance in the United Kingdom; such insurance is possessed by a little more than 10 percent of the population (Tuohy, Flood, and Stabile 2004). Other advantages include choice of specialist and more comfortable accommodations for hospital care (Smee 2000). In Australia, where private insurance is more common, those with private coverage can still receive government reimbursement toward the cost of stays in public hospitals.

Letting people opt out or supplement public coverage provides two possible advantages. First, it reduces government expenditures. A person who has private coverage does not need to use as many public resources. Some governments have found this argument compelling. Australians, for example, receive a 30-percent premium rebate from the government when they purchase private insurance. In 2003, 43 percent of the Australian population had private insurance (Palangkaraya and Yong 2005). Whether public expenditures are indeed reduced depends, however, on the extent to which private coverage is supplemented by the public sector.

Second, it allows individuals to use their own resources to purchase the coverage and services that they wish to have. People are allowed to purchase fancy homes and cars, advocates argue, so why should they be precluded from purchasing the best health coverage available? A counterargument, however, is that if those opting out are not required to purchase private coverage, they could re-enter the public system when they become ill, raising overall costs.

Allowing a large role for private insurance has two major disadvantages. First, as the percentage of the population with private coverage grows, those with public coverage may no longer have access to adequate care. When well-funded private plans compete with strapped public ones, members of the former tend to get the better providers and facilities and shorter waits. (The U.S. Medicaid program offers a good example of this.) As a result, a correlation between quality of coverage and income can develop—quite contrary to the notion of solidarity, in which care is dispensed according to need rather than ability to pay. Second, with multiple payers, selection bias becomes an issue. The worry is that sicker and poorer people will stay in the public system, while the healthier and wealthier gravitate toward the private sector.

Another issue is whether insurers can compete against each other. Under managed competition, insurers compete with each other on the basis of price, benefit offerings, service, and quality. As Alain Enthoven (1978a, 1978b, 1980), who is credited with developing the concept, envisioned, insurers would offer the best product possible to attract enrollees. To keep premiums manageable, they would also pressure providers to keep their fees low. A key to successful managed competition is preventing insurers from selecting a favorable (i.e., healthy) selection of enrollees. Requiring *open enrollment* so that anyone can join any insurance plan and *risk adjusting* premiums so that insurers are not disadvantaged if they have sicker enrollees can help.

Although it has not been fully implemented anywhere, managed competition's major characteristic—competing insurance plans—is being tested in more and more countries. (Volumes have been written both in favor of and against the concept, so a comprehensive treatment will not be attempted here.) While some choice of insurer has been common in the United States for some time, this is a fairly new concept in Europe. Citizens of Switzerland, Germany, and the Netherlands can now choose between sickness funds and insurers (Zweifel 2000; Pfaff and Wassener 2000), although the success of this choice is difficult to determine. In 2000, 5 percent of Germans changed sickness funds (Worz and Busse 2005). In the early 1990s in the Netherlands, sickness funds were permitted to compete against each other (partly on the basis of premiums) to try to attract subscribers. Previously, individuals had been required to join the fund in their particular region. Another important change was that rather than being paid retrospectively, sickness funds received a prospective, risk-adjusted capitation payment per enrollee, which might have provided them with a strong incentive to control costs. One of the major problems of this system has been determining an effective risk-adjustment payment formula so that plans compete on the basis of efficiency rather than trying to attract the healthiest enrollees (van Doorslaer and Schut 2000; Schut 1995; Saltman and Figueras 1998; Light 2001a).

With the implementation of the Health Insurance Act in 2006, the Netherlands moved toward a more complete version of managed competition. It is too early to predict how successful this will be, either economically or politically. All Dutch citizens must purchase private coverage that covers a particular set of benefits. They may change insurers annually. Those with low incomes are subsidized. Insurers are responsible for either purchasing services from providers or actually integrating with them, which is akin to managed care in the United States. Insurers must accept all applicants and cannot charge more to those in poor health (Van de Ven and Schut 2008).

For the system to work as envisioned, Frederik Schut and Wynand Van de Ven (2005, S66) state that several things needed to occur:

> First, an adequate system of risk adjustment had to be developed to prevent risk selection. Next, an adequate system of product classification and medical pricing had to be developed to give providers appropriate incentives for efficiency and to prevent cherry picking and stinting on the delivery of services. Third, an adequate system of outcome and quality measurement was necessary to enable full specified contracts between health insurers and health-care providers and to prevent competition focusing only on price. Fourth, an adequate system of consumer information about the price and quality of health insurers and health-care providers had to be developed to enable effective consumer choice. Finally, a successful implementation of the Dekker plan required the development of an adequate governance structure . . . and an effective competition policy to protect competition.

A potential advantage of managed competition in general and competition among health plans in particular is that competition on the basis of keeping premiums down may control costs. Insurers can attempt to do this by choosing providers who have proven themselves efficient, paying them in a way that gives them an incentive to conserve resources, and implementing programs that control the use of unnecessary and costly services. This can enhance quality as well if consumers can compare different plans' quality measures, an issue discussed in detail in Chapter 4. Finally, access can be ensured if generous subsidies are provided to low-income persons that allow them to "buy into" mainstream health plans.

However, concerns include the potential for

- plans to consolidate and monopolize certain markets, leading to higher prices and a reduced incentive to provide a good product;
- difficulties when individuals attempt to use comparative plan information about quality (see Section 4.1);

- difficulties in adequately risk adjusting plan premiums to help ensure that plans do not attempt to control costs by selecting healthier patients; and
- perceived inequities arising when some individuals and population groups have perceptibly worse coverage than others.

All countries provide hospital and physician services as benefits of their universal coverage programs. Countries vary, however, in the other services offered. Long-term care is often financed through a system parallel to that of health services. Pharmaceuticals, while often covered to some extent and nearly always provided to the poor, are likely to be subject to substantial patient cost sharing as a way of controlling usage. Dental coverage is commonly provided through supplemental insurance.

Benefits in Publicly Mandated Systems

The two primary advantages of public programs covering more services are (1) enhanced equity, in that ability to pay is less of an impediment for receiving services, and (2) easier cost control in government coverage because cost shifting is more difficult (although some would debate this point). In Canada, for example, the largest growth by far in health expenditures has been for services not covered by provincial health plans (Evans 2000).

An extensive list of covered services is not without its disadvantages. The most obvious disadvantage is cost. The expenditures involved in wider coverage need to be paid for through taxes or social insurance funds. Second, more comprehensive coverage leads to more service usage. When these services are more discretionary and perhaps less necessary than others, costs may outweigh the services' benefits (although this point is disputed in Chapter 4).

Historically, most developed countries have not relied on heavy cost sharing for hospital and physician services. The United States is an exception in that respect, particularly in the area of physician services, where deductibles and 20-percent coinsurance rates or copayments each time care is sought have been standard in the fee-for-service sector. However, the percentage of U.S. health expenditures paid out of pocket declined from 25 percent in 1987 to 19 percent in 2004. This is due in part to greater enrollment in managed care plans, which, until recently, tended to charge relatively low copayments (ASPE 2007, 387).

Cost-Sharing Requirements

Canada has eschewed patient cost sharing. One of the five overall requirements that provinces must meet to obtain full federal funding is "accessibility." Provinces must ensure "reasonable access to insured health care services . . . unprecluded or unimpeded, either directly or indirectly, by charges (user charges or extra billing) or other means" (Health Canada 2008b). As a result, provinces are prohibited from levying any cost-sharing requirements for covered services (Deber 2000). Other countries with relatively low levels of patient cost sharing include Germany and the United Kingdom.

Some countries, notably France, Switzerland, and Australia, do have significant cost-sharing requirements. In general, however, these do not apply to many services, and most of the population has supplemental insurance to provide protection. In France, for example, many procedures are exempt from the cost-sharing requirements, and 85 percent of the population has supplemental insurance that covers most of the costs of the services that are not exempt (Bellanger and Mosse 2005). Direct payments for health services exceed 10 percent of health-related financing in France, Switzerland, and the United States. In contrast, the figures for Germany, the United Kingdom, the Netherlands, and Sweden are 10 percent or less (Wagstaff et al. 1999).

We will forgo the discussion of the advantages and disadvantages of patient cost sharing here since they have been covered extensively in other parts of the book.

How Physicians Are Paid

Through the 1980s, the predominant method of paying physicians in most countries was fee-for-service. One exception was the British National Health Service, which provided its physicians an annual capitation payment that covered all of their office visits for the year for each patient registered in their practice. Another exception was that many countries paid salaries to specialists who practiced exclusively in the hospital. Most countries that use fee-for-service employ fee schedules. Usually, the fee schedules are negotiated between medical associations and sickness funds or insurers (Glaser 1991).

Recent years, however, have seen an increase in incentive-based payment systems, not just in the United States but in several European countries as well. Reforms in some countries have been aimed at integrating primary and hospital care. The United Kingdom allowed primary care physicians to register as "fundholders." Under this system physicians received, for each patient in their practice, financing that covered all primary care services and a budget for pharmaceutical and surgery services. Physician fundholders could retain their surpluses and use them to improve their facilities (Le Grand 1999). When the Labour Party came into power in 1997, fundholding was replaced by a similar system of Primary Care Trusts (PCTs) (Enthoven 2000) consisting of larger regional groups of primary care providers that provide or commission services for individuals in their areas. If PCTs underspend their budgets, they can spend the surplus on additional services or practice facilities (Koen 2000). Over time, it was predicted that these trusts "will absorb increasing amounts of financial risk and clinical responsibilities for managing not only primary care but also the specialty and public health care of their populations" (Bindman and Weiner 2000, 121–22). Indeed, they control over three-fourths of the total budget of the National Health Service (Oliver 2005). Nevertheless, Oliver (2005, S80) concludes that "the basic structure of the health service—that is, centrally regulated small area-based financing and planning of health care—is similar now to what it was in 1979."

The United States probably exhibits the greatest variation in physician payment. Under the Medicare program, 77 percent of enrollees are in the traditional fee-for-service program, with the remaining 23 percent in Medicare HMOs and a variety of other assorted plans (KFF 2008a). In contrast, the majority of working Americans with health insurance are in some form of managed care—either HMOs (20 percent in 2008), preferred provider organizations (PPOs, 58 percent), or point-of-service plans (POSs, 12 percent), with just 2 percent in conventional fee-for-service plans and 8 percent in high-deductible plans with a savings option (Claxton et al. 2008).[5]

Although most PPOs pay physicians on a fee-for-service basis, compensation methods are more diverse for HMO and POS plans. In paying for primary care, these health plans use fee-for-service 25 percent of the time, capitation 61 percent of the time, and salary 14 percent of the time. To pay specialists, the figures are 75 percent of the time for fee-for-service, 13 percent for capitation, and 11 percent for salary (MedPAC 2000).

The advantage of fee-for-service systems for physicians is that they may help prevent underprovision of care. They are costly, however, and can also lead to the provision of too much care. In contrast, capitation-type systems can save money but could lead to the underprovision of services unless some forms of mediating incentives are provided. For example, capitation payments could be adjusted based on quality or satisfaction scores, or they could be coupled with fee-for-service for services society wants to encourage, such as immunizations or preventive care. No matter what system of physician compensation is used, monitoring and safeguards are still required.

Choice of Providers

Free choice of a primary care physician is the norm in nearly all developed countries. Patients in countries that rely on competing health plans, such as the United States, are often limited to the primary care physicians in their plan, but they can usually choose any physician within the plan (unless, of course, the physician's practice is already full). In contrast, choice of specialist varies a great deal among countries. In a review of policies in 19 European countries, Saltman and Figueras (1998) state that, "There is no clear consensus among [European] countries as to whether patients should be allowed to refer themselves to specialist care or whether general practitioners should serve as gatekeepers to specialty care" (89). In U.S. HMOs, a patient normally cannot see a specialist without a referral from his or her primary care physician—although this is changing as HMOs move away from "heavy-handed" managed care practices. In contrast, patients in Japan generally can see any specialist that they like (Ikegami and Campbell 2004).

Because it is difficult to see any advantage to not allowing free choice of primary care provider, it is not surprising that almost all countries do provide this choice. The issue of free choice of specialist is not quite as straightforward, however. Because individuals often have less experience with and understanding of the procedures that specialists perform, they may choose a specialist poorly.

The advisability of offering free choice of hospital is even less clear. Such a choice is characteristic of the U.S. fee-for-service system, but is less true elsewhere. In Germany, for example, hospital referrals usually must be obtained from a primary care physician (Worz and Busse 2005), and normally the patient must go to the closest hospital appropriate for the medical condition (Brenner and Rublee 2002). However, one can argue that the choice of hospital has never been truly free even in the United States. Some years ago Paul Ellwood stated, "Hospitals don't have patients; doctors have patients and hospitals have doctors" (Fuchs 1983, 58). Indeed, U.S. doctors treat, on average, 90 percent of their patients in a single hospital (Miller, Welch, and Englert 1995).

Allowing consumers to choose a hospital places them in the best position to weigh the trade-offs among proximity, convenience, costs, and perceived quality. In addition, if the consumer researches quality sufficiently, he or she can (at least in theory) insist on a hospital with excellent medical outcomes. Presumably, this would apply only to elective admissions, where time to conduct sufficient research is available.

Conversely, free choice of a hospital might not be best for individuals or for society as a whole for three reasons. First, patients may choose hospitals that provide poor quality because they do not know which hospitals perform better for particular procedures. Second, economies of scale may be associated with concentrating volumes of particular services in a single hospital (Finkler 1979). If every hospital can perform every service, it may be impossible for such economies to be achieved. Third, if a particular service is concentrated in a single hospital, hospitals do not have to spend resources competing for patients and physicians. This must be weighed against higher costs that may accrue from giving hospitals more monopoly power.

Control of Expenditures

Governments must decide the extent to which they intervene in the marketplace to control health expenditures. Policies that set unit price, volume of services, or both can apply to hospitals, physicians, outpatient clinics, or pharmaceuticals. Alternatively, they can apply to the healthcare system as a whole or to large parts of it.

The box on the following page addresses the factors that lead some countries to spend more on healthcare than others.

Mandated fee schedules (also known as negotiated rates), global budgeting, and direct control of volume are three common ways to control expenditures. Each is discussed later in the context of healthcare markets and countries. Here we provide a brief overview of each.

Mandated fee schedules prospectively set the amount that a provider can receive for a particular service or episode of care. They may merely set the

Causes of High Healthcare Costs

Economists have suggested many reasons why some countries spend more than others on healthcare. We provide our personal opinions here, as well as ten key references for further reading. The theme mimics the remainder of the book: We do not believe that excessive consumer demand is the root cause of high healthcare costs, nor do we think that market-based policies such as increased consumer cost sharing and competition among for-profit insurers provide the best solutions for containing them. As noted throughout this chapter, countries that focus on direct control of supply and expenditures tend to achieve health outcomes more economically and equitably.

Here is our top-ten list of the primary causes of high healthcare expenditures. They are not mutually exclusive.

1. Lack of Power on the Purchasing Side
   Countries that take advantage of their purchasing power—that is, act as monopsonists (as described in Chapter 6)—are more successful at controlling costs. They have strong countervailing power in their negotiations with provider groups, which gives them greater price-setting power. Outside of monopsony—the hallmark of so-called single-payer systems—successful cost control is likely to occur only when there are many purchasers of care, all of whom pay providers the same rate—an "all-payers" system. Japan is an example.

2. High Unit Prices
   Expenditures are the product of price and quantity. The United States provides a relatively low volume of services but spends far more than other countries. This is because unit prices are high. Providers tend to be paid more in the United States than elsewhere, and basic services—hospital care, physician services, pharmaceuticals—cost more. This is where the first reason, market power on the purchasing side, fits in. With such power, public entities are better able to control unit prices.

3. Proliferation of Medical Technologies
   Medical advances tend to increase expenditures—not just through higher prices, but also because they tend to result in higher usage. This is not necessarily bad. Just because something costs a lot does not mean that it is a bad societal investment. Nevertheless, lack of control over the availability and use of new medical technology can lead to wastefulness—through prices that are higher than what can be justified by production costs, unnecessary utilization, or both. While markets have had little success in this area, a monopsonistic purchaser can control payment per use of a technology and even go so far as to not reimburse for technologies that it finds to be wasteful.

4. Lack of Universal Coverage
   Universal coverage might appear costly, but it can save in a number of ways. Most importantly, perhaps, is that it deters providers from charging healthier and wealthier patients more (although most countries do allow this to a certain degree to satisfy the desires of those who are economically better off to avoid waiting lists or public facilities). Universal coverage allows a country to target vulnerable populations for preventive and other primary care services. Finally, coverage can be provided for more cost-effective services, such as care in physicians' offices as opposed to emergency rooms.

5. Marketing and Administrative Costs

   When private insurers compete, associated marketing and administration costs tend to be high. Insurers use marketing to distinguish themselves from each other. They also need to monitor the health status of prospective policyholders to ensure that they do not have a particularly unhealthy set of enrollees. Finally, in the absence of a universal coverage system free of consumer copayments, they also must bill insurers and patients.

6. Regional Variation

   Most of the research on this topic has been conducted in the United States, but the phenomenon undoubtedly exists in most countries. Certain areas overprovide services but do not achieve better health outcomes, even controlling for population health status and demographic characteristics. New physicians coming into these areas tend to adopt the prevailing practices irrespective of where they trained. If all areas of the United States could adopt the utilization patterns of the more frugal areas, as much as one-third of healthcare costs could be saved.

7. Medical Specialization

   Countries that have more physicians in primary care and fewer in specialty care tend to spend less. Primary care physicians are less likely to utilize expensive technologies, and they tend to be paid less than specialists.

8. Fee-for-Service

   Most countries do employ fee-for-service reimbursement systems for physicians. This increases healthcare costs for two reasons. First, there is an economic incentive to induce demand for services (see Section 6.1). And second, other payment systems, such as global budgets, are designed with cost containment in mind.

9. Direct-to-Consumer Advertising for Prescription Drugs

   Few countries—mainly the United States and New Zealand—allow drug companies to advertise their products directly to consumers. Presumably the practice is profitable, since it continues to proliferate. Not only does this raise drug prices, but more importantly, it encourages patients to demand more expensive, brand-name drug prescriptions from their physicians.

10. Unhealthy Behaviors

    While health behaviors undoubtedly are a key factor driving healthcare costs, they do not stem directly from societal decisions about how to organize healthcare systems. Research has repeatedly shown that factors such as smoking, alcohol use, and obesity contribute significantly to healthcare costs. Public policies targeted at these behaviors can ameliorate their impact on costs.

Further Reading

Anderson, G. F., U. E. Reinhardt, P. S. Hussey, and V. Petrosyan. 2003. "It's the Prices, Stupid: Why the United States Is So Different from Other Countries." *Health Affairs* 22(3): 89–105.

Bodenheimer, T. 2005. "High and Rising Health Care Costs." Pts. 1–4. *Annals of Internal Medicine* 142 (10): 847–54; 142 (11) 932–37; 142 (12) 996–1002; 143 (1): 26–31.

Cutler, D. M., and M. McClellan. 2001. "Is Technological Change in Medicine Worth It?" *Health Affairs* 20 (5): 11–29.

Evans, R. G. 1990. "Tension, Compression, and Shear: Directions, Stresses, and Outcomes of Health Care Cost Control." *Journal of Health Politics, Policy and Law* 15 (1): 101–28.

Fisher, E. S., D. E. Wennberg, T. A. Stukel, D. J. Gottlieb, F. L. Lucas, and E. L. Pinder. 2003. "The Implications of Regional Variations in Medicare Spending." Pts. 1 and 2. *Annals of Internal Medicine* 138 (4): 273–87; 138 (4): 288–98.

Kuttner, R. 2008. "Market-Based Failure—A Second Opinion on U.S. Health Care Costs." *New England Journal of Medicine* 358 (6): 549–51.

Newhouse, J. P. 1993. "An Iconoclastic View of Health Cost Containment." *Health Affairs* 12 (Suppl.): 153–71.

New York Times. 2007. "The High Cost of Health Care." November 25.

Rice, T., and G. F. Kominski. 2007. "Containing Health Care Costs." In *Changing the U.S. Health Care System: Key Issues in Health Services Policy and Management,* ed. R. M. Andersen, T. H. Rice, and G. F. Kominski. San Francisco: John Wiley and Sons.

Thorpe, K. E., C. S. Florence, D. H. Howard, and P. Joski. 2004. "The Impact of Obesity on Rising Medical Spending." *Health Affairs* Web Exclusive. October 20: W4-480–W4-486.

price paid per resource use (e.g., per diem rates for hospitals or relative value scales for physicians), or they may pay a fixed amount irrespective of resource use (e.g., DRG payments for hospitals or capitation for physicians).

Global budgets are "prospectively set caps on spending for some portion of the healthcare industry" (Wolfe and Moran 1993, 55). They provide "macroregulation" of expenditures, in which little direct oversight is given to the provision of care, but strict controls are placed on how much money is paid out in total. Global budgets indirectly control volume by limiting how much can be spent on certain kinds of healthcare in a particular area over a particular time period. A study conducted in the early 1990s found that ten European countries had adopted some form of global budgeting (Wolfe and Moran 1993), mainly for the government portion of hospital and/or physician expenditures, but sometimes for total government health expenditures. Most countries that use global budgets administer them regionally (Jonsson 1989) and use them as one of several tools for controlling health expenditures.

Direct control of volume, in contrast, is a form of "microregulation" of expenditures. In the United States, volume is controlled through various managed care practices. Only occasionally—in the United States and elsewhere—has the explicit rationing of services occurred.

Hospital Fee Schedules and Global Budgeting

Some time ago, hospitals in most countries received per diem payments for each day of a patient's hospital stay, but this method was ineffective in controlling overall expenditures because it provided an incentive to keep patients longer (Glaser 1991) and was not based on the resource requirements of different types of patients.

The United States was the first country to pay hospitals a fixed amount for an entire patient stay. This practice, part of the DRG system first employed by the Medicare program and later by other private and public insurers, quickly shortened lengths of stay. Although concerns continue that DRGs threaten quality by encouraging early discharge, no systematic evidence indicates that this has occurred.[6] If DRGs have shortened stays without affecting quality, patients were probably staying in hospitals too long. Indeed, hospital lengths of stay in most developed countries have shortened in recent years. It is not clear whether this was due to evidence from the United States that shorter stays were indeed possible. Other factors, such as advances in certain medical techniques and pharmaceuticals, have also contributed to shorter stays.

The use of global budgets to pay hospitals is more common in other developed countries. In Canada, each hospital negotiates its own budget with provinces. If a hospital exceeds its budget, compensation is not guaranteed. In several European countries, hospital budgets are assigned based on historic costs but adjusted for case mix (Saltman and Figueras 1998). In countries with multiple payers, each must contribute to a hospital's global budget. This is usually done through negotiations between the hospital and either government or a consortium of sickness funds. Each of the funds then contributes a portion of the hospital's total budget based on how much its enrollees contribute to the hospital's overall utilization (Glaser 1991).

Each of the current payment methods—negotiated rates used by private health plans in the United States, DRGs, and global budgets—has advantages and disadvantages. The potential success of each system hinges, in part, on the ability of payers to adjust payments according to severity of illness so that hospitals are appropriately compensated. Nevertheless, some generalizations about each payment system are possible.

The use of competitive forces to set rates allows the market to equilibrate supply and demand, potentially enhancing economic efficiency. Critics, however, believe that hospital costs are impossible to control when multiple sources of payment exist. In addition, hospitals may end up favoring the patients of the more generous payers.

DRGs encourage hospitals to keep patients no longer than medically necessary. However, they have potential problems: Quality will suffer if stays become too short, so it must be continually monitored; hospitals may still favor the patients of one insurer over another if DRG payment rates vary; providers have an incentive to bill for more remunerative DRGs; and providers have an incentive to move care to sectors that are not paid on a DRG basis (e.g., outpatient departments). One might expect the effect of DRGs in the United States to be known by now, since they were implemented in 1983. However, because they were implemented nationally, isolating the effect of DRGs from other changes in the health system in the same time period (particularly the growth of managed care) is nearly impossible.

Hospital global budgets are difficult to evaluate in isolation because they are typically used in conjunction with other policies, such as controls on bed supply and medical technologies. The main advantage of paying hospitals a global budget is that it allows payers, be they government or private, to control overall hospital expenditures. It may also enhance efficiency because hospitals are free to allocate their budgets as they wish. Disadvantages include the difficulty of coming up with the appropriate total budget for each hospital, since this entails calculating how much the hospital would be spending if it were operating efficiently; concerns that hospitals will stint on hiring appropriate staff, since they are given a fixed budget; and the potential for keeping beds filled with patients who use fewer resources to keep budgets up but costs down (a problem that can be ameliorated by adjusting payments to patient severity).

As noted earlier, fee-for-service payments remain the most common method of compensating physicians in developed countries, though hospital-based physicians are sometimes salaried, and primary care physicians in the United Kingdom are paid using capitation (discussed in Chapter 6). In the typical system, physicians are paid based on a fee schedule, which is simply a list of procedures with a fee associated with each. In the U.S. Medicare program, fees are the product of a set of relative values[7] and a *conversion factor*. The relative values indicate the ratio of payment rates between different procedures. A conversion factor then converts these relative values into actual fee-for-service payment rates. For example, if a follow-up office visit has a relative value of 10, and the conversion factor is $8, total payment for the service would be $80. Other countries relying on fee-for-service generally do not use relative values and conversion factors. Rather, fees are negotiated between government or a consortium of sickness funds and provider organizations.

Physician Fee Schedules

Fee-for-service has been criticized for its inability to control costs and for the incentives it provides for overutilization of services. Some countries, notably Germany, the United States through its Medicare program, and most of the Canadian provinces, have dealt with these criticisms by attempting to control total expenditures for physicians—that is, the product of unit prices and the volume of services provided.

In the early 1990s the U.S. Medicare program began to use volume performance standards (VPSs). This was later replaced by a similar system called the sustainable growth rate (SGR). Under the VPS system, each year Congress set a target rate of increase in Medicare Part B physician expenditures. If actual spending exceeded the target, the next year's physician fee update was normally reduced by that amount (although Congress could do whatever it chose when the time came). Conversely, if the growth in spending was less than the target, physicians would get more. Suppose, for example, that the target for a particular year was a 10 percent increase in spending. If actual spending increased by 12 percent, the target would have been exceeded. Most likely, the overage would be extracted the next time Congress updated Medicare physician fees. If physicians were due a 5-percent cost-of-living increase, they would likely be granted only 3 percent.

The main difference between the SGR system, implemented in 1998, and the VPS system was that the SGR system set a target expenditure rate of "sustainable growth." One factor in setting the rate was the projected change in real gross domestic product (GDP) (MedPAC 2000). Essentially, this limited overall expenditure growth to the growth rate of the economy as a whole. As a result, a problem has arisen: The SGR formula results in a reduction in physician fees because healthcare volume is growing faster than the GDP. Because of the political fallout resulting from the prospect of falling physician payments, Congress has, for several years, overridden the formula so that fees would not decrease.

The VPS system (and by analogy, SGR) has been criticized as too blunt an instrument to affect individual physician behavior. Because the system applies nationally, individual physicians who increase the volume of the services they provide are not penalized by experiencing a decline in fees. The decline would happen only if all physicians behave this way. If a physician does not increase her volume but other physicians do, that physician would suffer. Her volume is constant, but the behavior of other physicians will cause the fee to fall. The VPS system may therefore contain a perverse incentive to increase the volume of services, which is exactly what it was supposed to prevent. One way to improve the incentives would be to target smaller groups of physicians by having separate targets for each specialty, state, or state-specialty combination (Rice and Bernstein 1990; Marquis and Kominski 1994).

Most of the Canadian provinces also adopted expenditure caps or targets in response to difficult economic times beginning in the late 1980s (Barer, Lomas, and Sanmartin 1996; Bodenheimer 2005), although few such programs are still in place now. As of the mid-1990s, eight of the ten provinces had established "hard" caps in which fees were reduced in proportion to the extent to which the caps were exceeded. One of the more interesting side effects is that the medical profession sought to reduce the supply of physicians as a way of stabilizing fees—the idea being that more physicians would result in more billings, which in turn would reduce payment rates.

The U.S. Medicare targets and the Canadian provincial caps apply at the aggregate level. As of the mid-1990s, five of the ten Canadian provinces had adopted some form of individual income cap as well. Typically, this entails reducing unit fees after a physician has exceeded a certain income threshold. In Ontario, for example, fees were reduced by 33 percent after annual income reached $404,000, and by 67 percent after it reached $454,000 (Canadian dollars) (Barer, Lomas, and Sanmartin 1996).

Two other examples come from Germany and Japan. Ambulatory care physicians in Germany are paid on a fee-for-service basis according to a fee schedule that is based on a uniform relative value scale. (Physicians providing inpatient care are typically salaried.) The total budget for ambulatory physician care rises with growth in wages. If the number of services rises faster than the budget, unit fees decline. As in the United States under the VPS and SGR systems, this leads to a perverse incentive for the individual to increase the quantity of services provided. To prevent this, a limit was put on reimbursable "points" or reimbursements per patient in the late 1990s (Worz and Busse 2005). A similar situation exists in Japan. According to Ikegami and Campbell (2004, 28), "prices are revised individually, adjusted for each procedure and drug [and] prices of procedures that show large increases in volume tend to be decreased." As an example, they note that the price of a magnetic resonance imaging (MRI) test of the head fell from $151 to $104 as a result of rising volumes.

With the exception of the United States, which has a history of utilization controls, most countries do not focus on direct volume controls or the microregulation of expenditures. They focus instead on regulating prices and indirectly controlling volume, through fee schedules or the global budgets discussed above, or on the supply of inputs. In spite of what is sometimes heard in the United States, other countries seldom explicitly ration services. Rather, they prioritize services on the basis of medical need, which can result in implicit rationing if there is not enough budget or capacity to treat those whose needs physicians perceive as lower.

Direct Regulation of Volume

In contrast, the United States continues to directly regulate volume. Examples include requiring certification before insurers pay for hospital stays, requiring second opinions before surgery is paid for, and profiling physician practices. Managed care plans also use direct volume controls. One example is preadmission certification of hospital stays, which requires the physician to contact a health plan employee for the stay to be covered. If the plan disagrees with the physician's assessment, a cumbersome appeals process can ensue. Another example is requiring that patients see a primary care gatekeeper before going to a specialist. To enforce this, health plans must examine every case. If the claim is denied, the patient can appeal, which results in more administrative costs. In general, microregulation means that someone is watching over a large percentage of physician and patient activities.

The advantage of direct control of volume is that it can reduce the waste in the system. For example, if a particular procedure is inappropriate for a patient with a given diagnosis, such procedures can, in theory, be prevented. The major disadvantage, however, is that it is often cumbersome from an administrative standpoint, involving much bureaucracy, paperwork, and undue oversight over the practice of medicine.

Control of Input Supply

Developed countries vary with respect to hospital ownership. Those that are privately owned vary regarding whether they are for-profit or nonprofit institutions. In the United Kingdom, for example, about 90 percent of

The Hospital

inpatient beds are in public facilities (Smee 2000). In contrast, the majority of acute care hospitals in the United States and Canada are private, not-for-profit facilities.

Controlling the supply of hospital beds is a strategy most developed countries use, particularly in the public sector. The logic goes back to Roemer's law, which states that in a well-insured population, "a bed built is a bed filled" (Shain and Roemer 1959). This "law" was consistent with empirical evidence until the advent of DRGs and the movement away from fee-for-service medicine.

The Physician

Most countries actively control the supply of physicians, usually because of the supposition that more physicians will result in higher health expenditures (see the discussion on physician-induced demand in Section 6.1). More recent years, particularly in the United States, have seen an emphasis on augmenting the supply of generalists at the expense of specialists (see Chapter 8 for a discussion of this issue in the United States). One way to change these distributions, at least in the long run, is to provide a financial incentive to physicians who choose to become general or family practitioners, internists, or OB-GYNs. In the United States, the Medicare fee schedule that was implemented in the early 1990s resulted in a substantial redistribution of fees away from specialists toward generalists (Ginsburg, LeRoy, and Hammons 1990). Nevertheless, income differences by specialty in the United States remain large. In 2008, U.S. cardiologists earned an average of $380,000 and radiologists over $400,000, compared to $200,000 for internists and $190,000 for family practitioners (American Medical Group Association 2008).

Countries have attempted to control physician supply using a variety of techniques. The most common are limiting medical school enrollment and reducing the number of foreign-trained physicians allowed to practice in a country (Schroeder 1984). Some of the Canadian provinces have been particularly active in this regard as a result of the financial difficulties that began in the late 1980s. Additional strategies one or more provinces used include paying new physicians only 50 percent of their usual fees unless they practice in particular geographic areas, not providing billing numbers (which are needed to obtain payment), and allowing older physicians to "buy out" their billing numbers to encourage retirement (Barer, Lomas, and Sanmartin 1996). The restrictions in billing numbers have not been terribly successful. Barer and colleagues (1996, 223) note that "despite the best intentions of the ministers of health in declaring their commitment to a national physician resource strategy, in reality provinces have pretty much done their own thing to keep others' graduates from their borders."

Most countries regulate physician supply to have some control over total health expenditures and to help plan for the desired distribution of health personnel. The major disadvantage is that government planners may mistakenly perceive shortages or surpluses of physicians and may make inappropriate policy decisions as a result. Given the lead time it takes to train physicians, it may take years to correct such mistakes.

With the exception of the United States, developed countries actively control the dissemination and use of expensive medical technologies. Table 10.2 shows the availability of two medical technologies—CT scanners and MRIs—across the ten countries in number of units per million population.[8] Japan has by far the most technologies. Yoshikawa and Bhattacharya (2002, 259–60) summarize the probable reason:

Capital and Medical Technology

> Under Japanese fee-for-service medicine with the uniform fee schedule, hospitals cannot engage in price competition. With such market conditions, hospitals tend to engage in nonprice competition to attract patients. When there are legal restrictions on advertising, a hospital's options are quite limited. Hence, many hospitals may purchase high-technology medical equipment to signal a level of medical sophistication that will attract more patients. Hospitals located in markets with a high level of local competition have an incentive to quickly acquire high-technology medical equipment to compete with their rivals.

Other than Japan, few clear patterns are evident in Table 10.2, except that the United States ranks second or third in both technologies. Interestingly, several of the countries have only about one-eighth as many CT scanners and MRIs per million population as Japan does.

The methods by which countries control these technologies vary. In Canada, provinces finance most capital equipment, and hospitals do not receive increases in their global budgets for the use of medical equipment that has not been approved by provincial governments. After studying the considerable differences in the utilization of cardiovascular procedures between Canada and the United States, Verrilli, Berenson, and Katz (1998, 481) found that lower rates in Canada, particularly for older individuals, are

> accomplished both by implicit, discretionary rationing by physicians and by more formal restriction on the availability of services through resource constraints. Canadian provincial governments strictly control both the number of hospitals performing cardiovascular procedures and the funding for these procedures.

The advantages and disadvantages of explicit supply controls are similar, whether they apply to hospitals, physicians, or medical technology. The advantages mirror those mentioned for budget controls, including the potential for cost control and greater ability of governments to provide necessary services to the population. The two main disadvantages are the inability of policymakers to determine the appropriate amount of inputs to produce, and

TABLE 10.2: Availability of Selected Medical Technologies*
(units per million persons)

	CT Scanners	MRIs
Australia	51.1	4.9
Canada	12.0	6.2
France	10.0	5.3
Germany	16.7	7.7
Japan	92.6	40.1
Netherlands	8.2	6.6
Sweden	NA	NA
Switzerland	18.7	14.4
United Kingdom	7.6	5.6
United States	33.9	26.5

SOURCE: Data from OECD (2008).

*Data are from the most recent year available between 2002 and 2006, which varies by country.

NA = data not available.

concern that controls will stifle life-enhancing or efficiency-producing innovations.

10.2 Cross-National Data on Health System Performance

This section provides recent data on the performance of different countries' health systems. It is divided into five subsections, each of which examines a particular aspect of performance: access, utilization, expenditures, quality/satisfaction, and equity of financing. The focus is on the ten countries discussed earlier and described in the Appendix: Australia, Canada, France, Germany, Japan, the Netherlands, Sweden, Switzerland, the United Kingdom, and the United States. Because comparable data are scarce, some categories compare only a subset of countries. Short descriptions of each country's system appear in the Appendix.

The World Health Organization (WHO) (2000) did attempt an assessment of the performance of the health systems of its 191 member states in 2000. Performance was based on five indicators: overall level of population health, health inequalities within the population, two measures of health system responsiveness, and the distribution of the health system's financial burden within the population. For the sake of completeness, the rankings are noted here: Australia (thirty-second), Canada (thirtieth), France (first), Germany (twenty-fifth), Japan (tenth), the Netherlands (seventeenth), Sweden (twenty-third), Switzerland (twentieth), the United Kingdom (eighteenth), and the United States (thirty-seventh). Curiously, Italy was ranked second in the world, in spite of the fact that "only 20 percent of Italians rate their health care system as satisfactory" (Jamison and Sandbu 2001, 1595).

This chapter does not rely on the WHO rankings because they appear fraught with methodological problems. Some of these include failure to control for confounding variables other than national education levels and health expenditures, assuming that all differences in outcomes are the result of health system performance, extreme sensitivity of the results to changes in specification of the statistical model, ignoring such measures as satisfaction and health promotion and preventive care in the ratings of performance, and assuming that every country has the same goals for its system (Jamison and Sandbu 2001; Robbins 2001; Mooney and Wiseman 2000). Until such an analysis can adequately deal with these issues, it is premature to rank different countries' health systems' performance.

Access

This section presents data on three different aspects of access to care: coverage rates, individuals' beliefs that they can obtain care when they need it, and waiting times for obtaining procedures. The first of these is a measure of potential access, whereas the second and third gauge realized access (Aday, Andersen, and Fleming 1980).

Unfortunately, comparable cross-national data on coverage rates are not available. Although most developed countries have systems with universal coverage, in some cases a subset of the population receives coverage through private rather than public sources. The first column of Table 10.3 shows eligibility for health benefits under *public programs* (OECD 2008). In eight of the ten countries, more than 98 percent (and often 100 percent) of the population is covered in this manner. The figures are lower in Germany (89.9 percent) and the United States (27.4 percent). As the second column indicates, in the case of Germany, almost everyone who does not have public coverage has private insurance. The only country with an uninsurance rate greater than 2 percent is the United States, at 16 percent.

Table 10.4 shows the prevalence of uninsurance in the United States in 2006. During this year, 43.9 million people were uninsured (ASPE 2007). Rates are higher for certain subgroups: 30 percent of those aged 18 to 24, 35 percent of Hispanics or Latinos, and about 30 percent of those below 150 percent of the poverty level.

One limitation of the data in Table 10.4 is that they do not address the availability of medical care. Although access to care is supposed to be related to health insurance coverage, this is not necessarily the case. Uninsured individuals can pay for care themselves, or they can use the safety net of facilities and providers designed to serve the poor and uninsured. Similarly, insured

TABLE 10.3: Eligibility for Healthcare Benefits Under Public Programs and Uninsurance

	Population Covered Under Public Programs	Population Uninsured, 2007
Australia	100%	0%
Canada	100%	0%
France	99.9%	NA
Germany	89.5%	<1%
Japan	100%	NA
Netherlands	98.7%	<2%
Sweden	100%	NA
Switzerland	100%	NA
United Kingdom	100%	0%
United States	27.4%	16%

SOURCES: (1) Data for population covered from OECD (2008). (2) Data for population uninsured used with permission from Schoen, C., R. Osborn, M. M. Doty, M. Bishop, J. Peugh, and N. Murukutla. 2007. "Toward Higher-Performance Health Systems." *Health Affairs* 26 (6): W717–W734.

NOTE: Data for population covered are from the most recent year available, either 2005 or 2006, which varies by country.

individuals may still face access barriers if, for example, the supply of medical personnel, facilities, and technologies is insufficient to serve the population. Still, uninsured Americans are far more likely than the insured to say that they are not able to get the medical care that they need (Donelan et al. 1999). Studies indicate that compared to the insured, the uninsured are more likely to forgo recommended treatments because of cost, to receive fewer preventive services, to be hospitalized for "avoidable conditions," and to be diagnosed with cancer when the disease has reached a more advanced stage (Hoffman and Schlobohm 2000).

Table 10.5, which is based on data collected from telephone surveys of adults with chronic conditions in several countries, examines indicators of access, costs, and quality among these countries (Schoen et al. 2008). Focusing on patients with chronic conditions is useful because they have the most contact with healthcare systems. The table shows that the British, Dutch, and Germans had the best success in getting care outside of the emergency room during nights, weekends, or holidays. Americans reported the most difficulty. Similarly, Americans were the most likely to report a medical mistake or a medication error, although Canada and Australia were not too far behind. The biggest difference among the countries is the extent to which high costs impeded access. At least 36 percent of Americans with chronic

TABLE 10.4: Number of Uninsured in the United States and Percentage Insured by Selected Characteristics, 2006

Total Number of Uninsured (millions)	43.9

Percentage Uninsured by Characteristic

Age	
Under 6 years	7.5%
6–17 years	10.5%
18–24 years	29.9%
25–34 years	27.2%
35–44 years	18.8%
45–54 years	15.0%
55–64 years	10.8%
Sex	
Male	18.8%
Female	15.3%
Race	
White	16.7%
Black	18.1%
Asian	15.0%
Hispanic or Latino	35.0%
Percentage of Poverty Level	
Below 100 percent	30.2%
100–149 percent	31.2%
150–199 percent	28.0%
200 percent or more	10.5%
Geographic Region	
Northeast	11.2%
Midwest	13.4%
South	21.1%
West	18.8%
Location of Residence	
Within MSA	16.6%
Outside MSA	19.3%

SOURCE: Data from ASPE (2007). Table 139.

MSA = metropolitan statistical area.

TABLE 10.5: Reports on Indicators of Access, Cost, and Quality of Care Among Those with Chronic Conditions, 2008

	Australia	Canada	France	Germany	Netherlands	United Kingdom	United States
Difficulty Getting Care Nights, Weekends, Holidays Without Going to ER							
Very difficult	34	33	29	15	15	20	40
Somewhat difficult	28	23	27	21	15	24	20
Very or somewhat easy	36	39	42	63	65	53	36
Reported Medical Mistake or Medication Error	22	21	14	16	14	15	23
Access Problems Because of Cost in the Last Two Years							
Did not fill a prescription	20	18	13	12	3	7	43
Did not visit a doctor when sick	21	9	11	15	3	4	36
Did not get recommended test or follow-up	25	11	13	13	3	6	38

SOURCE: Data used with permission from Schoen, C., R. Osborn, S. K. H. How, M. M. Doty, and J. Peugh,. 2008. "In Chronic Conditions." *Health Affairs* 28 (1): W1–W16.

illness reported problems with the following due to costs: filling a prescription, visiting a doctor when sick, and getting recommended tests or follow-up care. The countries in which these indicators were rarely a problem were the Netherlands and the United Kingdom.

Waiting lists, particularly for obtaining surgical care and tests, have received a great deal of attention internationally. Unfortunately, compiling comparable cross-national data on waiting lists is nearly impossible. Countries rarely keep consolidated lists of patients who are waiting for treatment.

Perhaps a better way to approach the problem is to examine waiting time. This gets around the problem that people may be on several lists at once. Unfortunately, no objective data are available on waiting time. A reasonable alternative is to ask consumers about their experiences, as was done in the Schoen and colleagues (2005) study. Table 10.6 shows the results. Germans had the shortest average waits for elective surgery, with the United States and

TABLE 10.6: Self-Reported Waiting Times, 2005

	Australia	Canada	Germany	United Kingdom	United States
Waiting Times for Elective Surgery (percentages):					
Less than 1 month	48	15	59	25	53
1–3.9 months	33	52	35	34	39
4 months or more	19	33	6	41	8
Waiting Time for Specialist Appointment					
Less than 1 week	11	10	27	11	20
1–4 weeks	43	33	51	29	57
4 weeks or more	46	57	22	60	23

SOURCE: Data used with permission from Schoen, C., R. Osborn, P. T. Huynh, M. M. Doty, K. Zapert, J. Peugh, and K. Davis. 2005. "Taking the Pulse of Health Care Systems." *Health Affairs* Web Exclusive (July–December, Suppl.); W5-509–W5-525.

Australia not far behind. Nearly 60 percent of Germans waited less than a month. In contrast, only 25 percent of Britons and 15 percent of Canadians waited a month or less. Over 40 percent of Britons waited four months or longer for elective surgery. In most countries, those with higher incomes are able to avoid waiting times by obtaining services through private insurance or self-payment. Indeed, in some countries, physicians have an incentive to make public patients wait—they can obtain more lucrative fees through the private market.

The second half of Table 10.6 shows waiting time for specialist appointments. Again, Germany performs best and the United States second best. The other three countries reported considerably longer waits for specialist appointments.

Another, somewhat older survey examined a related question: how many patients needing elective cataract surgery in three countries were willing to pay to reduce waiting time (Anderson et al. 1997). One finding was that few—12, 15, and 24 percent of respondents in Spain, Canada, and Denmark, respectively—were in favor of higher income taxes to eliminate waiting times. Furthermore, relatively few were willing to pay market prices to avoid waits in public facilities. The authors conclude that "in spite of expressed public dissatisfaction with waiting lists in all three sites, a majority of the respondents did not support the actions that could have reduced their own wait" (Anderson et al. 1997, 181).

Utilization

Utilization is not a measure of a country's health system performance. It is simply a measure of the use of various types of healthcare. We discuss it here briefly because utilization figures provide a glimpse into how different countries manage their resources.

Table 10.7 shows four measures of usage: inpatient care (acute care bed days per capita), outpatient care (physician consultations or visits per capita), and two measures involving cardiovascular care (coronary artery bypass and coronary angioplasty operations per 100,000 population) (OECD 2008). Most countries have comparable rates of inpatient utilization. Exceptions include the United States and the Netherlands, whose rates are somewhat lower, and Japan and Germany, whose rates are considerably higher than the rest. Physician consultation rates show more variation, with Sweden lower than the others and Japan substantially higher. Japan's rate is roughly double (or higher) that of any other country. This is attributable to a low fee schedule, which encourages physicians to see many patients for short visits, and historically high levels of prescription drug use. A large proportion of physician visits in Japan are simply to obtain prescriptions (Ikegami and Campbell 1999).

The table shows extremely high rates of use of the two coronary procedures in the United States. The U.S. rate is almost twice the average of the other countries' for bypass operations and about three times as high as every country but Germany for angioplasty, a finding confirmed by a more systematic cross-national study of heart attack care around the world (TECH Research Network 2001). These differences are, in part, a result of explicit supply-side rationing and the use of strict global budgets in several of the other countries (Saltman and Figueras 1998; McClellan and Kessler 1999; TECH Research Network 2001).

Another explanation is that U.S. use of cardiovascular procedures is especially high for the "oldest old." A study of 1992 data from the United States and Canada found that the difference in usage between the two countries rose dramatically with patient age. For example, among coronary artery bypass procedures, the ratio between U.S. and Canadian usage was 1.4 for those aged 65 to 69, 2.6 for those aged 70 to 74, 4.2 for those aged 75 to 79, and 7.2 for those aged 80 or older. The pattern for angioplasty (1.9, 3.2, 4.9, and 7.7, respectively) was similar (Verrilli, Berenson, and Katz 1998, 482). The authors conclude that

> As a result of both resource constraints and societal and physician attitudes towards care of the elderly, physicians in Canada appear to use age as a basis for limiting the provision of technologically oriented medical care. In contrast, since the threshold for providing cardiovascular services to the elderly is higher in the U.S. than it is in Canada, it appears that U.S. physicians consider age a less

TABLE 10.7: Utilization of Select Services

	Acute Care Bed Days per Capita	Physician Consultations per Capita	Coronary Artery Bypass Operations per 100,000	Coronary Angioplasty Operations per 100,000
Australia	1.0	6.1	70	168
Canada	0.9	5.9	87	138
France	1.0	6.4	41	156
Germany	1.7	7.0	78	353
Japan	2.0	13.7	NA	NA
Netherlands	0.7	5.6	57	93
Sweden	NA	2.8	54	173
Switzerland	1.1	3.4	34	113
United Kingdom	0.9	5.1	43	101
United States	0.7	4.0	145	434

SOURCE: Data from OECD (2008).

*Data are most recent available:
   Acute care bed days: 2005 or 2006
   Physician consultations: 2004–2006 except 2002 for Switzerland
   Coronary artery bypass operations: 2004–2006 except 2001 for France
   Coronary angioplasty operations: 2003–2006 except 2001 for France

NA = data not available.

important factor in determining who receives cardiovascular services. In the general absence of budgetary constraints, whether this encourages profligate service use or whether it contributes to improved outcomes among elderly persons in the U.S. is uncertain.

These differences in usage rates do not appear to affect mortality much. In another study, Tu and colleagues (1997) found that angiography was five times as common among seniors in the United States as in Ontario, Canada, and angioplasty and coronary artery bypass surgery were seven times as common. In spite of this, 30-day mortality rates were only slightly lower in the United States (21.4 percent vs. 22.3 percent), and one-year mortality rates were nearly identical (34.3 percent in the United States vs. 34.4 percent in Ontario).

These stark differences in utilization, especially among older patients, are undoubtedly related to the way costs are controlled in the two countries. In the U.S. Medicare program, costs are controlled mainly through limited physician fees and DRG payments and aggregate expenditure targets for all physician services. In contrast, Canadian cost controls center on hospital global budgets and regulation of the diffusion of medical technology. As a result, most provinces lack the capacity to provide as many surgeries to older patients as the United States does.

Expenditures

The first column of Table 10.8 shows per capita expenditures on health in each of the ten countries during 2005 (OECD 2008). These figures have been adjusted by "purchasing power parities," which account for different price levels across countries so that a given amount of money will purchase the same market basket of goods and services. The second column shows the ratio of expenditures in the United States compared with each other country. The 2.12 figure for Australia, for example, means that per capita expenditures were a little more than twice as high in the United States. The final column shows the percentage of GDP devoted to health in each country during 2005.

The United States, at $6,347, is far above all others, with Switzerland a distant second at $4,069. The U.S. level is particularly noteworthy given that about 16 percent of the population is uninsured. Japan spends the least on health at $2,474, with the United Kingdom a bit higher at $2,580. The percentage of GDP spent on health shows a similar pattern, although the range among countries is narrower.

Because wealthier countries can devote a larger share of national income to health, it is useful to control for this factor when comparing countries. Figure 10.1 shows the relationship between wealth and health expenditures for all Organisation for Economic Co-operation and Development

TABLE 10.8: Total Healthcare Expenditures, 2005

	Per Capita Expenditures in U.S. Dollars	Ratio of Expenditures to the U.S. Level	Gross Domestic Product Spent on Health
Australia	$2,999	2.12	8.8%
Canada	$3,460	1.83	9.9%
France	$3,306	1.92	11.2%
Germany	$3,251	1.95	10.7%
Japan	$2,474	2.57	8.2%
Netherlands	$3,192	1.99	9.2%
Sweden	$3,012	2.11	9.2%
Switzerland	$4,069	1.56	11.4%
United Kingdom	$2,580	2.46	8.4%
United States	$6,347	1.00	15.3%

SOURCE: Data from OECD (2008).

FIGURE 10.1: Relationship Between Health Expenditures and
National Wealth

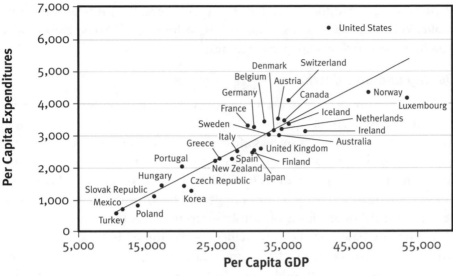

SOURCE: Data from OECD (2008). Trend line provided by the authors (ordinary least squares regression).

(OECD) countries in 2005. In almost every case, a country's health spending can be predicted quite accurately by the level of per capita GDP; almost all fall on the diagonal line. The main exception is the United States, which spends far more on health than would be predicted based simply on its income.

A comparison of these figures with the utilization patterns shown in Table 10.7 shows that care is more expensive in the United States, given that its overall usage rates for hospital and physician services are low by international standards. One explanation is the higher usage rates for the two cardiac procedures shown, which likely indicates a pattern for other procedures. Another explanation, not shown in these tables, is differences in unit prices between countries. Researchers have compared unit prices for medical care in the United States and Canada. One study, using data from the mid-1980s, found that the ratio of U.S. private insurance physician fees to those paid by the Canadian provinces averaged 2.4, with ratios exceeding 3.0 for surgery (Fuchs and Hahn 1990). Although Americans may be getting more for their fees, these differences may not reflect differences in the quality of care delivered (an issue we address later). Differences in provider incomes are more likely. Physician incomes are far higher in the United States than anywhere else—almost twice as high as those of Canadian physicians and more than twice as high as those in the other countries examined here (OECD 2001).

However, higher unit costs are not necessarily a reflection of waste; the services being priced might not be comparable in terms of quality. A day in the hospital in the United States, for example, might entail better quality or more desirable amenities than a day in a Canadian hospital. Similarly, U.S. physicians could produce more for their higher fees. This is why comparing quality and satisfaction across countries is so important. Some comparative data on these outcomes are presented next.

Quality and Satisfaction

In spite of the importance of quality in policy discussions on health system reform, little cross-national quality information is available. The most common data concern vital statistics such as life expectancy and infant mortality. While important, these figures are more reflective of a country's sociodemographic conditions than the quality of its medical care systems. Perhaps a better way of assessing quality across countries might be to *ask* individuals about their perceptions, although this is obviously subjective. Another flaw is that people's tastes are based on their experience (as we argued in Chapter 5). Consequently, rigorous studies of important health outcomes across countries, controlling, as much as possible, for differences in population characteristics, would be better. Unfortunately, few such studies have been conducted.

Satisfaction is easier to evaluate across countries. Satisfaction is sometimes criticized, however, as being overly subjective and not targeted on aspects of quality that most interest policymakers. Furthermore, compared to objective measures of quality, satisfaction measures based on survey responses tend to shift more over time.

Beginning with the vital statistics, Table 10.9 shows average life expectancy, infant mortality rates, and potential years of life lost (due to deaths prior to age 70) for the ten countries (OECD 2008). Life expectancy shows relatively little dispersion. Among the small differences, the averages are higher in Japan and lower in the United States than elsewhere. A much greater difference, however, is found in infant mortality rates. Rates for Sweden (2.4) and Japan (2.8) are less than half the U.S. rate (6.9). The much higher infant mortality rates in the United States are due, in part, to lack of insurance and poorer living conditions among poorer residents. The pattern in the last column, which examines potential years of life lost, is similar to that of the other two, with the United States performing far worse than the other countries.

Finally, we move to data that more directly address the quality of healthcare across countries. We begin with two older studies that simply compare Canada and the United States.

Roos and colleagues (1990) compared postsurgical mortality in the New England states and Manitoba. The researchers divided procedures into low, moderate, and high mortality, and looked at mortality rates 30 days, one

TABLE 10.9: Life Expectancy, Infant Mortality, and Potential Years of Life Lost

	Life Expectancy at Birth (years)	Infant Deaths per 1,000 Live Births	Potential Years of Life Lost per 100,000 Population*
Australia	80.9	5.0	3,228
Canada	80.4	5.4	3,365
France	80.2	3.8	3,611
Germany	79.4	3.9	3,360
Japan	82.0	2.8	2,757
Netherlands	79.4	4.9	3,103
Sweden	80.6	2.4	2,929
Switzerland	81.4	4.2	2,952
United Kingdom	79.1	5.1	3,549
United States	77.8	6.9	4,934

SOURCE: Data from OECD (2008).

*Potential years of life lost is a measure of premature mortality, calculated by adding up deaths occurring at each age and multiplying this by the number of remaining years to live until age 70.

Life expectancy and infant deaths for 2005.

Potential years of life lost for 2004 except 2003 for Australia.

year, and three years after surgery. After adjusting the best they could for case-mix differences, they found mortality rates to be lower in Manitoba for low-risk and moderate-risk procedures over all three time intervals. Thirty-day mortality rates were lower in New England for high-mortality procedures, but these differences subsided over time (Roos et al. 1992).

The second study examined cancer survival rates in the United States and Ontario (U.S. Government Accountability Office [GAO] 1994). Specifically, it examined survival of a large sample of patients from 1978 to 1990 for four types of cancer: breast, lung, colon, and Hodgkin's disease. In general, the study found similar survival rates for three of the cancers, but higher survival rates in the United States for breast cancer patients. Ten years after diagnosis, 65 percent of U.S. breast cancer patients were still alive, compared to 60 percent of Canadians. The study, however, was not able to determine whether the better survival rates in the United States were due to better outcomes or simply earlier detection, concluding that, "Until the effect on survival of differences in detection practices can be determined, the implications of these results for assessing quality of care in the two locations are unclear" (GAO 1994, 5). In general, though, most experts believe that early detection does increase chances of survival.

The largest recent comparison of quality between countries was conducted by the Commonwealth Fund (Davis et al. 2006). The researchers conducted a telephone survey of a representative sample of adults in 2004, and a sample of "sicker adults" in 2005, in the countries listed in Table 10.10. The results were then grouped into six categories developed by the Institute of Medicine, National Academy of Sciences: patient safety, effectiveness, patient-centeredness, timeliness, efficiency, and equity. Table 10.10 also lists per capita health expenditures in each country.

To give an idea of what was being measured, here are the specific criteria that were used to determine the efficiency rankings:

- Visited emergency department for a condition that could have been treated by a regular doctor, had one been available
- Medical records/test results did not reach MD office in time for appointment in past two years
- Sent for duplicate tests by different healthcare professionals in past two years
- Hospitalized patient went to emergency room or was rehospitalized for complications after discharge

The results show that the U.S. ranked at the bottom of the six countries in overall quality and in four of the six specific groupings, in spite of the fact that spending per capita was so much higher. Germany had the best results by far and New Zealand the second best.

TABLE 10.10: Rankings of Healthcare Quality, Selective Countries, 2005

	Australia	Canada	Germany	New Zealand	United Kingdom	United States
Overall Rankings	4	5	1	2	3	6
Patient safety	4	5	2	3	1	6
Effectiveness	4	2	3	6	5	1
Patient-centeredness	3	5	1	2	4	6
Timeliness	4	6	1	2	5	3
Efficiency	4	5	1	2	3	6
Equity	2	4	5	3	1	6
Health Expenditures						
Per capita	$2,903	$3,003	$2,996	$1,886	$2,231	$5,635

SOURCE: Data used with permission from Davis, K., C. Schoen, S. C. Shoenbaum, A. J. Audet, M. M. Doty, A. L. Holmgren, and J. L. Kriss. 2006. "Mirror, Mirror on the Wall," p. 4. New York: The Commonwealth Fund.

The OECD has ranked countries according to their success in achieving a number of quality measures; the U.S. rankings are shown in Table 10.11 (Anderson and Frogner 2008). The United States performed relatively well in cancer screening rates and survival rates for breast and colorectal cancers. It performed poorly, however, in vaccinations and asthma mortality rates.

Finally, Table 10.12 examines whether consumers in different countries believe that their healthcare systems should go through a major revamping (Schoen et al. 2007). U.S. citizens were most likely to believe that their system needed to be rebuilt completely, and least likely to say that only minor changes were necessary. Germans were the second unhappiest with their system, which is curious given that they gave the system such high marks on quality, as shown in Table 10.10.

Equity of Financing System

Each of the cross-national outcomes measures we discussed concerns the delivery of care—who has access to it, how much they use, how much it costs, and the resulting effects on quality and satisfaction. Here we examine a different issue: the equity of the system used to finance this care. A set of studies on this topic covers seven of the ten countries considered in this chapter—all except Australia, Canada, and Japan (Wagstaff et al. 1999; van Doorslaer et al. 1999).[9]

The authors first examine the sources for financing health services, dividing them into five types, the first three of which are public and the last two private: direct taxes, indirect taxes, social insurance, private insurance, and direct payments. Direct taxes are those paid directly by the taxpayer (e.g., income, sales, or property taxes). Indirect taxes are those that are borne, but not paid directly, by the consumer (e.g., value-added taxes[10]). Social insurance is direct contribution to welfare or health programs (e.g., payroll taxes for the U.S. Medicare program). Private insurance is premium payments by enrollees, while direct payments are out-of-pocket costs when services are used.

Table 10.13 shows the distribution of financing sources by country and indicates a large amount of cross-national variation. (Although this information is a bit dated now, we were unable to find comparable data from more recent periods.) Only two of the countries, Switzerland and the United States, rely mostly on private funding sources. In both countries, consumers of health services pay relatively high portions directly. The other five countries rely on public funding sources, primarily taxes (Sweden and the United Kingdom) or social insurance payments (France, Germany, and the Netherlands).

The authors then compared this information with income data from the countries to see whether these payments are regressive or progressive. If a system is progressive, wealthier people will pay more than their share, and

TABLE 10.11: Rank of United States Out of Total Number of OECD Countries' Most Recent Reporting of Selected Healthcare Quality Indicators

	U.S. Rank	*Total Number of Countries Reporting*
Avoidable Risk Indicators		
Smoking rate (percentage of total population)	2[a]	29
Asthma admission rate (discharges per 10,000 age 18 and older)	16[b]	17
Process Indicators		
Cervical cancer screening rate (percentage of women ages 20–69 screened)	1[c]	22
Retinal exams in diabetics (rate per 100 for diabetics ages 18–75)	5[b]	12
Influenza vaccination (percentage over age 65 offered vaccination)	9[a]	23
Mammography screening rate (percentage of women ages 50–69 screened)	12[c]	23
Coverage for basic vaccination program (percentage fully immunized at age 2)		
Overall	8[d]	11
Hepatitis	9[d]	14
Measles	15[d]	24
Pertussis	23[d]	24
Outcome Indicators		
Cervical cancer five-year survival rate		
Relative survival rate (crude rate)	8[e]	18
Observed survival rate (crude rate)	9[e]	19
Breast cancer five-year survival rate		
Relative survival rate (crude rate)	2[e]	18
Observed survival rate (crude rate)	5[e]	19
Colorectal cancer five-year survival rate		
Relative survival rate (crude rate)	2[e]	18
Observed survival rate (crude rate)	5[e]	20
Asthma mortality rate, per 100,000 ages 5–39	21[c]	25
Incidence of vaccine-preventable diseases per 100,000		
Measles	1[d]	23
Pertussis	14[d]	21
Hepatitis	15[d]	23

SOURCE: Data used with permission from Anderson, G. F., and B. K. Frogner. 2008. "Health Spending in OECD Countries." *Health Affairs* 27 (6): 1718–27.

NOTES: Relative survival rate numerator is the observed rate of women diagnosed with cancer surviving five years after diagnosis, and denominator is the expected survival rate of a comparable group from the general population. Observed survival rate numerator is the number of people diagnosed with cancer surviving five years after diagnosis, and denominator is the number of people with cancer.
[a]2005. [b]2002. [c]2003. [d]2004. [e]1998–2002.

TABLE 10.12: Consumers' Views of Their Healthcare System, 2007

	Australia	Canada	Germany	Netherlands	United Kingdom	United States
Only minor changes needed, system works well	24%	26%	20%	42%	26%	16%
Fundamental changes needed	55%	60%	51%	49%	57%	48%
Rebuild completely	18%	12%	27%	9%	15%	34%

SOURCE: Data from Schoen, C., R. Osborn, M. M. Doty, M. Bishop, J. Peugh, and N. Murukutla. 2007. "Toward Higher-Performance Health Systems." *Health Affairs* 26 (6): W717–W734.

poorer people, less. They find that Switzerland and the United States have the most regressive systems, and the United Kingdom the most progressive. France is mildly progressive, Sweden is moderately regressive, and Germany and the Netherlands are somewhat more regressive (Wagstaff et al. 1999). One reason that Switzerland and the United States are so regressive is their reliance on private insurance and out-of-pocket costs—systems in which people pay their own way, with little in the form of cross-subsidization. Tax-based systems such as the United Kingdom's tend to be more progressive because income tax rates are higher for wealthier people. The mixed findings for the countries relying mainly on social insurance are explained largely by the fact that in France (a progressive country) all individuals participate in the system, whereas in Germany, a regressive country, many wealthier individuals opt out of the public system.

TABLE 10.13: Sources of Funds for Health Sector Financing*

	Direct Taxes	Indirect Taxes	Social Insurance	Private Insurance	Direct Payments
France	0%	0%	74%	6%	20%
Germany	11%	7%	65%	7%	10%
Netherlands	6%	5%	65%	16%	8%
Sweden	64%	8%	18%	0%	10%
Switzerland	24%	5%	7%	41%	24%
United Kingdom	29%	35%	20%	7%	9%
United States	28%	7%	13%	29%	22%

SOURCE: Data used with permission from Wagstaff, A., et al. 1999. "Equity in the Finance of Health Care." *Journal of Health Economics* 18 (3): 263–90. Copyright © 1999, Elsevier.

*Data are from the most recent year available between 1987 and 1993, which varies by country.

Summary of Evidence

The differences shown in the tables and discussion presented earlier are difficult to summarize. Among ten countries, 45 comparisons of sets of two countries are possible. Some of the main findings (emphasizing differences between the United States and other countries) are:

- Access is higher or lower in the United States, depending on how it is defined. On the negative side, more U.S. citizens say that they are prevented from obtaining needed medical services because of costs. In contrast, access is better in the United States if one defines it in terms of waiting times for obtaining care.
- Overall hospital and physician usage rates are somewhat lower in the United States than in other countries, but rates are much higher for high-tech cardiac procedures. The United States also has far higher expenditures than other countries.
- Countries that rely on private insurance and out-of-pocket costs, such as the United States and Switzerland, have less equitable financing systems than others.
- Less information is available on quality and satisfaction among countries. The most recent data, which rely on surveys from a number of countries, finds that Germany provides the best quality overall among six countries surveyed, and the United States the worst. The Dutch were happiest with their systems (among six countries surveyed); Americans were least satisfied.

10.3 Ten Lessons on the Role of Government in Healthcare Systems

Fair comparisons between market and nonmarket alternatives are extremely difficult to make. Because there is no generally applicable formula for choosing between them, the results of such comparisons often depend more on the predispositions of the evaluators than on their analyses (Wolf 1993, 117).

Being objective is indeed difficult when drawing conclusions about whether one country's health system is superior to another's. Answers about which system is best are a matter of—informed, one would hope—opinion. Moreover, as illustrated in Section 10.2, good data comparing system outcomes in different countries are hard to find. Finally, and perhaps most important, different countries may not want the same things from their health systems. Some may want to emphasize access, others cost control, others efficiency over equity, and others the opposite. Even where goals are similar, different countries may prefer different methods of reaching those goals.

Because of these challenges, the ten lessons presented in this section should be considered cautiously. They are based on the authors' reading of cross-national literature, only a small amount of which could be presented in this chapter. While many will disagree with the lessons, others may find them fairly noncontroversial and not particularly bold.

Strategies that work in some countries often will not be successful in others. Furthermore, each country's system has its own strengths. The United States, for example, generally gets high marks for organizational innovation but does poorly with respect to equity, whereas the United Kingdom used to have the opposite reputation.

The advantage of these inquiries is that countries have the potential to learn something from each other (Hsiao 1992). The United Kingdom experimented with a system of internal markets, in part to improve organizational innovation (although undoubtedly part of a larger drive by the Thatcher government to privatize more of the economy), while the United States is gradually trying to enfranchise the uninsured through such initiatives as the State Children's Health Insurance Program.

Unfortunately, a number of impediments prevents some of the characteristics of a successful healthcare system from being easily transferable. For example, some analysts have concluded that parliamentary-style governments are less susceptible to regulatory capture than the presidential system used in the United States. (As discussed in Chapter 3, this refers to a situation where rather than serving the public, regulation serves those that it is designed to regulate.) In parliamentary-style governments, individual legislators tend to have less influence because they need to "toe the party line," thus, efforts of special interests to influence a few selected legislators will tend to be less effective (Weaver and Rockman 1993; Reinhardt 1994). In contrast, U.S. legislators have more freedom to deviate from their parties and therefore may be more sought after by special interests. Another example is that regulatory capture is probably also less likely when a cadre of dedicated, upper-management civil servants retain their positions after a change in government occurs—something that is truer in most other developed countries than in the United States. In both of these examples, there is little chance that the systems of one country could be imported to others; countries are entrenched either constitutionally or by long historic tradition. Little would be gained by turning these observations into lessons.

Lesson 1: Health Services Coverage Should Be Universal

Section 10.1 listed the advantages and disadvantages of universal health services coverage. Six major advantages, ranging from improving the health of the population to avoiding risk selection to reducing costs, were noted. The only disadvantage was that comprehensive coverage could result in the overuse of services, particularly those of marginal value.

Many methods, however, can address the problem of overuse and its resulting effect on expenditures within a framework of universal coverage. Much of the chapter has been devoted to the various ways different countries have attempted to keep costs manageable. These techniques include coordinating provider reimbursements across payers to avoid cost shifting, moving away from fee-for-service toward capitated payments, instituting patient cost-sharing requirements, establishing global budgets and controls on the diffusion of expensive medical technologies, and controlling the supply of hospitals and physicians.

No one template is best; different policies are used in different countries. The point is that most developed countries have managed to provide universal coverage while keeping their expenditures far lower than those in the United States—a country in which more than 16 percent of the under-65 population is uninsured.

Lesson 2: Coverage Should Be Financed Primarily from Public Sources or Government-Ensured Social Insurance Using Progressive Revenue Sources

The equity of a country's healthcare system is enhanced when revenues are generated from progressive sources. Some degree of equity is also maintained when everyone contributes a percentage of earnings to insurance pools. But equity is reduced when people must pay out of pocket for care, because this constitutes a larger proportion of poorer persons' income. Countries relying on private insurance and out-of-pocket costs and those allowing wealthier people to opt out of government-ensured coverage programs have less equitable financing systems.

Why should we care about the equity of a health financing system? The answer is somewhat philosophical and certainly open to debate: Poorer people, who also tend to be in poorer health, should not be doubly disadvantaged by paying more if they need health services. Although individuals have some control over their health through their actions and behaviors, much illness is the result of random events or of circumstances over which individuals have little control. Those who do incur illnesses and cannot afford care should have care subsidized by those who are better off. Requiring the already financially disadvantaged to pay more of their scarce incomes when they get sick is, in the view of many, unfair. As noted by Robert Evans and colleagues:

> [P]eople pay taxes in rough proportion to their incomes, and use health care in rough proportion to their health status or need for care. The relationships are not exact, but in general sicker people use more health care, and richer people pay more taxes. It follows that when health care is paid for from taxes, people with higher incomes pay a larger share of the total cost; when it is paid for by the users, sick people pay a larger share. . . . Whether one is a gainer or loser, then, depends upon where one is located in the distribution of both income . . .

and health. . . . In general, a shift to more user fee financing redistributes net income . . . from lower to higher income people, and from sicker to healthier people. The wealthy and healthy gain, the poor and sick lose. (Evans, Barer, and Stoddart 1993, 4)

Progressively based revenues that are largely unrelated to the actual usage of services is a remedy.

Lesson 3: The Delivery of Services Can Be Carried Out Privately Under the Oversight of Government, Which Acts as a Purchaser of Services

Universal coverage does not mean public ownership or even control of a country's health system. Although certain countries—the United Kingdom is the best-known example—rely more on the public ownership of health resources, this is not a precondition. Canadian researchers often point out that almost all health resources in that country are privately owned. Thus, government can choose to purchase services rather than provide them directly.

This is sometimes called a "make-or-buy" decision (Preker and Harding 2007). Although much of the attention on this topic has focused on developing countries, the concept can be applied to developed countries. In most instances, government can purchase services from the private market, taking advantage of competition among producers of these inputs. This competition can limit inefficiencies (Preker, Harding, and Travis 2000; Wolf 1993; Vining and Weimer 1990).

How does government decide whether to produce health-related goods and services itself or purchase them in the marketplace? One determinant is the "contestability" of the private market that would produce the input—that is, the potential for competition among suppliers (Vining and Weimer 1990; Preker and Harding 2007). If competition is likely, government purchase of a good or service has advantages over government production. A second determinant is the trustworthiness of private suppliers, which is determined in part by the degree to which potential suppliers can act opportunistically. When would opportunism likely be a major problem? The answer to this question leads to a third determinant of whether government should produce or purchase—measurability. If the quality of the outputs produced by private suppliers can be measured more easily, then there is less room for opportunism and more for reliance on buying rather than making. If, in contrast, the quality or quantity of inputs is hard to determine, then a stronger case for government control of the production process exists (Preker and Harding 2007).

Putting all this together, Preker and Harding (2007) argue that when the inputs and outputs of a particular health-related good or service are highly contestable and highly measurable, markets can function well. Examples they note in healthcare include retail drugs and equipment. Thus, if government wishes to ensure that poor people receive a particular service, they should purchase it from the private market. If, on the other hand, inputs or outputs have low contestability and low measurability, government itself may need to produce the good or service. Examples of these might include research, higher education, and policymaking. They go on to list a number of ways that government can make input and output markets both more contestable and measurable, which enhances the possibility that private markets can be used effectively (Preker and Harding 2007, 39–41).

Even if government's role in a health system is strong, competition can enhance efficiency. Separating the purchaser from the providers encourages competition among the latter—as long as the number of providers is adequate to avoid monopolization. Many developed countries are relying more on purchasing services and less on producing them. The United Kingdom, a country with a reputation of strong national control, offers a good example. As noted earlier, as part of the "internal markets" reform movement, hospital services were purchased by district health authorities, and specialty services were purchased by primary care physician "fundholders." As the United Kingdom moves away from the internal markets system, regional groups of primary care physicians are taking on expanded roles and purchasing specialty and other services for area residents (Oliver 2005; Enthoven 2000; Bindman and Weiner 2000).

Donald Light (2001b, 1164) argues that enhancing government's role as purchaser has several advantages. Government as purchaser can result in a greater focus on purchasing the types of services that enhance a population's health and in greater accountability on the part of providers. He writes,

> [W]e are in a transitional period of dislocation as we pass from providing medical services to purchasing for health gain. Thus, the enduring contribution of the managed competition policy movement is likely to be not so much competition per se but the transformation of state control from service administrator to strong purchaser or commissioner for evidence-based quality and health gain. That, it turns out, is what we have been wanting all along.

Lesson 4: Emphasis Should Be Placed on Containing Costs Through Supply-Side Methods

Most countries focus their cost-containment efforts on suppliers of services rather than on consumers. The supply-side cost-containment methods discussed in this chapter include global budgets, control of the diffusion of medical technologies, limits on the number of hospital beds and physicians, hospital and physician payment incentives, and utilization review.

Supply-side methods have two main advantages over those aimed at the demand side. First, informational problems often make demand-side policies less effective. For example, as we noted in Chapter 4, consumers often do not respond to information about health plan quality by choosing more cost-effective plans. Second, unlike demand-side policies such as increased patient cost sharing, those aimed at suppliers are not by nature regressive (Ellis and McGuire 1993).

Supply-side approaches do have their problems, however. Several of the methods just mentioned, especially limits on technologies and hospital beds and funding, may result in long waits for services. Conversely, reliance on price—the key market mechanism—tends to produce shorter waits because services are rationed by ability to pay. If waits are too long, prices will increase, shortening queues.

Some countries, notably the United States and Germany, report little in the way of waits for services. In contrast, the systems of the United Kingdom and Canada have been criticized for long waits, particularly for elective surgery and diagnostic testing, and the data show evidence of waiting lists for care in Australia (Willcox 2001), Japan (White 1995), the Netherlands (Laeven 2001), and Sweden (Hanning 2001) (see also Table 10.6). Research is currently being conducted in various countries on the extent of waits and how they can be reduced. No consensus has been reached yet, but researchers have found that in systems where there is a parallel private financing system to the public one, as in the United Kingdom, public waiting lists tend to be longer (Tuohy, Flood, and Stabile 2004).

The problem of patients waiting to receive services is largely one of equating supply and demand, so health systems that do not rely on price rationing often (but not always) have longer waits. Nevertheless, such systems can shorten waits by

- having a centralized information system that records waits throughout the system, allowing patients to be treated at more remote facilities when space is available;
- providing financial and nonfinancial inducements to hospitals and other facilities and physician specialists that are able to keep waiting time down; and
- making reasonable waits, however defined, an explicit policy goal, and perhaps even a right of citizens (Hurst and Siciliani 2003).

Lesson 5: Patient Cost-Sharing Requirements Should Be Kept Reasonably Low

Various parts of this book have stressed problems inherent to reliance on patient cost sharing. We have argued, for example, that high patient cost sharing dissuades patients from seeking services, whether useful or less so; discourages preventive care; may not be successful if providers respond by inducing demand; and is particularly difficult on lower-income persons, who also tend to have more health problems.

Not surprisingly, some countries rely more than others on user charges. Table 10.13 shows that France, the United States, and Switzerland relied on them far more than Germany, the Netherlands, Sweden, and the United Kingdom. User charges were also relatively low in Canada, but appear to be higher in Australia and Japan (Yoshikawa and Bhattacharya 2002; White 1995). In addition, user charges for prescription drugs and dental care are a common way in almost all countries of stemming unnecessary prescribing and utilization (except for the poor). On the whole, countries that rely more on user charges tend to have less progressive financing systems (Wagstaff et al. 1999).[11]

A compelling statement against high employee cost-sharing requirements is provided by UK economist Alan Maynard (2005, S257):

> Despite the evidence about user charges, libertarian policy advocates who oppose collectionist single-payer health care systems continue to promote such policies as a means by which "waste" will be reduced and the tax "burdens" of public health care can be reduced. The "waste" argument remains of dubious veracity: most patients consult a doctor because they believe they are ill, even though such demands and utilisation may not merit care on the basis of "need", i.e. capacity to benefit. If such demands are erroneously translated into utilization, this is a product of provider failure not patient deviance. To penalise "innocent" consumers with user charges because of provider profligacy remains a curious and inefficient policy loved by policy makers in Europe and worldwide.

When cost sharing is used, efforts should be made to insulate those who are least able to afford payments. Fortunately, this is done in most countries. In the United States, for example, Medicaid beneficiaries are exempted from cost-sharing requirements. In France, among those exempted are people with low incomes, the unemployed, and the disabled (Bellanger and Mosse 2005).

More research should be conducted on targeting lower cost-sharing requirements toward services that are more beneficial to patients with particular medical problems, so that financial barriers for the most-needed services can be kept low. Fendrick and colleagues (2001) argue for a system of "benefit-based copays," where cost-sharing requirements would be lower when expected clinical benefits are higher, and vice versa. Although the authors discuss this in the context of prescription drugs, it could be applied to any service where there is strong clinical evidence about what constitutes appropriate treatment. Such a system would be challenging from an administrative standpoint, since it involves tailoring different copays to individual patients based on the expectation of how much they can gain from that service.

Nevertheless, this sort of fine-tuning has the potential to enhance cost savings and potentially improve clinical outcomes, so long as the administrative costs don't outweigh the cost savings.

Lesson 6: To the Extent Possible, Payments to Providers Should Be Coordinated Among Payers

When there are multiple payers, a number of advantages can be achieved by coordinating payments—that is, having each payer provide the same amount. (This is a decidedly nonmarket approach; explicit payment coordination is the antithesis of markets.) These advantages include horizontal equity—all patients are worth the same to providers, so they are more likely to be treated equally well; better potential to control costs; and the inability of providers to shift costs from one payer to another. As noted earlier, the main disadvantage is that all-payer rates do not allow higher-quality providers to distinguish themselves. If a country wishes to provide financial incentives to enhance quality, it needs to reward providers in other ways. However, there is little evidence that providers in all-payer and single-payer countries provide poorer care than those in other countries.

According to Abel-Smith (1992, 414), all-payer systems have been quite successful.

> The key to Europe's success [in controlling costs] is the use of monopsony power whereby one purchaser dominates the market, and not just the hospital market. Where there are many purchasers, as in Germany, they are forced to act together. Because the insurers are not allowed more revenue, either from tax or contributions, and because what they can charge the insured in copayments is centrally determined, they are forced either to confront providers or to ration their allowable resources. In most countries this does not lead to lines of patients waiting for treatment.

Another advantage is that pricing regulations tend to be less intrusive than those aimed at controlling quantities.

Some countries, such as Australia and Germany, do allow wealthier individuals to opt out of the public system by purchasing private coverage. As a result, these patients tend to be worth more to providers and are likely to get favorable treatment. One key to preserving support of the public system is to keep the proportion of the population opting out of the public plan reasonably low. If too many people opt out of the public system, there will be greater inequality of treatment by providers and less cross-subsidization, since people tend to pay their own way when they have private insurance. The question, according to Morone (2000, 967) is, "Will people continue to see themselves as citizens, as members of a shared community? Or will they turn into shoppers looking for their own best deal?"

Lesson 7: Countries Should Proceed with Caution in Providing Consumers a Choice of Insurer

"Choice" has become a key buzzword in the "consumer revolution" in the health services area. Economists usually consider more choice desirable, but consumers can be given many types of choices. Examples include whether to have universal coverage or to allow individuals to choose whether or not to purchase coverage, whether to assign an insurer or permit consumers to choose from among them, whether patients can go to any provider they like, and the extent to which patients are able choose the medical services they prefer (Rice 2001).

From this list, perhaps the choice that has received the most recent attention is whether consumers should be able to choose their health insurer. Until recently, most countries did not allow this. Consumers received coverage through their national or regional public plan, or through the sickness fund to which they were assigned. The United States has been an exception; most working-age consumers have chosen their own health plans for many years.

Some European countries have begun to follow suit. In general, these countries have found it necessary to proceed slowly. Some of the adverse consequences have included:

- Insurers competing for healthier patients, in large measure because of difficulties involved in risk adjusting health insurance premiums (van Doorslaer and Schut 2000; Zweifel 2000)
- Consumer difficulties in obtaining and using comparative information on plan performance (van Doorslaer and Schut 2000)
- Political difficulties as the perception grows that government is moving away from a system of solidarity (Morone 2000; Pfaff and Wassener 2000)

This is not to suggest that a choice of insurers is necessarily undesirable. Rather, countries should proceed cautiously because the potential for experiencing these problems—and probably others—increases when consumers are offered a choice of health plans.

Lesson 8: Fee-for-Service Payment Should Be Reevaluated

Another trend among developed countries is the gradual movement away from fee-for-service medicine. Fee-for-service does have one major advantage—in most cases it gives providers an incentive to provide a sufficient quantity and intensity of services. The other side of the coin, however, is that too many services may be provided, potentially compromising quality and making it more difficult to control expenditures.

This trend is perhaps most obvious in Europe. Even in Canada, a country known for its total reliance on fee-for-service for physician payment, a movement away from the practice may be afoot. In a 2000 interview, Canada's minister of health, Allan Rock, stated that:

> If we're going to keep Canada's public health care system, primary health care reform—moving away from fee-for-service as the standard form of remuneration—has to occur. I'm encouraged by movement in that direction. . . . [T]here is now growing support for a rostered approach to primary care, delivered to a defined population by a team of family doctors. . . . This includes . . . a method of payment for a physician that is other than fee-for-service. . . . More and more of the provinces seem to be moving toward negotiating for this type of care approach as they sit down with their medical associations to work out compensation arrangements for the coming years. (Iglehart 2000, 136–37)

This movement away from fee-for-service is not isolated. It is part of a larger movement to establish regional budgets for the health services provided to populations (particularly in Europe). These budgets are capitated, in that regions receive a fixed amount of medical resources per service. This should not be construed as implying that providers are paid on a capitation basis; in some places they are, and in others, they are not. Within that context, Nigel Rice and Peter Smith (2001, 107) write:

> Capitation is, without doubt, here to stay. There is a remarkable degree of agreement that—whatever the structure of the health care system—a policy of cost containment and devolved responsibility for health care requires setting prospective budgets on the basis of capitation payments. The question is therefore not *whether* to set capitations, but *how* to do so.

Interestingly, this exists in countries that are moving toward markets and those that are not.

Lesson 9: Government Should Fund Impartial Research on and Analysis of Health System Performance

No country's health system is ideal; reforms have the potential to improve efficiency and equity. Moreover, a static system will be unresponsive to changes in medical technology, demographics, the economic environment, and even people's tastes.

In most areas of the economy, markets are relatively efficient in terms of the distribution of information on prices and quality. However, information problems in the health services area are often severe. Individuals have trouble determining such things as the most appropriate health plan when they have a choice of insurer, the best provider given their needs and associated costs, and even whether to seek care in the first place. Therefore, the government should monitor population health and quality, financing, access, and outcomes in the health services system.

Most countries already invest resources into areas where private companies have less incentive to conduct research (as in the case of monitoring the prevalence of disease in the population) or the payoffs are uncertain (as in the case of basic medical research). The quality of policymaking is improved when sophisticated, impartial analyses of alternative options and rigorous research of the state of the system are available. Research generated by private for-profit organizations (e.g., prescription drug companies), while often useful, raises concerns about potential bias. Even if objective researchers carry out the work, concern remains that only projects likely to result in benefits to the funding organization will be carried out in the first place. Government should play a major role in the funding of such research.

In this respect, the United States performs well compared to many other countries. In addition to funding basic clinical medical research that results in new pharmaceutical and technological breakthroughs, government agencies fund universities and research firms to conduct health services research. Because government has invested heavily in research, we know, for example, the true number of the uninsured in the United States. The Agency for Healthcare Research and Quality funds research concerning quality and efficiency in the health sector. Other agencies, such as the Centers for Medicare & Medicaid Services, the Centers for Disease Control and Prevention, the Veterans Administration, and the National Institutes of Health, also provide critical data and analyses of these issues. In 2007 these agencies received almost $1.5 billion in federal funding directed toward health services research (Coalition for Health Services Research 2008).

One of the largest efforts of any country in using health services research to improve organization performance is the National Institute for Health and Clinical Excellence (NICE) in the United Kingdom. NICE "is the independent organisation responsible for providing national guidance on the promotion of good health and the prevention and treatment of ill health" (NICE 2008). It focuses on public health initiatives, the assessment of medical technologies, and the appropriate use of health technologies, services, and medications. Australia is a leader in developing and applying health technology assessment. What's unusual about Australia's system is that not only are quality, safety, and efficacy required for a service to be covered under public insurance, but its cost-effectiveness is considered as well (Jackson 2007).

Research and analysis of health systems is not necessarily easy. Health services research is costly and requires a longer-term commitment to establishing systems and organizations of data collection and analysis, without an immediate payoff. Research may not be in the political interest of governments. Government might *claim* that it wants impartial information on the inputs and outputs of a national health system, but the actual process of scrutiny often reveals flaws that are embarrassing to a country's health leadership or even an entire government. A further problem is that the ruling parties in certain countries are reluctant to fund studies that might reach conclusions that are inconsistent with their philosophies and party platforms. This is unfortunate, because it makes the development of appropriate reform policies a "data-free" exercise.

While investing domestically in research, countries should also share information through institutions such as the OECD, the World Bank, and the WHO to facilitate reliable cross-national comparisons of health systems. Adequate funding of health services research through independent or depoliticized government agencies and international consortia is essential for improving the efficiency and equity of health systems.

Lesson 10: A Greater Reliance on Market Forces Does Not Necessarily Improve the Performance of Healthcare Systems

The key question is not whether countries should use markets or government to organize, deliver, and finance health services. Rather, it is how to determine the most appropriate roles of each and the balance between them. This chapter has discussed the various choices that countries must make concerning this balance and presented some evidence that indicates—albeit inexactly—the relative success that ten countries have had.

Can the evidence presented earlier indicate the most successful balance between markets and government? Unfortunately, the answer is no, for at least four reasons.

1. Different countries may not want the same things from their health systems. Some may want to emphasize access, others cost control, others efficiency over equity, and others equity over efficiency. Moreover, historical and cultural factors are critical determinants in the development of health services systems, making it risky to suggest that any one country's system be replicated by others.

2. Creating an agreed-on set of weights among the different outcomes would probably be impossible. How does one weigh, for example, short waits (a characteristic of the U.S. system) against the equity of health system financing (a characteristic of the UK system)?

3. Characterizing countries according to the reliance of each on markets versus government is difficult. Germany offers a good example. Although government involvement in health services financing (which is largely left up to the sickness funds) is not explicit, a great deal of government oversight and direction occurs, particularly on the supply side. Further complicating matters is that countries' healthcare systems change, sometimes fairly rapidly. Both the United Kingdom and the

Netherlands, for example, went from fairly non-marketlike systems to reliance on competition. The United Kingdom has stepped back somewhat, but in the Netherlands the emphasis on more choice between and competition among sickness funds continues.

4. Although cross-national measures of access and costs are reasonably good, we still do not know enough about the quality of care provided in different countries.

10.4 Chapter Summary

This chapter first discussed some of the decisions countries must make in organizing their healthcare systems. This was followed by evidence as to which countries have the best access to high quality care, and at what cost. We concluded with ten lessons on the role of government in healthcare systems. Among our conclusions are that coverage should be universal and that it should be financed mainly from either public sources or government-ensured social insurance with revenue raised through progressive taxes—but that the actual delivery of services can be carried out privately, subject to government oversight. Throughout the book, we have emphasized various advantages of containing costs through supply-side methods. In that regard, we suggest that patient cost-sharing requirements be kept reasonably low. One way to control these costs is through coordination of payment to providers among insurers and other payers.

Notes

1. The European Observatory on Health Systems and Policies defines a sickness fund as a "third-party payer in social health insurance system, covering the community as a whole or sections of the population." Generally, they are distinguished from private health insurers in that they are nonprofit, quasi-public entities and are subject to strict government rules and regulations. Some of these rules may include regulations on pricing practices such as requiring risk adjustment or community rating—that is, charging everyone the same premium—or requirements that everyone have the right to enroll in the groups that they serve. See www.euro.who.int/observatory/Glossary/Top Page?phrase =Sickness%20fund.

2. Universal coverage does not eliminate adverse selection because different people may be covered by different plans. It does ensure, however, that sicker individuals are not excluded from obtaining coverage.

3. The primary distinction between employer and employee "contributions" versus "taxes" is that in the cases of taxes, the revenue passes through government hands. Sickness funds usually are not considered part of government, although they often must conform to strict governmental regulations.

4. Nearly all countries allow for the sale of supplemental insurance. Such coverage is sometimes provided through employment (as in Canada and France) and other times purchased individually (as in Australia). It tends to cover services that are excluded from the public plan (e.g., dentistry, private hospital rooms) or all or part of patient cost-sharing requirements. Because of the ubiquity of this coverage, it is not listed here as an explicit societal choice.

5. PPOs typically contract with provider groups to provide care to enrolled patients. PPO patients receive discounts if they go to these participating providers, but may still use nonparticipating providers. Unlike HMOs, PPOs do not normally pay providers with incentive-reimbursement systems such as DRGs and capitation. POS plans are similar to PPOs, but usually exhibit several differences: Patients must see a gatekeeping primary care physician before seeking specialist care; cost-sharing requirements are higher (often 40 percent higher) for care provided outside of the network (but unlike HMOs, enrollees *can* receive care from out-of-network providers); and like HMOs, POS plans often employ incentive-reimbursement techniques.

6. One study on the impact of DRGs during their first three years found no overall diminution in quality (Kahn et al. 1990), although another component of the study found that more patients were being discharged in a clinically unstable condition (Kosecoff et al. 1990).

7. The relative values used by the Medicare program were established using a different procedure. They were originally based on a research study conducted at Harvard University and were then modified by a congressional agency. The American Medical Association and various specialty groups, however, participated in and contributed to the findings. See Hsaio and colleagues (1988).

8. CT or "CAT" scans, short for computed tomography scans, provide three-dimensional images of parts the human body based on computer syntheses of a series of X-rays. MRIs, short for magnetic resonance images, provide three-dimensional body images through the use of magnets and radio waves, avoiding the use of radiation. Radiation therapy uses high-energy rays to treat disease, especially cancer. Lithotriptors use intense sound waves to destroy kidney stones. These procedures were chosen because they constitute four of the five reported by the OECD (2001). The other measure, hemodialysis stations (for kidney dialysis), was not available for three of the ten countries.

9. More recent data are no longer publicly available because the OECD now uses a different categorization.

10. Value-added taxes (VAT) are sometimes difficult for Americans to understand because they are rarely used. They can be contrasted with sales taxes, where the consumer directly pays a proportion of the final selling price. Those firms that produce inputs that are not sold directly to the consumer but are instead used as inputs by the firm that ultimately sells the consumer good do not pay sales taxes. A VAT, in contrast, taxes each component of production so that every firm involved in the production process pays a tax based on how much

estimated value it added. The consumer then only pays a portion of the total tax—the value added by the ultimate seller.

11. The one exception is France, which Wagstaff and colleagues (1999) found to be mildly progressive. In their study, progressivity was determined not only by out-of-pocket costs but by whether premiums were collected from all workers (as in France) or alternatively, whether individuals can opt out of the system (as in Germany).

CONCLUSION

The theme of this book is different from that of a traditional health economics text. Other texts generally accept, without strong evidence to the contrary, that relying on market competition will result in the best outcomes, at least with regard to efficiency. For example, one book that the authors regard highly notes:

> The use of our economic tools may lead to predictions that turn out to be different than what we observe. . . . When predictions differ from what we observe . . . it does not mean that the theory is wrong or not useful. Instead, it is an indication that one or more of the assumptions underlying the theory have been violated. . . . When the underlying assumptions are different from what is expected, there is a possible role for public policy. (Feldstein 1988, 593–94)

This statement appears—at least to most economists—to be eminently reasonable. Since economic theory shows that market competition will lead to Pareto-optimal outcomes, why not allow market forces to operate unencumbered by government interference, unless we have solid evidence that such intervention will improve outcomes?

This book has taken (and justified, we hope) an entirely different approach. The previous quotation illuminates this approach. Paul Feldstein allows government a role, but *only* if we observe that the predictions of economic theory differ from our observations. In particular, we must keep in mind that

- the onus is on those who contend that market forces will not result in the best outcomes, and
- to justify government involvement, it is necessary to demonstrate that reality differs from the predictions of the theory.

Feldstein's view, which pervades economic thought, is the wrong approach to the study of health economics and the formulation of health policy. There is no reason to suppose that a competitive marketplace will result in superior health outcomes, so demonstrating that the outcomes of a hypothetical competitive market will be different from what theory would predict is unnecessary.

Why is there no reason to believe that a competitive marketplace will automatically result in the best outcomes? This book examined over a dozen of the assumptions that need to be fulfilled to ensure that a free market results in the best outcomes for society; none of them was even close to being met in the health services. If these assumptions are not met, economic theory provides no basis for the superiority of competitive approaches. Thus, the burden of proof should not fall on those who profess the need to explore alternative approaches to the reliance on markets.

Suppose a country is deciding whether to limit how much it will spend each year on health-related goods and services. The Feldstein quotation implies that such a policy should be considered only if costs under a truly competitive marketplace are higher than theory predicts. But even if this is true, it would be very difficult to demonstrate, because it involves trying to answer a counterfactual[1] question: How much would a perfectly competitive market spend on health services? Because an answer to this question is hardly obvious and would be the subject of much dispute, the competitive mind-set makes it nearly impossible to justify government involvement in healthcare.

A better approach to policymaking spares believers in government intervention the burden of proof. Instead, all alternative policies being considered would start on an equal basis. Then empirical evidence would be gathered to determine the likely effect of each alternative. In the global budget example, one would need to predict the effect of enacting (versus not enacting) such a policy on costs, quality and outcomes, waiting times, and so on, and then compare these various effects to determine which policy is superior. Such an analysis might find that global budgets are not a good idea, but only after conducting the research. Competitive (i.e., noninterventionist) approaches would not be *presumed* superior.

This distinction may seem niggling to some, but it is fundamental. If we view competition as one possible policy alternative rather than as the superior policy, any number of possible policies could show themselves to be superior. Many such examples were given throughout the book. Furthermore, one of the main conclusions of Chapter 10 was that empirical evidence contradicts the superiority of a market-based system (to which the United States comes closest) when resource expenditures are considered—not only from an equity standpoint, but with respect to efficiency and health outcomes as well.

In the conventional model, few levers are actually available to policymakers who are interested in health services. Because this model is driven by consumer demand, the primary tools involve influencing demand, either by changing out-of-pocket price or by providing additional information to consumers. Influencing supply is less viable because the model presumes that suppliers will simply produce those things that are demanded.

Health policy throughout the world, however, relies on supply-side policies. Policy tools include capitation, diagnosis-related groups, utilization review, practice guidelines, comparative effectiveness research, technology controls, and global budgets, just to name a few. None of these policies arise from the competitive model, nor would economic theory show them to result in superior outcomes. Nevertheless, most countries rely on supply-side policies, and many analysts would argue that they have resulted in superior outcomes in the health services marketplace.

Determining which policies are superior, however that may be defined, is a challenging task. The answers, of course, will vary depending on the particular circumstances (e.g., the disease, the population group, the country). Health services and health policy researchers worldwide are key participants in this undertaking and provide critical information. But to prescribe the best possible set of policy options, these researchers must employ tools that expand rather than narrow the set of options.

The challenges health policymakers face—ensuring that costs are kept manageable and quality remains acceptable in a world of limited budgets but expanding technological capabilities—are daunting. New and innovative ideas are essential. If analysts misapply economic theory to health by assuming that market forces are necessarily superior to alternative policies, they will blind themselves to policy options that might actually better enhance social welfare.

Note

1. See Section 4.1 for a discussion of counterfactual questions.

APPENDIX:
OVERVIEW OF THE HEALTHCARE SYSTEMS OF TEN DEVELOPED COUNTRIES

Miriam J. Laugesen* and Thomas Rice

Australia

All Australian citizens and permanent residents are covered by the country's national health insurance program, called Medicare. The Medicare program provides comprehensive coverage, including primary care, hospital care, and pharmaceuticals. Responsibility for the health service is shared among federal government, six states, and two territories, although the federal government spends more than twice as much as the states and territories on health services.

In 2005 Australia spent $3,179 per person on health, which was 8.8 percent of its gross domestic product (GDP). The public sector financed 67 percent of this expenditure, and 33 percent was financed by private payers, including private insurers (7.4 percent) and out-of-pocket expenditures (18.2 percent) (OECD 2008). The federal (commonwealth) government finances 46 percent of total health expenditure (Healy, Sharman, and Lokuge 2006, 67) and exerts considerable influence over the health sector through financial grants to states and territories, regulation of private insurers, direct financial grants to organizations providing health services, and national priorities and programs (Hall 1999). It also finances and regulates pharmaceuticals and long-term care and provides grants to various organizations for major capital equipment, rural health services, Aboriginal health, and mental health services. Australia's six state governments spend around 22 percent of national health expenditures. The states' major responsibility in health is for acute and psychiatric services, although they also regulate health professionals. The federal government and the states negotiate five-year funding contracts that establish their respective obligations.

*Miriam J. Laugesen is an assistant professor at the UCLA School of Public Health, Department of Health Services. She received her PhD in political science from the University of Melbourne in 2000, and she also trained in health policy at Harvard University. She is a political scientist, and her research interests include Medicare physician payment, state health insurance coverage and regulatory policies, and comparative health policy. Her work has appeared in *Health Services Research*, *Inquiry*, and *Journal of Health Politics, Policy and Law*.

Historically, private and government roles in the Australian health system have oscillated between systems of public and private insurance and between systems of free, fee-based, and means-tested hospital care (Gray 1996). Today, private health insurers operate as an optional supplement to Medicare rather than as an alternative payer for health services (Commonwealth Department of Health and Aged Care 1999). Private insurance accounted for just 7.4 percent of health expenditure in 2005 (OECD 2008), although almost half of all Australians have private insurance: In 2008, 44.7 percent of Australians were enrolled in private health insurance plans (Private Health Insurance Administration Council 2008). The role of private insurance is essentially to provide patients a choice of hospital physician, faster access to hospital treatment, and greater privacy and comfort while in the hospital.

After private health insurance enrollment declined in the 1990s, the government introduced policies to encourage enrollment in private health insurance. Individuals receive a tax rebate of between 30 and 40 percent (older people receive 40 percent rebates) for premiums paid for private health insurance. In 2000, the Australian government introduced a policy to encourage lifelong insurance enrollment. The government was concerned that individuals were buying insurance when they needed hospital care and canceling it after they received treatment. Lifetime Cover allows insurers to charge a late-entry fee to people older than 30 who are buying insurance for the first time. The late-entry fee is 2 percent of the premium for each year a member is older than 30 if she did not sign up before the age of 31 or before July 2000. Individuals can change insurers without penalty, but if they go without insurance for a defined period they lose their lifetime coverage status. A 50-year-old with no history of private health insurance coverage in July 2000 would pay 38 percent over the base rate premium, up to a maximum fee of 70 percent, which applies to those older than 65. However, people born before 1934 are exempt.

The federal government's Private Health Insurance Administration Council, which is funded by insurance industry levies, corrects insurance market failures through such actions as regulating the prices of premiums and the benefits that insurers can offer. Insurers are required to have minimum levels of financial reserves. Private health insurers are prohibited from charging fees based on risk and are required to provide community rating, or uniform insurance premiums, to all enrollees. A reinsurance system transfers funds from insurers with a low proportion of claims by aged and chronically ill members to insurers with a high proportion of such claims (Commonwealth Department of Health and Aged Care 1999, 63).

Hospital care is perhaps the best example of the Australian mix of public and private roles. Australia has a free public hospital system managed by the states, while Medicare subsidizes physician fees in private hospitals. Medicare pays 75 percent of the Medicare benefit schedule fee for in-hospital treatment. Public hospitals provide quality care at no cost to the patient, but the public hospital system does not provide immediate access to nonurgent surgery or treatment, nor does it allow choice of physician. Nevertheless, waits are relatively short. In 2005, fewer than one-fifth of respondents (19 percent) reported having to wait more than four months for elective surgery (see Table 10.6 in Chapter 10).

In private hospitals around 42 percent of private hospital stays involve out-of-pocket charges for physician fees. The average out-of-pocket charge in 2007 was US$787 (Ipsos 2008, 12). These fees result from the lack of price regulation of physician fees above the fee schedule. A policy called Closing the Gap allows insurers to offer policies to cover the gap between the Medicare fee-schedule benefit and the actual physician charge in private hospitals. Insurers can only offer "gap cover schemes" by agreement with Medicare.

Medicare has a more significant role in outpatient services, partly because of regulations limiting private health insurance coverage. Medicare covers physicians, optometrists, and some dental surgery services in full or in part. It pays for specialist treatment referred through a gatekeeper physician. Physicians are paid on a fee-for-service basis, and patients can choose their own physician. As the U. S. Medicare system does, Australia uses a fee schedule, which lists fee amounts and benefits for medical services, to pay its providers. Unlike the U.S. Medicare, Australian Medicare payments are sometimes less than 100 percent of the fee schedule. For example, an outpatient physician consultation is paid at 85 percent of the fee schedule.

Primary care services are largely free for patients as a result of government incentives to limit out-of-pocket charges to patients. Medicare encourages primary care physicians to bill Medicare directly for services—through a system known as "bulk billing"—rather than billing patients directly. Bulk billing offers advantages for physicians, who are ensured payment for their services, while reducing out-of-pocket costs for patients. A provider who is bulk billing Medicare cannot charge patients additional fees. Around 70 percent of services for which Medicare benefits pay are bulk billed and are therefore free to the patient (Commonwealth Department of Health and Aged Care 2000). Patients receiving care from providers who are not bulk billing are likely to pay higher out-of-pocket costs, because federal law does not restrict the fees physicians charge. Private insurers cannot offer coverage for the difference between the schedule and the fee paid.

Out-of-pocket expenditure for health services in Australia is relatively modest at US$579 per person in 2005, representing 18.2 percent of national health expenditure (OECD 2008). Cost sharing, which is generally limited to prescribed medicines, private hospital care, and some outpatient services, accounted for 4.6 percent of total health expenditure at US$147 per person in 2005 (OEDC 2008). Welfare beneficiaries, the elderly, veterans, and low-income patients are eligible for reduced copayments, and an annual safety-net deductible limits the total amount of out-of-pocket charges. After the deductible is met, patients pay reduced copayments or no copayments, depending on their eligibility status.

Medicare is funded by general tax revenue and a compulsory 1.5 percent levy on taxable income for taxpayers above defined income thresholds, although this was being debated as of 2008. An additional 1 percent surcharge on taxable income is imposed on people who earn more than the thresholds of $50,000 (single) or $100,000 (couple/family). Higher-earning taxpayers are exempt from the additional 1 percent levy if they purchase private insurance (Commonwealth Department of Health and Aged Care 2000). The Medicare levy contributes just over a third of the revenue for Medicare.

Canada

Canada provides universal coverage for all medically necessary hospital and physician services. Each of the 13 provinces and territories (henceforth referred to as provinces) administers its own system, but each provincial system adheres to five national principles included in the federal government's Canada Health Act. The federal government can influence the provincial systems, because it helps fund them and can withhold a portion of funding to a provincial system in violation of the principles. There is some dispute about how much funding the federal government contributes, with provinces sometimes claiming as little as 16 percent. The federal government asserts that the proper figure is between 33 and 40 percent, depending on which federal programs are considered (Health Canada 2008a).

The following are five principles that must be met for a province to receive the maximum federal contribution (Health Canada 2008b):

1. Public administration: The system must be "administered and operated on a non-profit basis by a public authority."
2. Comprehensiveness: All necessary hospital and physician services must be covered.
3. Universality: All residents must be covered.
4. Portability: Coverage must be provided to residents traveling in another province, and urgent care is covered when traveling outside of the country.
5. Accessibility: Covered services must be accessible to all residents on the same terms and conditions with no direct financial costs such as user charges or extra billing by physicians.

The Canadian provinces are the sole payers for medically necessary physician and hospital services the act covers. This prevents providers from shifting costs or charges between payers and gives provinces a great deal of leverage in negotiations with providers. However, a number of healthcare services—including prescription drugs and dental care—are not included in the act, and provinces cover these at their discretion.

Each province provides coverage for outpatient prescription drugs for selected population groups, generally those on social assistance (the poor) and the elderly. Some patient cost sharing is usually required. Many of the provinces also provide drug coverage to the general population, but cost-sharing requirements tend to be substantial. Dental coverage is limited and is provided mainly to poor persons (Goldsmith 2002).

Private health insurance coverage has traditionally been effectively prohibited for services that are covered by the provincial health plans. Consequently, there is no private insurance for medically necessary hospital and physician services. Private insurance is common, however, for other care (e.g., drugs, dentistry, optometric services), with two-thirds of the population having some form of supplemental private insurance in 2006 (OECD 2008). Premiums are subsidized by employers and the government as part of a fringe benefit package or are paid out of pocket by consumers.

The prohibition against private coverage for services provided by hospitals and physicians may change, however. A June 2005 Supreme Court ruling, *Chaoulli v. Quebec (Attorney General)*, sided with the plaintiff (who had waited a year for hip-replacement surgery) that the provincial prohibition against private health insurance was unconstitutional. The problem, according to the court, was the waiting lists for services, which could lead to "suffering or even dying" (Krauss 2006). Similar rulings in other provinces could pave the way for private insurance in those provinces as well—which in turn would make it more feasible for private clinics to establish themselves, since insurance reimbursement may be possible. The development of private clinics is most extensive in Alberta, British Columbia, and Quebec. Moreover, the case appears to have spurred action to reduce waits for services (Steinbrook 2006).

Almost all hospitals are nonprofit. They directly negotiate a global budget for their operating expenses with the provincial government. This has resulted in a strong incentive for hospitals to keep down these expenses, most of which are labor related. In that regard, one study from the 1980s found that there were twice as many hospital employees per filled hospital bed in the United States as there were in Ontario (Newhouse, Anderson, and Roos 1988). Data from 2005 indicate that total hospital employment per 1,000 population is 25 percent higher in the United States than in Canada (OECD 2008). In contrast, most capital expenditures, including expensive medical equipment, is funded by the provinces. In general, provinces need to approve such hospital expenditures, irrespective of the source of funding, or additional funding to operate the equipment will not be covered under the global budget. In most provinces this has resulted in less diffusion of such equipment compared to many other countries (see Table 10.2 in Chapter 10).

About half of Canadian physicians provide primary care, a much higher proportion than in the United States. The majority of primary care physicians do not have hospital privileges (White 1995). In general, they are also responsible for specialist referrals (Goldsmith 2002; White 1995). Physicians tend to practice privately and are paid on a fee-for-service basis, though alternative blended payment systems that include capitation, fee-for-service, and programmatic funding are growing. There is little managed care in Canada, though some government officials would like to see a movement in that direction (Iglehart 2000).

The medical profession establishes relative fee levels, and the provinces mainly determine conversion factors (i.e., actual payment levels). Monopsonistic power and low economic growth rates caused physician fees in Canada to fall about 60 percent relative to those in the United States over a 20-year period (White 1995). Because fees are low and provinces are the only payer, there is a built-in financial incentive for physicians to induce demand. In the early 1990s several provinces responded by enacting expenditure caps on physician services (Barer, Lomas, and Sanmartin 1996), but these are no longer in effect, except in Quebec. During that time period, some provinces also tried to control the number of physicians practicing, through limits on medical school enrollment, but as in the case of expenditure caps, this is no longer the case. Medical school enrollment has increased during the 2000s in response to a perceived shortage of physicians (Hurley 2008).

The system is financed by a variety of sources. These include federal and provincial taxes paid by individuals and corporations; employer payroll taxes; other governmental taxes; premiums paid by employers and individuals for services not covered by the provinces; and out-of-pocket costs for these services. The proportion of total expenditures paid from public sources declined from 74.5 percent to 70.2 percent between 1990 and 2000, largely because the cost of services not publicly covered increased faster than the cost of publicly covered services, but in part because of budget cutting by provinces (Goldsmith 2002; Evans 2000). Since that time, however, the proportion has been stable at around 70 percent (OECD 2008). The source of the 30 percent of expenditures from private sources varies across provinces and may include prescription drugs, long-term care, dental services, home care, and cosmetic surgery (Steinbrook 2006).

France

The French population is almost universally covered by health insurance funds that are largely organized on the basis of professional sectors in the labor market. A second comprehensive universal coverage known as CMU (Couverture Maladie Universelle), which has been operating since 2000, covers the poor, those without stable employment, and legal migrants without coverage (Imai, Jacobzone, and Lenain 2000, 11). In 1999, 300,000 legal residents of France—about half of 1 percent—were without insurance (Poullier and Sandier 2000, 899; Lancry and Sandier 1999).

The French health system aims to balance freedom of choice with social solidarity. Some analysts have described it as a hybrid Bismarckian-Beveridge system (Poullier and Sandier 2000) or a compromise between Britain's National Health Service and the health system of the United States (Rodwin and Le Pen 2004). The system is based on three tenets that reflect this balance of choice and solidarity: French residents have access to the physician or healthcare professional of their choice, there is no limit on goods or services reimbursed, and the only limitations on prescribing are requirements that physicians follow practice guidelines (Sandier, Paris, and Polton 2004, 38).

Health insurance funds come from a payroll tax contributed by employers and a "social contribution" levy of 5.25 percent by individuals. Employers contribute about half of the budget for sickness funds, and individuals' social contribution levy funds make up 34.6 percent. The remaining portion comes from excise taxes, taxes on insurers, and employee contributions (Sandier, Paris, and Polton 2004, 38).

The national government regulates the expenditures and distribution of hospital resources and the prices of pharmaceuticals and medical fees and determines the level of financing for public hospitals (Poullier and Sandier 2000). For over a decade, central government has sought more control over health expenditure through a national global budget target. Under the 1996 Juppé Plan, Parliament adopted an annual national health expenditure objective for physician, prescription, public hospital, and private clinical expenditures (Imai, Jacobzone, and Lenain 2000). This measure's effectiveness is questionable, since total reimbursements are not capped. In practice, it has foundered due to the political difficulties of imposing cost restraints on providers, especially physicians (Rochaix and Wilsford 2005). Cost containment has been, and will likely continue to be, France's most significant challenge.

Regional levels of the health system took on new responsibilities in the 1990s, and devolution is increasing (High Committee on Public Health 1998). Regional hospitalization agencies distribute global budgets, coordinate regional health services, and work with the regional sickness funds. The directors who manage these authorities are appointed by the cabinet restructuring to allow more devolution. A wider range of responsibilities for regional health agencies is proposed for 2009.

The National Health Insurance Agency for Salaried Workers, the main national health insurance fund, covers 80 percent of the population. Various other funds cover smaller, professionally based groups. Insurance funds are governed by employer representatives and employees. Levels of insurance coverage vary according to the type of service, from full coverage of major surgery to around 75 percent coverage for physician consultations.

Funds from employers and individuals and other fees are counted as public sources of financing and account for around 80 percent of total health expenditures. Social insurance sickness funds pay around 75 percent of total health expenditure (US$2,937 per person in 2006), and the government contributes around 5 percent. Private insurance in France paid for 12.8 percent of health expenditure in 2006 and user fees around 6.7 percent (OECD 2008). Individuals buy supplementary insurance to cover compulsory copayments such as per diem hospital charges. Supplementary insurance also pays for the difference between the insurance benefit and the fee schedule or fee charged by physicians. However, not all supplementary insurance funds will reimburse patients for the difference between the fee schedule amount and the amount the patient paid (Costich 2002). Private insurers act as secondary payers but rarely cover services excluded by public insurers (Couffinhal and Paris 2001). CMU pays the coinsurance and copayments of its members directly (Costich 2002). Eighty-eight percent of the population has complementary insurance from for-profit and nonprofit insurance companies (OECD 2008). Many employees receive or purchase this coverage through their employers.

The areas with the largest share of direct payments within each expenditure category are dental care (30 percent), other medical goods (29.8 percent), and pharmaceuticals (17.1 percent). Inpatient care is largely paid for by sickness funds, with users contributing just 3.7 percent of expenditures and complementary insurers 4.2 percent. In the area of outpatient physician consultations, sickness funds finance 71.8 percent of the cost, 20.2 percent is financed by complementary insurance, and users pay 8 percent (Couffinhal and Paris 2003).

Almost two-thirds of physicians in the ambulatory care sector in France work in private practice. Physicians in public hospitals are salaried. Payments for physicians in private practice are based on a fee schedule, which will eventually resemble the Resource-Based Relative Value Scale used by the U.S. Medicare program. Patients can visit specialists without referrals. In 2004, direct access to specialists was modified so that patients pay a higher share of the cost (50 percent compared to 70 percent with referral) if they access a specialist without a referral.

The fee schedule is negotiated between a government-appointed representative of the public sickness funds and physicians' unions. The minister of health must approve the fee schedule before it can be adopted. The relationship between physicians and insurance funds has always been strained (Couffinhal and Paris 2001). Physicians can, however, increase their fees above the reimbursement level of the insurance funds, because supplementary insurance or out-of-pocket payments will cover the charges (Imai, Jacobzone, and Lenain 2000).

Hospitals are managed by the public sector (45 percent), nonprofit organizations (15 percent), and the private sector (35 percent). Hospitals receive global budgets, and local hospital managers and boards are responsible for management and staffing decisions within the hospitals. Central government determines hospital allocations, but the sickness funds distribute the money Historical costs and estimates of future operating costs determine individual hospital allocations. Since 1996, hospitals have reported to regional hospitalization agencies (World Health Organization 1997).

Regional planning has a long tradition in France through a map called the Carte Sanitaire, which is used to measure and plan the distribution of hospital services. The Schéma Régional d'Organisation Sanitaire is used to plan the regional distribution of equipment and services. The Carte Sanitaire has limited the growth of hospital beds, but it has not addressed the other costs that contribute to increased hospital expenditure (Lancry and Sandier 1999).

Germany

Germany has a compulsory national health insurance system that covers close to 90 percent of the population, who are enrolled in approximately 200 nonprofit sickness funds (Busse 2008). Additionally, around 10 percent of the population—including civil servants, self-employed people, and those with high incomes—was enrolled with private insurers in 2006. Around 200,000 people (one-quarter of a percent of the population) were uninsured in 2007 (Bundesministerium für Gesundheit 2007). Recent reforms address the issue of the uninsured. Starting in 2009, health insurance will be compulsory for all residents, including higher-income individuals, although Germany has long mandated statutory insurance for all those below a certain income and has required employers to pay half the contribution. For those who are employed, employers will continue to finance nearly half of the contribution rate.

Seventy-seven percent of total health expenditure is public. Of this amount, 68 percent is accounted for by nonprofit health insurance funds and 9 percent by state and local governments (Statistisches Bundesamt 2008a). Households account for 13 percent of total health expenditure, and private insurance funds, 9 percent. Overall, Germany spent 10.6 percent of its GDP on health in 2006 (US$3,718 per person) (OECD 2008).

A key feature of the German health system is the corporatist dispersal of decision making among different tiers of government (federal and state) and nongovernmental organizations (see Wilhelm-Schwartz and Busse 1997). In other words, doctors' associations and sickness funds jointly administer the health insurance system on behalf of the government by implementing federal policy through negotiated collective agreements. As a result, German health policy has tended toward stability because of the veto power of multiple interest groups in the health system (Giaimo and Manow 1997).

Since the mid-1990s, the German federal government has engaged in health sector reforms. The post-2000 period has seen many health policy changes, including the extension of mandatory insurance requirements after 2009 to all residents of Germany, including those who are privately insured. In 2009, fundamental changes directed toward the improvement of medical care quality and the reform of private health insurers and the sickness funds are likely (Bundesministerium für Gesundheit 2007). For the first time, the level of insurance premiums or contributions in the private and sickness fund markets will be regulated.

The federal government regulates long-term care, health professionals, and the health insurance funds, including compulsory health insurance benefit packages, the organizational structure of the funds, the scope of negotiations between the funds and providers of health services, and the financing of health services (Busse 1999). The 16 states (Länder) are responsible for regional hospital planning, regulating the professions, public health, and emergency services. State-level, corporatist associations of insurers and doctors implement federal laws through collective agreements.

Historically, Germans' choice of statutory insurer depended on their occupational status, as there were different funds for different occupations. After 1997, Germany allowed individuals to choose their statutory insurer to increase competition. The transition to full-scale competition—allowing funds to offer different benefit packages and selective contracting with providers—was never made, partly because greater differentiation across insurers would result in an erosion of solidarity (Brown and Amelung 1999). In the late 1990s, policy changes increased the level of government health funding and reduced patient copayments (European Observatory on Health Systems and Policies 2000a, 19–20).

Private insurance is generally concentrated in the higher-income and self-employed groups. As we noted, private insurance funded 9 percent of 2006 health expenditures (OECD 2008). Supplementary insurance plans provide better hospital accommodation and cover copayments. Although comprehensive private insurance has not been heavily regulated, changes starting in 2009 are designed to redistribute the risk across private insurers and reduce premiums for older and sicker enrollees. Providers treating private patients have more discretion in setting their own fees.

The Länder and the federal government jointly finance hospital capital budgets from taxation, but the Länder plan hospital investments (European Observatory on Health Systems and Policies 2004, 8). The hospital sector in Germany shifted from global budgets to a DRG payment system in 2004. Fifty-four percent of all hospitals in Germany are in the public sector, 38 percent are not for profit, and around 8 percent are in the private sector (European Observatory on Health Systems and Policies 2004, 6).

Physicians are paid through a reimbursement system based on relative values for different services. The system, established at the national level, is called the uniform valuation scale (EBM—Einheitlicher Bewertungsmaßstab).

Actual payment rates, volume, and expenditure caps are determined by negotiations between physicians and the sickness funds at the state level. Physician associations distribute payments from health insurance funds to their members.

Health insurance is financed by payroll taxes shared between employees and employers. In 2008, the average contribution rate was 15 percent of pretax wages, split between employers (7 percent) and employees (8 percent) (Busse 2008). Beginning in 2009, the contributions will depend on health insurers' ability to contain costs within each fund: If their costs exceed their revenues, they will be able to require additional contributions from members (within a ceiling). Funds will have an incentive to limit their increases in contributions—to avoid a decrease in enrollment.

Funds charge different prices (although the differences are not dramatic), so individuals pay different amounts. Contributions depend on income and are limited by a contribution ceiling. Maximum contribution rates are determined annually. People who do not earn wages, such as the retired, also make contributions, but in these cases the retirement or unemployment fund people are enrolled in assumes the employer role (European Observatory on Health Systems and Policies 2000a, 40). People who contribute to the health insurance funds receive coverage for dependent family members within certain income limits. As of 2009, the German government will regulate contribution rates. All health insurance contributions are to be pooled and redistributed to funds based on a risk-adjustment formula (Busse 2008). In addition, healthcare for children will no longer come out of payroll-based contribution rates. Instead, the federal government will pay for this out of taxation, making payments directly to the Central Fund (Bundesministerium für Gesundheit 2007).

Out-of-pocket expenditures for those insured through the statutory health insurance funds are low compared to U.S. out-of-pocket expenditures, with an annual average expenditure of US$121 per member (Statistisches Bundesamt 2008b), and exemptions from copayments are available once members spend more than 2 percent of household income or, if they are chronically ill, 1 percent of household income (Busse 2008).

Japan

Japan's universal compulsory health insurance system was established in 1961 and covers the entire population. In 2005, Japan spent 8.2 percent of its GDP on health, or US$2,908 per person. Almost 83 percent of health expenditure is funded from public sources. Out-of-pocket charges finance 14 percent of total health expenditure (OECD 2008).

There are two basic types of health insurance in Japan. Employee insurance, for those people working for firms, covers 59 percent of individuals, (including dependents). The remaining 41 percent are enrolled in National Health Insurance (Statistics Bureau of Japan 2008, 637). In contrast to some European countries, people in Japan do not have a choice of funds; they are assigned based on employment status and location.

Employees of large companies and public-sector organizations are enrolled in plans managed by the Health Insurance Society (32.58 million subscribers within 1,584 insurers). A second insurance scheme called the Government-Managed Health Insurance (GMHI) plan covers employees of small to medium-sized companies (35.62 million subscribers within a single plan). The employee sector also has insurance plans for specific groups, such as seamen, national public service employees, local public service employees, and teachers and staff employees of private schools (9.71 million enrolled within 76 insurers). All other individuals—self-employed people, farmers, the unemployed, retirees and their dependents, and anyone else who does not otherwise qualify for health insurance—are covered by National Health Insurance, which is managed by municipal governments (51.58 million enrolled in 2,697 insurers) (Okamoto 2008; Yoshikawa and Bhattacharya 2002). Premiums for employed individuals are around 8.2 percent of income, and employers contribute half of this amount (Okamoto 2008).

Japan's system combines a social insurance and national health insurance, with social insurance contributing the majority of funding (64.3 percent). However, general taxes also contribute a higher proportion of funding (20 percent) than would occur under a pure social insurance system (OECD 2008). Funds receive different levels of tax subsidies from government. For example, National Health Insurance receives 43 percent of total benefits from government, while the Government-Managed Health Insurance scheme receives 13 percent of its revenues from government (Okamoto 2008, 53).

Government has a long-established role as both payer and policymaker in this hybrid system (Ikegami and Campbell 1999). The system features an employer- or municipality-based insurance system, private provision, close involvement of interest groups in decision making, and government regulation of the insurance industry and the global health budget. Japan gives municipalities a larger role than they have in many European systems. Benefits are standardized, and risk selection is regulated. Premium prices are not regulated outside of the GMHI plan. A compensation scheme for the higher health service costs of the elderly, called the Roken system, is managed by municipalities and financed through transfers from all insurers and the government (Yoshikawa and Bhattacharya 2002). The government uses supply-side regulation of medical school enrollment and hospital bed numbers to restrict costs (Imai 2002).

The most distinctive feature of the Japanese health system is the national medical fee schedule for physician services. The schedule and the delivery of health services are inseparable; "each shapes the other" (White 1995,

115). The government's fee-schedule decisions affect all insurers. A council of 20 members representing professionals, business, government, labor, and experts reviews the schedule every two years. An innovative feature of the schedule is the use of varying payments for procedures the government considers overused. For example, payments for MRI (magnetic resonance imaging) were reduced from US$138 to US$95 in 2002 to discourage use of these services. Government is thus able to "micro-manage physician practice patterns" (Ikegami and Campbell 2008, 111–12).

Given this aggressive approach to cost containment, Japan's record in restraining costs over the last two decades has been relatively successful. One contributing factor may be the fixed rate of subsidy from the government to funds such as the GMHI. This creates the means and an incentive for the government to limit cost growth in the private sector. However, while cost containment was successful, it did not compensate for diminishing resources. For almost two decades, health costs were increasing faster than firms' revenues and employees' wages. The ongoing challenge for Japan is containing rising healthcare costs within a declining national income (Ikegami and Campbell 2004).

The hospital system in Japan is made up of private, university, prefectural, and municipal hospitals. Eighty-one percent of Japanese hospitals are privately owned and 19 percent are in the public sector, but almost half of all beds are in the public sector (Okamoto 2008, 47). Most acute and costly inpatient care is provided in university and public hospitals, and some care is provided in 294 hospitals and sanatoriums owned by the Department of National Hospitals. These nationally owned hospitals provide services such as organ transplants and positron radiation therapy. Sanatoriums provide services for conditions such as muscular dystrophy and mental health services.

Private hospitals and clinics are typically owned by private medical corporations that are prohibited from paying dividends. For-profit investor-owned hospitals are not permitted (Okamoto 2008, 47). Physician-owned clinics provide outpatient and inpatient services. Japan has 14.59 acute care beds per 1,000 people, which is one of the highest ratios among developed countries (Economic and Social Research Institute 2006, 64). This is mainly a function of the fluidity between the hospital and outpatient sectors. Whereas in some countries outpatient, long-term care, and primary care services are highly differentiated, in Japan these services are often provided in the same institution.

Japan introduced prospective payment in 1994 and developed its own payment system, the Diagnosis Procedure Combination (DPC), in 2003. The DPC is a case mix–based system that mixes prospective payment (71 percent of the fee) with fee-for-service methods for hospital physician fees (28 percent of the fee) (Economic and Social Research Institute 2006, 63). The hospital DPC is a prospective payment that pays a defined rate based on average length of stay for each diagnosis group (Economic and Social Research Institute 2006, 63).

Physicians work mainly in private practice, and nearly all physicians are in sole practice due to legal restrictions on sharing equipment and staff (Campbell and Ikegami 1998, 81). The healthcare system relies on a large number of primary care physicians. Of the 249,574 physicians in Japan in 2002, almost 30 percent (74,704) were in internal medicine (Ministry of Health, Labour, and Welfare 2008). General practice medicine is not clearly established as a separate discipline, so specialist doctors are not differentiated from general practitioners, and doctors in private clinics try to treat all problems their patients have (Imai 2002). Physicians are reimbursed through the fee schedule. Outpatient primary care, including pharmacy services, is reimbursed at the same rate as hospital treatment. Revenue from pharmaceuticals allows physicians to offset fee-schedule reductions (Ikegami and Campbell 1999). As a result, pharmaceutical consumption is extremely high, the number of consultations per capita per year is more than twice the OECD average, and inpatient admission rates to general beds is well below the OECD average (Imai 2002).

The Netherlands

Under the Health Insurance Act of 2006, residents of the Netherlands must enroll in plans covering a standardized set of benefits from not-for-profit health insurers (Ministry of Health, Welfare, and Sport 2008). Half of the health expenditures the act covers are paid by income-related contributions (collected through taxation), 45 percent are paid by community-rated premiums (directly paid to the chosen health insurer), and the remaining 5 percent are paid by tax money (to cover the cost for children aged 17 or younger, who are exempted from paying premium contributions). In addition, about two-thirds of Dutch households receive an income-related tax credit from the government to make health insurance more affordable. Employers and individuals may purchase supplementary coverage. Around 90 percent of individuals are enrolled in one of four health insurers (van de Werd 2008).

A second type of insurance, called exceptional medical expenses (AWBZ—Algemene Wet Bijzondere Ziektekosten), covers nursing home care, residential care for the elderly, home health care, hospital care that lasts longer than 12 months, inpatient and outpatient treatment for physical and mental disorders, and long-term mental health services for the entire population. Enrollment in the AWBZ is also mandatory. The AWBZ is financed by income-related contributions and income-related copayments and is administered by regional offices mandated by health insurers.

The Netherlands spent 9.3 percent of its GDP, or US$3,391 per person, on health in 2006. Social insurance financed 78 percent of health expenditures in 2006, general tax revenues financed 4 percent, supplementary health insurance financed 5.9 percent, and out-of-pocket payments financed 8 percent. Historically, out-of-pocket payments for curative health services in the Netherlands have been relatively low, but the government recently introduced a small annual deductible of €150. Individuals can voluntarily buy supplementary health insurance for benefits that are not included in the mandatory coverage, such as dental care for adults, eyeglasses, physical therapy, and alternative medicine (Van de Ven and Schut 2008).

Past analyses of the Dutch health system stressed the unique mix of public and private financing through health insurance funds, private insurance, and corporatist decision making involving health insurers, providers, and government (Schut 1995). However, this structure changed in the 1980s and 1990s when the Netherlands gradually increased the level of competition in the healthcare system and moved away from corporatism. For example, people were given the freedom to choose their insurer in the annual open-enrollment period, price competition among sickness funds was introduced, and any-willing-provider laws were abolished.

The Health Insurance Act of 2006 blurred prior distinctions between sickness funds and private insurers in the Netherlands. Previously, only the wealthy could enroll in private health insurance plans, but now all individuals can enroll in the fund of their choice. The act also gave insurers more negotiating freedom with providers. However, choice for consumers and funds' greater autonomy to negotiate with providers are balanced by strong regulation of benefits and risk adjustment. Insurers must provide "a duty of care" for their enrollees, and they cannot turn applicants away, although they can decline applicants for add-on supplementary insurance plans (Ministry of Health, Welfare, and Sport 2008).

Regulation of health insurers reduces incentives for cream-skimming. A redistribution scheme compensates funds with enrollees who have higher expected healthcare costs. About half of all healthcare costs are paid by a system called the Risk Equalization Fund (REF) that compensates insurers for enrollees with predictably high medical expenses. Since insurers are now obliged to charge each applicant a community-rated rather than an individual-rated premium, they receive high risk-adjusted equalization payments from the REF for high-risk members. Conversely, insurers pay into the REF for low-risk members (Van de Ven and Schut 2008).

All hospitals in the Netherlands are nonprofit, and they receive a global budget for 80 percent of their operating expenses. For the remaining 20 percent (primarily routine care), hospitals are free to negotiate prices with health insurers. Prices are set per Diagnostic Treatment Combination, a Dutch variant of a DRG. The government retrospectively reimburses the capital costs of the regulated segment, provided the hospital has a legal building license. In 2009, the freely negotiable part of hospital expenditure will be raised from

20 to 34 percent. In addition, the government plans to publish comparative quality indicators to encourage patients to compare hospitals (Hoogervorst 2007). Some quality indicators have already been made public.

General practitioners are paid using a mixture of capitation and fee-for-service payment. Members of the insurance funds register with a general practitioner of their choice and may only receive services from that physician. Patients can switch or be referred to other physicians. Whereas primary care physicians previously had pro-forma contracts with sickness funds, since 2006 the providers have negotiated contracts with insurers through regional groups. This resulted in improved healthcare for patients with chronic illnesses and some gains in practice payments for physicians (Knottnerus and ten Velden 2007).

Sweden

Sweden has a publicly operated, locally led health system that provides healthcare services to all residents. Its national health expenditure is slightly less than that of most Western European countries at US$3,973 per person in 2006, or 9.2 percent of its GDP. Eighty-two percent of health expenditure in Sweden is financed publicly (OECD 2008), with around 15 percent coming from out-of-pocket sources (Diderichsen 2000). Private insurance finances less than 1 percent of health expenditure. Of the public health expenditure, 71 percent is financed at the local level by income taxes, and 16 percent is financed from national sickness insurance and central government grants.

National government writes the broad framework legislation of the healthcare system, while county councils or larger regional governments (one in each of the three large metropolitan areas) are responsible for financing and management, since almost all services are provided and funded by county councils. County councils collect taxes from residents to finance health services and manage local hospitals and health centers. Access to healthcare is defined by the Health and Medical Services Act (1982), which requires care to be prompt and of good quality and establishes the responsibility of counties to offer "good health and medical services to those living within its boundaries" (Ministry of Health and Social Affairs 2003). Under the healthcare guarantee agreement signed between counties and the national government in 2006, counties are legally required to provide access to health services within three months, after which an individual can request that the county pay for care in another county. In general, county facilities operate as monopolies within each county, although counties have allowed patients to choose their own hospital since the 1990s (Anell 1996). Almost all services are provided at the county level, but more complicated and rarer services are treated at regional centers (Glenngård et al. 2005).

Central government institutions are involved in evaluation of new technologies, public health, professional licensing and regulation, and oversight of the health sector. The Ministry of Health and Social Affairs (Socialde-partementet) and the National Board of Health and Social Welfare (Social-styrelsen) supervise the county councils by developing national-level health legislation and evaluating the services county councils provide (Glenngård et al. 2005).

The county councils are usually divided into health districts, and these are divided into primary care districts. Elected board members govern the health districts. County councils are elected every four years, so voters can hold local politicians accountable for the delivery of health services (Calltorp 1999). Some districts act as purchasers for their populations. Districts were traditionally organized around providers, such as a hospital and a primary care center. Within each district there is often a primary health district that follows the geographic contours of the municipality. Interspersed within the subregional level are Sweden's 290 municipalities, which are responsible for long-term care and nursing home care.

Sweden followed other countries in introducing some market-based reforms in the late 1980s and 1990s. Managed competition was pursued within the traditional Swedish framework of decentralization and largely public provision of health services. In most counties reforms focused on patient choice of provider and managerial independence of hospitals, but they were not uniformly adopted (Saltman and Bergman 2005). Where a purchase–provider split was adopted to increase the managerial independence of hospitals, new purchasers simply overlaid previous geographic areas and council structures. The separation of providers and purchasers was weak compared to that found in the United Kingdom (Anell 1996).

Compared to many other European countries, Swedish reforms were relatively minor since purchasers continued to have a monopoly in each district. Purchasers had few opportunities to control costs. For example, free choice of hospital meant that purchasers were required to pay the fee the hospital charged for a service (Andersen, Smedby, and Vågerö 2001). However, one durable aspect of this reform is the purchaser–provider split, in which many councils purchase hospital services through contracts with public and private hospitals.

The Swedish hospital system is organized around 65 district hospitals and 8 regional hospitals that provide more specialized care. Approximately 95 percent of general hospital beds are in the public sector. Hospitals often are managed by a combination of elected public officials and hospital managers, who are civil servants (Glenngård et al. 2005). County hospitals are responsible for acute care, but municipalities are responsible for longer-term care. Municipalities are discouraged from shifting costs to counties for their patients in longer-term and nursing care through reimbursements to county councils for the post-acute care expenses for municipal geriatric and disabled patients (Andersen, Smedby, and Vågerö 1197). Sixteen out of 21 health authorities (counties) use the DRG system to pay hospitals. The DRG payment system was introduced in some counties in the 1990s to address waiting times for hospital treatment and the perceived lack of incentives for hospitals to increase their output. Some hospitals introduced volume caps to balance these incentives (Anell 1996), while other counties returned to fixed or global budgets (Diderichsen 2000). Regional hospitals are commonly reimbursed through retrospective fee-for-service payments (Glenngård et al. 2005).

Physician care is mainly provided through 1,000 health centers financed by the county councils and by private practitioners. The Health and Medical Services Act requires counties to "organize primary care in such a way that everybody living within the county council area will have access and be able to choose a permanent medical contact" (Health and Medical Services Act, Section 5). This general requirement is fulfilled differently in each county. In some counties, publicly employed physicians predominate, while other counties have a larger proportion of private practice physicians. Most are employed in the public sector and receive salaries (Glenngård et al. 2005), but they also receive some payments depending on the number of patients they treat. Approximately 8 percent of physicians work on a fee-for-service basis in private practice. Private practitioners account for 26 percent of all physician visits (specialists and general practice) (Swedish Federation of County Councils 2001). Private providers are paid through councils. The National Social Insurance Board pays councils for care from private-sector providers. The board also regulates private-sector payment rates.

The county councils' total health services budget is determined by general income tax revenues, state grants, patient fees, and reimbursements from other sources outside the county council (Glenngård et al. 2005). Employee and employer contributions also pay for health services. Private and public employers pay a contribution per employee to the health insurance system, which in 2004 was 11 percent of the employee's salary (Glenngård et al. 2005, 45).

Switzerland

Switzerland established compulsory health insurance in 1996, but a system of voluntary health insurance combined with premium subsidies dates to 1911. Every citizen is required to purchase health insurance, with employer-sponsored insurance programs limited to supplementary coverage. Switzerland's health system is notable for the absence of a government-controlled social insurance fund and for its high levels of health expenditure compared to other European countries (11.3 percent of GDP in 2006 or US$5,877 per person). The public sector finances 60.3 percent of total health expenditure, of which compulsory insurance financed 43 percent in 2006 and general government financed 17.2 percent (OECD 2008).

Switzerland's federal structure delineates roles for the Confederation, 26 cantons, and local government. The Confederation funds premium subsidies, public health, research, safety, and professional accreditation and contributes less than 1 percent of total health expenditure. Cantons pay for around 15 percent of total health expenditure and provide matching subsidies for low-income individuals and subsidies to hospitals (OECD 2006, 37). Cantons are responsible for regulating and training health professionals, public health, and implementing federal laws (European Observatory on Health Systems and Policies 2000b). Local government funds 1.5 percent of health expenditure.

Most European countries use taxes or social insurance payroll contributions to finance health services, but individuals and households in Switzerland make direct premium payments to insurance companies. Compulsory health insurance is individually purchased and provided by nonprofit health insurance funds that are regulated by the Federal Office of Public Health. The average number of insurers in each canton is 56 (Frank and Lamiraud 2008). Insurers must accept all individuals who apply for coverage. Each insurer sets its own rates. Insurers are allowed to have up to three rating bands for different areas of the canton, but within those geographic bands they must charge uniform premiums to all subscribers. All insurers are required to offer the same package of benefits. The benefits package encompasses all services received from a doctor, medical treatment in general hospital wards, and prescribed generic pharmaceuticals from a drug specialty list (Colombo 2001). Although the insurance market is highly regulated, individuals can choose policies that have a higher deductible with lower premiums, bonuses for no claims, and managed care plans that reduce their premium (WHO 2001).

Cantons subsidize the cost of health insurance for people whose premiums exceed 8–10 percent (depending on the canton of residence) of their taxable incomes. About one-third of the population received this assistance in 2004 (OECD 2006, 36). Each canton fixes the allowable proportion, and the federal government matches these contributions (Zweifel 2000, 940). A risk-adjustment scheme redistributes funds to insurers with higher-cost enrollees (Colombo 2001); however, Zweifel (2000) argues that the payments do not fully compensate for risk differences.

Supplementary private insurance policies cover hotel costs and other benefits not provided by compulsory insurance. Supplementary insurance cannot be used to pay coinsurance for the mandatory benefits package. This type of insurance is regulated less strictly, and insurers are free to set premiums. Private insurance financed 8.5 percent of total health expenditures in 2006 (OECD 2008).

Hospitals receive subsidies from cantons and payments from health insurance funds and private insurers. In 2004, almost 44 percent of the total inpatient care expenditures were funded from cantonal subsidies (OECD 2006, 54). Many of the cantons operate their own hospitals. Payment methods vary in each canton. Most payments are per day, but in some cantons global budgets are standard. There is movement toward developing a national DRG system that will increase uniformity among cantons (OECD 2006, 55). The federal health insurance law requires cantons to plan hospital provision and to limit the range of providers who will be reimbursed by compulsory insurance programs (European Observatory on Health Systems and Policies 2000b). This is essentially a control on the supply of hospitals.

In the ambulatory care sector, Switzerland has a national fee schedule that establishes relative values for each service. It replaced cantonal schedules negotiated between health insurers and physician associations (European Observatory on Health Systems and Policies 2000b). However, since the 1996 insurance reforms, insurers have created modified physician payment arrangements such as preferred provider networks and health maintenance organizations. Managed care plans pay their physicians through a mix of capitation and global budgets. Physicians working in hospitals are mostly salaried.

United Kingdom

All residents of the United Kingdom receive care through the National Health Service (NHS). The United Kingdom spent 8.4 percent of its GDP on health (US$3,332 per person) in 2006 (OECD 2008). Eighty-seven percent of health expenditure is financed from public sources (OECD 2008) and almost 13 percent by the private sector.

The United Kingdom consists of four countries: England, Scotland, Northern Ireland, and Wales. Scotland and Wales have achieved greater independence from England in recent years. Health sector arrangements in these areas have been similar to the NHS in England with some variation in the organization and number of purchasers. England is responsible for 80 percent of health expenditures within the United Kingdom.

The English NHS is made up of national and local organizations. The national Department of Health is responsible for public health and health policy and for overseeing the NHS. In 2009, the Care Quality Commission (2008) will be responsible for regulating healthcare and social care in England. The National Institute for Health and Clinical Effectiveness provides evidence-based guidelines and technology assessments that inform all levels of the NHS. The Department of Health determines the allocation of funding to ten strategic health authorities. Strategic health authorities are responsible for monitoring the performance of local primary care trusts (PCTs) and NHS trusts. At the local level, 152 PCTs provide and commission services and develop health services plans for the populations they serve. In the hospital sector, 290 NHS trusts manage 1,600 NHS hospitals and specialist care centers; 105 foundation hospitals also offer care.

The NHS has a reputation for providing a high standard of care at a relatively low cost. However, since the mid-1980s, the NHS has been the target of repeated reforms. England developed an internal market for NHS

health services in 1991. These reforms established local purchasing organizations to buy health services from primary care providers and hospitals.

Purchasers and providers, however, did not function as anticipated in
the internal market. Rather than negotiating highly specific contracts with
the lowest cost provider, purchasers and providers formed stable relationships
that resulted in less specificity in contracts and reduced information and transaction costs (Tuohy 1999). Smee (2000) argues that the internal market was
not effective because it was difficult to develop purchasers powerful enough
to counter the information advantage of providers. In addition, there were
serious capacity constraints. Hospitals had a long history as local monopolists,
and there was little information on cost or quality of care.

After six years of attempting a provider–purchaser split and competition among providers, the 1997 Labour government introduced reform plans
that deemphasized competition. However, since 2004 the government has
emphasized competition and choice, and has committed to increasing NHS
quality and levels of funding. Past reform plans have focused on the absence
of national standards or clear incentives to improve performance, overcen-
tralization, and poor responsiveness to patients (Secretary of State for Health
2000).

A reform plan announced in 2000 promised more ambitious improvements to the NHS than previous reform plans. Supported by the largest sus-
tained increase in funding ever planned for the NHS, the secretary of state
for health promised major improvements, such as increases in health funding and in the number of hospitals, physicians, and nurses. Reforms in this
decade have focused on three strategies (Stevens 2004). First, government
has supported providers by increasing the supply of physicians, modernizing
the infrastructure, and offering opportunities for lifelong learning. A second
strategy was to develop comprehensive national standards with targets, performance indicators, and inspection and regulatory mechanisms. Finally, reforms that began in the late 1990s were aimed at increasing local control of
healthcare through the PCTs, providing greater patient choice, and widening
the range of private providers. By December 2008, the agency charged with
measuring performance of the healthcare system suggested that the NHS has
improved significantly since 2003 (Healthcare Commission 2008).

Private insurance has not played a major role in financing health services
in England, especially compared with countries such as Australia. Around 11
percent of the population, or 6.8 million people, had private insurance coverage in 2006 (OECD 2008). The majority (around 5 million) of the privately
insured are covered through their employers, while the remaining 1.8 million
purchase private insurance (Koen 2000). Most insurance policies cover hospital inpatient stay, outpatient service, and day treatment in a private hospital or
a private ward in an NHS hospital; drugs; and X-rays. Policies do not generally
cover the treatment of chronic or long-term illnesses that cannot be cured,

such as asthma, diabetes, or multiple sclerosis. Private insurance requires patients to be symptom-free and does not cover preexisting symptoms for two years, nor does it cover primary care services, treatment for HIV/AIDS, or pregnancy (Foubister et al. 2006).

Hospitals in England are largely publicly owned and provide care free of charge, excluding small charges for amenities. Unless a patient needs emergency treatment, hospital treatment requires a referral from a primary care provider. Waiting times for nonemergency care traditionally have been long, but in recent years the government has made efforts to reduce them. Reduced waiting times for hospital and doctor appointments, cleaner wards, better food and facilities in hospitals, and improved health services for older people were promised starting in 2000 (Secretary of State for Health 2000). The Department of Health promised that by 2008 no one would wait longer than 18 weeks from first outpatient appointment to be treated. One indication of the NHS's responsiveness is that in the quarter concluding September 30, 2008, 85 percent of those on the waiting list had waited no longer than six weeks for an outpatient appointment with a specialist following referral (authors' calculation based on Department of Health 2008).

Hospitals in the NHS are categorized as acute trusts or foundation trusts. Under the Health and Social Care (Community Health and Standards) Act of 2003, hospitals can convert their status to NHS foundation trusts if they meet certain performance criteria. Foundation trusts are independent public-benefit corporations with fewer central government restrictions on their operation, but they continue to receive public funding for their services.

Specialists and general practitioners are paid differently. Specialists are employed on salaries within public hospitals. Publicly employed hospital specialists can and often do have limited part-time private practices. Physicians outside of hospitals are mainly self-employed. Most primary care physicians are paid according to an annual national contract between the government and the British Medical Association. The contract specifies a mix of fixed allowances for practice expenses, capitation fees (which provide around half of physicians' income), and fee-for-service payments (European Observatory on Health Systems and Policies 1999).

Primary care is the first point of access for nonemergency care in the NHS. Around 90 percent of patient contacts with the NHS are with primary care physicians (European Observatory on Health Care Systems and Policies 1999, 53). Primary care is provided free of charge to patients. Patients register with a general practitioner. Most primary care physicians work in individual or group practices.

Reform is gradually transforming the primary care sector, and the role of primary care physicians is increasing. In April 1999, Labour introduced a new system of funding primary physician care through primary care groups, which later evolved into PCTs. PCTs provide all primary care and purchase much hospital care (except some forms of tertiary and long-term care and some high-cost procedures) for their enrolled patients. PCTs are groups of self-employed primary care practices in geographic areas covering 50,000 to 250,000 people (European Observatory on Health Systems and Policies 1999). PCTs receive a fixed payment per patient and are allowed to retain budget surpluses. Surpluses can be spent on services or facilities that benefit patients (Koen 2000).

Health services are mainly financed by general government revenue, although around 12 percent of expenditure is financed by an earmarked tax called the national health insurance contribution. The amount of funding available for health services is determined by Cabinet and distributed by the Treasury to the Department of Health and to the NHS.

United States

The United States does not provide universal coverage for healthcare services, although at the time of this writing, healthcare reform is once again on the agenda. Government does, however, have an important role as insurer of the elderly, the disabled, and the poor. Nearly all Americans aged 65 or older have some coverage through the Medicare program, and 46 percent of those below the poverty level have Medicaid coverage (ASPE 2007). In total, about 27 percent of Americans were covered by one or both of these two programs in 2006. Another 60 percent had private coverage through an employer, and 9 percent had other private coverage, which is usually purchased individually. Nevertheless, during 2006, 16 percent of Americans were uninsured at any one point during the year (ASPE 2007). In spite of these major gaps in coverage, the United States spent 15.3 percent of its GDP ($6,347 per person) on health services in 2005—a figure that far exceeds any other country's healthcare spending. It is 56 percent higher than the spending of the second-place country, Switzerland, and is nearly double that of most developed countries (OECD 2008).

Since 1965, senior citizens have been covered by the federal Medicare program, which was later expanded to cover disabled individuals. All Americans who need a kidney transplant or renal dialysis because of chronic kidney disease are also entitled to Medicare benefits regardless of their age. Medicare provides hospital, physician, and some nursing home and home health services. In 2006, the program started covering prescription drugs. Medicare is divided into four parts. Part A is a social insurance program financed primarily through payroll deductions of 2.9 percent and mainly covers hospital (and some nursing home) care. The deduction is split between the employer and employee, with self-employed individuals paying both contributions. Part B mainly covers physician services in and out of the hospital and other outpatient services. Three-quarters of its costs come from general (federal) revenues, with the remaining 25 percent paid through beneficiary premiums. In 2008 the premium was $96.40 per month per person. Part D is the new prescription drug program, where beneficiaries purchase drug coverage from private insurers. In 2008, premiums (which are subsidized by the program) averaged about $25 per month. Part C (called "Medicare Advantage"), an alternative to Parts A, B, and D, provides similar coverage through managed care organizations.

Medicare, however, has a number of gaps in coverage. There are substantial coinsurance and copayment requirements, including 20 percent of all Part B costs, as well as various uncovered services, including most long-term care. As a result, about 90 percent of Medicare beneficiaries have supplemental insurance coverage—32 percent through former employees, 29 percent through individual "Medigap" insurance policies, 15 percent through private Medicare managed care plans like HMOs, and 14 percent through the Medicaid program (America's Health Insurance Plans 2008). About 90 percent of seniors have some prescription drug coverage through Part C, Part D, Medicaid, or an employer or former employer. But there are gaps in drug coverage. Most notable is the famous "doughnut hole"—a gap in Part D coverage where patients pay 100 percent of costs. This gap, which starts anew each calendar year, begins after the Medicare beneficiary has spent a total of $2,700 on drugs and ends when she has incurred $4,350 in out-of-pocket costs (in 2009). Nearly all drug costs are covered after that.

Medicaid coverage is more comprehensive, but, unlike Medicare, the program is administered by the states (and financed jointly with the federal government). As a result, eligibility requirements and benefits are not standardized. Eligibility tends to be "categorical"—to be covered, individuals must meet certain requirements, which vary among states. Most beneficiaries have low incomes and are either dependent children, pregnant women, seniors, or disabled. Whereas some states cover nearly all poor persons, others cover only a fraction of the poor. As noted earlier, 46 percent of those below the poverty level have Medicaid coverage (Centers for Disease Control and Prevention 2001), although many others do have private insurance coverage through their own or a family member's employer. Some Medicaid benefits are mandatory in all states (e.g., inpatient, outpatient, and physician services), but others are optional (e.g., prescription drugs, dental care). About one-third of Medicaid spending goes toward long-term care, particularly—although not entirely—for low-income seniors (Kaiser Commission on Medicaid and the Uninsured 2008). Because these individuals often spend most of their incomes and assets on nursing home care, once they become poor they are often eligible for Medicaid coverage.

Private insurance for those aged 64 or younger is provided largely through employers. Coverage is usually extended to the employee's dependents and spouse, and most employers offer a choice of insurance plans. Employers purchase insurance on behalf of their employees through contracts with insurance carriers or managed care companies that are usually negotiated annually. Individually purchased coverage represents only about one-tenth of the total. There are many reasons for this, including the following:

- Historically, coverage provided through the workplace has benefited from substantial tax advantages.
- Groups can often elicit discounts from insurers as a result of economies of scale.
- Workers tend to be healthier (and therefore less risky) than those not in the workforce.
- Coverage through the workplace protects against adverse selection, in particular, people obtaining coverage specifically because they expect to incur substantial health service costs.

One of the main problems with this patchwork system of insurance coverage is that many people remain uninsured, either because (1) they are not employed, (2) they are employed by a firm that does not offer coverage, (3) their firm offers coverage but they are not eligible for it, (4) they are eligible for employer-sponsored coverage but cannot afford it, or (5) they are denied insurance when they try to purchase it on the individual market. While each of these reasons is important, the last one is most responsible for the upward trend in uninsurance. The number of uninsured in the United States rose from 33 million in 1989, to 39 million in 1998, to 47 million in 2006 (Centers for Disease Control and Prevention 2001; ASPE 2007). For some groups, however, there has been an increase in insurance coverage. For example, coverage among low-income children has expanded as a result of state initiatives.

In addition to insuring the most vulnerable members of the population, the federal government and some state governments regulate insurers. For example, federal legislation known as COBRA (Consolidated Omnibus Budget Reconciliation Act) requires employers to offer employees the option of continuing their insurance coverage if they leave their job and have no coverage, either because it is not provided or because they are not working. Some states require all health insurers to cover certain services, although most large employers are exempt from this because they self-insure and by law are not subject to state health insurance regulation. State and federal regulatory mechanisms are relatively weak, however, and pale in comparison to the regulations or protections under which insurers operate in nearly all other developed countries. Although COBRA coverage may provide a safety net for people between jobs, the price of premiums is not regulated and employees must pay them out of pocket. This cost places COBRA insurance beyond the reach of many individuals.

Most U.S. hospitals are nonprofit. Seventy percent of beds in community hospitals are in nonprofit facilities, 14 percent are in for-profit facilities, and the remaining 16 percent are under the jurisdiction of state or local government. By international standards, occupancy rates are low, averaging 69 percent in 2005 (ASPE 2007). The Medicare program pays hospitals on the basis of DRGs—that is, a fixed amount per admission based on the patient's diagnosis. Other payers, however, use a variety of methods, including DRGs, per diems, and discounted usual charges.

The United States has a greater proportion of specialist physicians than most other countries do. U.S. physicians are paid in different ways. The majority of Medicare beneficiaries receive their care from physicians who are paid on a fee-for-service basis according to the Resource-Based Relative Value Scale. About 23 percent are in Medicare Advantage plans, which include HMOs, and therefore are not part of the Medicare fee-for-service system (KFF 2008a). Private insurers use a combination of methods to pay physicians, including salary, capitation, and fee-for-service. Bonuses or "withholds" for meeting or not meeting certain productivity or cost-containment goals can affect payment. Most HMOs pay their primary providers using capitation, but an even larger majority base specialist payment on fee-for-service. More than 40 percent of plans use bonuses or withholds for primary care physicians, and about 30 percent use them for specialists (MedPAC 2000).

While there have been many calls for fundamental reform and the introduction of a national health insurance program, most changes thus far have been incremental in scope. The major significant development in recent years was the establishment of the State Children's Health Insurance Program in 1997, aimed at covering a large proportion of the country's uninsured children. With a new president and a supportive Congress, there will be even stronger calls for universal coverage.

REFERENCES

Aaron, H. J. 1994. "Public Policy, Values, and Consciousness." *Journal of Economic Perspectives* 8 (2): 3–21.

Aaronson, W., J. Zinn, and M. Rosko. 1994. "Do For-Profit and Not-for-Profit Nursing Homes Behave Differently?" *The Gerontologist* 34 (6): 775–86.

Abel-Smith, B. 1992. "Cost Containment and New Priorities in the European Community." *Milbank Quarterly* 70 (3): 393–422.

Abramson, J. 2004. *Overdo$ed in America: The Broken Promise of American Medicine.* New York: HarperCollins.

Aday, L. A., R. Andersen, and G. V. Fleming. 1980. *Health Care in the U.S.: Equitable to Whom?* Beverly Hills, CA: Sage.

Adler, D. 2006. "P4P's Promise." *Employee Benefit News*, June 1: 24–25.

Agency for Healthcare Research and Quality. 2008. National Guideline Clearinghouse. [Online database; retrieved 4/6/09.] www.guideline.gov/about/about.aspx.

Agodoa, L. Y. C., R. A. Wolfe, and F. K. Port. 1998. "Reuse of Dialyzers and Clinical Outcomes: Fact or Fiction." *American Journal of Kidney Disease* 32: S88–S92.

Ahern, M. M., M. S. Hendryx, and K. Siddharthan. 1996. "The Importance of Sense of Community in People's Perceptions of Their Health-Care Experiences." *Medical Care* 34 (9): 911–23.

Aiken, L. H. 2007. "U.S. Nurse Labor Market Dynamics Are Key to Global Nurse Sufficiency." *Health Services Research* 42 (3, Pt. II): 1299–1320.

Aiken, L. H., S. P. Clarke, R. B. Cheung, D. Sloane, and J. H. Silber. 2003. "Educational Levels of Hospital Nurses and Surgical Patient Mortality." *Journal of the American Medical Association* 290 (12): 1617–23.

Aiken, L. H., S. P. Clarke, D. M. Sloane, J. Sochalski, and J. H. Silber. 2002. "Hospital Nurse Staffing and Patient Mortality, Nurse Burnout, and Job Dissatisfaction." *Journal of the American Medical Association* 288 (16): 1987–93.

Akerlof, G. A., and W. T. Dickens. 1992. "The Economic Consequences of Cognitive Dissonance." *American Economic Review* 72 (3): 307–19.

Alexander, D. L., J. E. Flynn, and L. A. Linkins. 1994. "Estimates of the Demand for Ethical Pharmaceutical Drugs Across Countries and Time." *Applied Economics* 26 (8): 821–26.

Altenstetter, C., and R. Busse. 2005. "Health Care Reform in Germany: Patchwork Change Within Established Governance Structures." *Journal of Health Politics, Policy and Law* 30 (1–2): 121–42.

Altman, S. H., D. Schactman, and E. Eliat. 2006. "Could U.S. Hospitals Go the Way of U.S. Airlines?" *Health Affairs* 25 (1): 11–21.

American Academy of Family Physicians. 2007. "Statement of the American Academy of Family Physicians." [Online information; retrieved 4/2/09.] www.aafp.org/online/etc/medialib/aafp_org/documents/policy/fed/congress testimony/healthinsur.Par.0001.File.dat/SmallBusinessImpactHealthIns Consol.pdf.

American Association of Colleges of Nursing. 2008. "Fact Sheet: Nursing Shortage." [Online information; retrieved 4/6/09.] www.aacn.nche.edu/Media/Fact Sheets/NursingShortage.htm.

American Hospital Association. 2008. *TrendWatch Chartbook 2008: Trends Affecting Hospitals and Health Systems,* Chart 4.6. Chicago: American Hospital Association.

———. 2007a. "Fast Facts on U.S. Hospitals." [Online information; retrieved 4/6/09.] www.aha.org/aha/resource-center/Statistics-and-Studies/fast-facts .html.

———. 2007b. "The 2007 State of America's Hospitals: Taking the Pulse." [Online PowerPoint presentation; retrieved 4/6/09.] www.aha.org/aha/content/ 2007/PowerPoint/StateofHospitalsChartPack2007.ppt.

American Medical Group Association. 2008. "2008 Physician Compensation Survey." [Online information; retrieved 4/6/09.] www.cejkasearch.com/ compensation/amga_physician_compensation_survey.htm.

American Nurses Credentialing Center. 2008. "Magnet Recognition Program." [Online information; retrieved 4/6/09.] www.nursecredentialing.org/Magnet .aspx.

America's Health Insurance Plans (AHIP). 2008. "Medigap: What You Need to Know." [Online information; retrieved 4/6/09.] www.ahipresearch.org/ pdfs/MedigapWhitePaper.pdf.

Andersen, R. M., B. Smedby, and D. Vågerö. 2001. "Cost Containment, Solidarity and Cautious Experimentation: Swedish Dilemmas." *Social Science and Medicine* 52 (8): 1195–1204.

Anderson, G., C. Black, E. Dunn, J. Alonso, J. Christian-Norregard, T. Folmer-Anderson, and P. Bernth-Peterson. 1997. "Willingness to Pay to Shorten Waiting Time for Cataract Surgery." *Health Affairs* 16 (5): 181–90.

Anderson, G. F., and B. K. Frogner. 2008. "Health Spending in OECD Countries: Obtaining Value per Dollar." *Health Affairs* 27 (6): 1718–27.

Anderson, G. F., B. K. Frogner, and U. E. Reinhardt. 2007. "Health Spending in OECD Countries in 2004: An Update." *Health Affairs* 26 (5): 1481–89.

Anderson, R. I., D. Lewis, and J. R. Webb. 1999. "The Efficiency of Nursing Home Chains and the Implications of Non-Profit Status." *Journal of Real Estate Portfolio Management* 5 (3): 235–45.

Anell, A. 2005. "Swedish Healthcare Under Pressure." *Health Economics* 14: S237–S254.

———. 1996. "The Monopolistic Integrated Model and Health Care Reform: The Swedish Experience." *Health Policy* 37 (1): 19–33.

Angell, M. 2004. "Excess in the Pharmaceutical Industry." *Canadian Medical Association Journal* 171 (12): 1451–53.

Antonazzo, E., A. Scott, D. Skatun, and R. F. Elliott. 2003. "The Labor Market for Nursing: A Review of the Labor Supply Literature." *Health Economics* 12: 465–78.

Aronson, E. 1972. *The Social Animal.* San Francisco: W. H. Freeman.

Arrow, K. J. 1983. "Some Ordinalist-Utilitarian Notes of Rawls's Theory of Justice." In *Social Choice and Justice: Collected Papers of Kenneth J. Arrow*, 96–117. Cambridge, MA: Belknap Press.

———. 1963a. *Social Choice and Individual Values.* New York: John Wiley.

———. 1963b. "Uncertainty and the Welfare Economics of Medical Care." *American Economic Review* 53 (5): 940–73.

Askildsen, J. E., B. H. Baltagi, and T. H. Holmas. 2003. "Wage Policy in the Health Care Sector: A Panel Data Analysis of Nurses' Labor Supply." *Health Economics* 12: 705–19.

Association of American Medical Colleges (AAMC). 2006. "AAMC Statement on the Physician Workforce." [Online information; retrieved 4/6/09.] www.aamc.org/workforce/workforceposition.pdf.

Atherly, A., B. E. Dowd, and R. Feldman. 2004. "The Effect of Benefits, Premiums, and Health Risk on Health Plan Choice in the Medicare Program." *Health Services Research* 39 (4, Pt. I): 847–64.

Baicker, K., and A. Chandra. 2004. "Medicare Spending, the Physician Workforce, and Beneficiaries' Quality of Care." [Online article; retrieved 4/6/09.] http://content.healthaffairs.org/cgi/reprint/hlthaff.w4.184v1.pdf.

Baker, C., P. Messmer, C. Gyurko, S. E. Domagala, F. M. Conly, T. Eads, K. S. Harshman, and M. Layne. 2000. "Hospital Ownership, Performance, and Outcomes: Assessing the State-of-the-Science." *Journal of Nursing Administration* 30 (5): 227–40.

Baker, J. B. 1988. "The Antitrust Analysis of Hospital Mergers and the Transformation of the Hospital Industry." *Law and Contemporary Problems* 51 (2): 93–164.

Bamezai, A., J. Zwanziger, G. A. Melnick, and J. M. Mann. 1999. "Price Competition and Hospital Cost Growth in the United States (1989–1994)." *Health Economics* 8: 233–43.

Bander, S. J., J. M. Lazarus, and S. M. Lindenfeld. 2000. "Ownership of Dialysis Facilities and Patients' Survival." *New England Journal of Medicine* 342 (14): 1054.

Barer, M. 2002. "New Opportunities for Old Mistakes." *Health Affairs* 21 (1): 169–71.

Barer, M. L., R. G. Evans, and R. J. Labelle. 1988. "Fee Controls as Cost Controls: Tales from the Frozen North." *Milbank Quarterly* 66 (1): 1–64.

Barer, M. L., J. Lomas, and C. Sanmartin. 1996. "Re-Minding Our Ps and Qs: Medical Cost Controls in Canada." *Health Affairs* 15 (2): 216–34.

Barr, M. D. 2001. "Medical Savings Accounts in Singapore: A Critical Inquiry." *Journal of Health Politics, Policy and Law* 26 (4): 709–26.

Bator, F. M. 1958. "The Anatomy of Market Failure." *Quarterly Journal of Economics* 52 (3): 351–79.

Becker, G. S. 1979. "Economic Analysis and Human Behavior." In *Sociological Economics*, edited by L. Levy-Garboua. Beverly Hills, CA: Sage.

———. 1964. *Human Capital.* New York: Columbia University Press for the National Bureau of Economic Research.

Becker, G. S., and K. M. Murphy. 1988. "A Theory of Rational Addiction." *Journal of Political Economy* 96 (4): 675–700.

Bellanger, M. N., and P. R. Mosse. 2005. "The Search for the Holy Grail: Combining Decentralised Planning and Contracting Mechanisms in the French Health Care System." *Health Economics* 14: S119–S132.

Ben-Nur, A., and B. Gui. 1993. *The Nonprofit Sector in the Mixed Economy.* Ann Arbor: University of Michigan Press.

Bentham, J. 1968. "An Introduction to the Principles of Morals and Legislation." In *Utility Theory: A Book of Readings,* edited by A. N. Page, 3–29. New York: John Wiley.

———. 1791. *Principles of Morals and Legislation.* London: Doubleday.

Berk, M. L., and A. C. Monheit. 2001. "The Concentration of Health Expenditures, Revisited." *Health Affairs* 20 (2): 9–18.

Berkowitz, C. 2004. "Projecting, Predicting, Shaping: The Challenge of Workforce Models." *Pediatrics* 113 (4): 918–19.

Bindman, A. B., and J. P. Weiner. 2000. "The Modern NHS: An Underfunded Model of Efficiency and Integration." *Health Affairs* 19 (3): 120–23.

Biviano, M., S. Tise, M. S. Fritz, and W. Spencer. 2004. "What Is Behind HRSA's Projected Supply, Demand, and Shortage of Registered Nurses?" [Online article; retrieved 4/6/09.] ftp://ftp.hrsa.gov/bhpr/workforce/behindshortage.pdf.

Blackstone, E., and J. Fuhr Jr. 2007. "Specialty Hospitals: The Economics and Policy Issues They Pose." *Journal of Health Care Finance* 34 (2): 1–9.

Blendon, R. J., and J. M. Benson. 2001. "Americans' Views on Health Policy: A Fifty-Year Historical Perspective." *Health Affairs* 20 (2): 33–46.

Blendon, R. J., J. Benson, K. Donelan, R. Leitman, H. Taylor, C. Koeck, and D. Gitterman. 1995. "Who Has the Best Health Care System? A Second Look." *Health Affairs* 14 (4): 220–30.

Blendon, R. J., M. Brodie, J. M. Benson, D. E. Altman, L. Levitt, T. Hoff, and L. Hugick. 1998. "Understanding the Managed Care Backlash." *Health Affairs* 17 (4): 80–94.

Bloch, M. G. 2007. "Consumer-Directed Health Care and the Disadvantaged." *Health Affairs* 26 (9): 1315–32.

Bloom, J. R., J. A. Alexander, and B. A. Nuchols. 1997. "Nurse Staffing Patterns and Hospital Efficiency in the United States." *Social Science and Medicine* 44 (2): 147–55.

Blumenthal, D. 2004. "New Steam from an Old Cauldron: The Physician-Supply Debate." *New England Journal of Medicine* 350 (17): 1780–87.

Bodenheimer, T. 2005. "High and Rising Health Care Costs. Part 1: Seeking an Explanation." *Annals of Internal Medicine* 142 (10): 847–54.

Booton, L. A., and J. I. Lane. 1985. "Hospital Market Structure and the Return to Nursing Education." *Journal of Human Resources* 20 (2): 184–96.

Born, P., and C. Simon. 2001. "Patients and Profits: The Relationship Between HMO Financial Performance and Quality of Care." *Health Affairs* 20 (2): 167–74.

Boulding, K. E. 1969. "Economics as a Moral Science." *American Economic Review* 59 (1): 1–12.

Boyd, C. M., J. Darer, C. Boult, L. P. Fried, L. Boult, and A. W. Wu. 2005. "Clinical Practice Guidelines and Quality of Care for Older Patients with Multiple Comorbid Diseases: Implications for Pay for Performance." *Journal of the American Medical Association* 294 (6): 716–24.

Bradbury, R. C., J. H. Golec, and F. E. Stearns. 1991. "Comparing Hospital Length of Stay in Independent Practice Association HMOs and Traditional Insurance Programs." *Inquiry* 28: 87–93.

Brandolini, A., and T. M. Smeeding. 2007. "Inequality Patterns in Western-Type Democracies: Cross-Country Differences and Time Changes." [Online working paper; retrieved 4/6/09.] www.lisproject.org/publications/liswps/458.pdf.

Brennan T. A., D. J. Rothman, L. Blank, D. Blumenthal, S. C. Chimonas, J. J. Cohen, J. Goldman, J. P. Kassirer, H. Kimball, J. Naughton, and N. Smelser. 2006. "Health Industry Practices that Create Conflicts of Interest: A Policy Proposal for Academic Medical Centers." *Journal of the American Medical Association* 295 (4): 429–33.

Brenner, G., and D. Rublee. 2002. "Germany." In *World Health Systems: Challenges and Perspectives*, edited by B. J. Fried and L. M. Gaydos, 121–36. Chicago: Health Administration Press.

Brewer, C., and P. Frazier. 1998. "The Influence of Structure, Staff Type, and Managed-Care Indicators on Registered Nurse Staffing." *Journal of Nursing Administration* 28 (9): 28–36.

Brody, H. 2007. *Hooked: Ethics, the Medical Profession, and the Pharmaceutical Industry*. Lanham, MD: Rowman & Littlefield.

Brook, R. H., J. E. Ware Jr., W. H. Rogers, E. B. Keeler, A. R. Davies, C. A. Donald, G. A. Goldberg, K. N. Lohr, P. C. Masthay, and J. P. Newhouse. 1983. "Does Free Care Improve Adults' Health? Results from a Randomized Controlled Trial." *New England Journal of Medicine* 309 (23): 1426–34.

Brooks, R. G., M. Walsh, R. E. Mardon, M. Lewis, and A. Clawson. 2002. "The Roles of Nature and Nurture in the Recruitment and Retention of Primary Care Physicians in Rural Areas: A Review of the Literature." *Academic Medicine* 77 (8): 790–98.

Brouwer, W. B. F., A. J. Culyer, N. J. A. van Exel, and F. F. H. Rutten. 2008. "Welfarism vs. Extra-Welfarism." *Journal of Health Economics* 27: 325–38.

Brown, L. D., and V. E. Amelung. 1999. "Manacled Competition: Market Reforms in German Health Care" *Health Affairs* 18 (3): 76–91.

Brown, M. P., M. C. Sturman, and M. J. Simmering. 2002. "The Benefits of Staffing and Paying More: The Effects of Staffing Levels and Wage Practices for Registered Nurses on Hospitals' Average Lengths of Stay." *Advances in Health Care Management* 3: 45–57.

Buchanan, J. M. 1977. "Political Equality and Private Property: The Distributional Paradox." In *Markets and Morals*, edited by G. Dworkin, G. Bermant, and P. G. Brow. Washington, DC: Hemisphere.

Buchmueller, T. 2006. "Price and the Health Plan Choices of Retirees." *Journal of Health Economics* 25: 81–101.

Buchmueller, T. C. 1998. "Does a Fixed-Dollar Premium Contribution Lower Spending?" *Health Affairs* 17 (6): 228–35.

Budetti, P. P. 2008. "Market Justice and U.S. Health Care." *Journal of the American Medical Association* 299 (1): 92–94.

Buerhaus, P. I. 1991. "Economic Determinants of Annual Hours Worked by Registered Nurses." *Medical Care* 29 (12): 1181–94.

Buerhaus, P. I., D. I. Auerbach, and D. O. Staiger. 2007. "Recent Trends in the Registered Nurse Labor Market in the U.S.: Short-Run Swings on Top of Long-Term Trends." *Nursing Economics* 25 (2): 59–66.

Buerhaus, P. I., K. Donelan, B. T. Ulrich, L. Norman, and R. Dittus. 2006. "State of the Registered Nurse Workforce in the United States." *Nursing Economics* 24 (10): 5–12.

Buerhaus, P. I., and D. O. Staiger. 1996. "Managed Care and the Nurse Workforce." *Journal of the American Medical Association* 276 (18): 1487–93.

Buerhaus, P. I., D. O. Staiger, and D. I. Auerbach. 2008. *The Future of the Nursing Workforce in the United States: Data, Trends and Implications.* Sudbury, MA: Jones and Bartlett.

———. 2000a. "Implications of an Aging Registered Nurse Workforce." *Journal of the American Medical Association* 283 (22): 2948–54.

———. 2000b. "Why Are Shortages of Hospital RNs Concentrated in Specialty Care Units?" *Nursing Economics* 18 (3): 111–16.

Bufalino, V., E. D. Peterson, G. L. Burke, K. A. LaBresh, D. W. Jones, D. P. Faxon, A. M. Valadez, L. M. Brass, V. B. Fulwider, R. Smith, and H. M. Krumholz. 2006. "Payment for Quality: Guiding Principles and Recommendations." *Circulation* 113: 1151–54.

Bundesministerium für Gesundheit 2007. "Wilkommen in der Solidarität! Informationen zur Gesundheitsreform 2007." [Online information; retrieved 4/6/09.] www.bmg.bund.de/cln_110/nn_1168682/SharedDocs/Standard artikel/DE/AZ/G/Glossarbegriff-Gesundheitsreform.html.

Bunker, J., and B. Brown. 1974. "The Physician-Patient as an Informed Consumer of Surgical Services." *New England Journal of Medicine* 290 (19): 1051–55.

Buntin, M. B., C. Damberg, A. Haviland, K. Kapur, N. Lurie, R. McDevitt, and M. S. Marquis. 2006. "Consumer-Directed Health Care: Early Evidence About Effects on Cost and Quality." *Health Affairs* 25 (6): W516–W530.

Bureau of Health Professions. 2006a. *The Registered Nurse Population: Findings from the 2004 National Sample Survey of Registered Nurses.* [Online report; retrieved 4/6/09.] bhpr.hrsa.gov/healthworkforce/rnsurvey04.

———. 2006b. "Physician Supply and Demand: Projection in 2020." [Online article; retrieved4/6/09.]ftp://ftp.hrsa.gov/bhpr/workforce/PhysicianForecasting Paperfinal.pdf.

———. 2002. "Projected Supply, Demand, and Shortages of Registered Nurses: 2000–2020." Washington, DC: Bureau of Health Professions, Health Resources and Services Administration, U.S. Department of Health and Human Services.

Bureau of Labor Statistics. 2008. "Household Data Annual Averages." Table 9. [Online information; retrieved 4/6/09.] www.bls.gov/cps/cpsaat9.pdf.

Burgess, J. F., Jr., K. Carey, and G. J. Young. 2005. "The Effect of Network Arrangements on Hospital Pricing Behavior." *Journal of Health Economics* 24 (2): 391–405.

Burns, L. R., R. M. Anderson, and S. M. Shortell. 1990. "The Effect of Hospital Control Strategies on Physician Satisfaction and Physician-Hospital Conflict." *Health Services Research* 25 (3): 527–60.

Burns, L., R. DeGraaff, and H. Singh. 1999. "Acquisition of Physician Group Practices by For-Profit and Not-for-Profit Organizations." *Quarterly Review of Economics and Finance* 39 (4): 465–90.

Busse, R. 2008. "The German Health Care System." [Online information; retrieved 4/6/09.] www.commonwealthfund.org/topics/topics_show.htm?doc_id=674975.

―――. 1999. "Priority-Setting and Rationing in German Health Care." *Health Policy* 50 (1–2): 71–90.

Butler, T. W., and L. Li. 2005. "The Utility of Returns to Scale in DEA Programming: An Analysis of Michigan Rural Hospitals." *European Journal of Operational Research* 161: 469–77.

Cafferty, P. 2005. "Big Pharma Behaving Badly: A Survey of Selected Class Action Lawsuits Against Drug Companies," 4th ed. [Online information; retrieved 4/6/09.] http://familiesusa.org/assets/pdfs/Rx_Lawsuits_Survey_4th_edition_pmdabc2.pdf.

Calem, P. S., A. Dor, and J. A. Rizzo. 1999. "The Welfare Effects of Mergers in the Hospital Industry." *Journal of Economics and Business* 51: 197–213.

Callahan, D. 1999. "Medicine and the Market: A Research Agenda." *Journal of Medicine & Philosophy* 24 (3): 224–42.

Calltorp, J. 1999. "Priority Setting in Health Policy in Sweden and a Comparison with Norway." *Health Policy* 50: 1–22.

Campbell, J. C., and N. Ikegami. 1998. *Art of Balance in Health Policy: Maintaining Japan's Low-Cost, Egalitarian System.* Cambridge, UK: Cambridge University Press.

Campbell, R. J., A. M. Ramirez, K. Perez, and R. G. Roetzheim. 2003. "Cervical Cancer Rates and the Supply of Primary Care Physicians in Florida." *Family Medicine* 35 (1): 60–64.

Cantril, H. 1965. *The Pattern of Human Concerns.* New Brunswick, NJ: Rutgers University Press.

Capps, C. S., and D. Dranove. 2004. "Hospital Consolidation and Negotiated PPO Prices." *Health Affairs* 23 (2): 175–81.

Care Quality Commission (United Kingdom). 2008. *State of Healthcare 2008.* [Online report; retrieved 4/6/09.] www.cqc.org.uk/publications.cfm?widCall1customDocManager.search_do_2&tcl_id=2&top_parent=4513&tax_child=4514&tax_grand_child=4568&tax_great_grand_child=4569&search_string=.

Carlsen, F., and J. Grytten. 1998. "More Physicians: Improved Availability or Induced Demand?" *Health Economics* 7: 495–508.

Carlson, M., W. T. Gallo, and E. H. Bradley. 2004. "Ownership Status and Patterns of Care in Hospice: Results from the National Home and Hospice Case Survey." *Medical Care* 42 (5): 432–38.

Castle, N. G. 2005. "Nursing Home Closures, Changes in Ownership, and Competition." *Inquiry* 42: 281–92.

Castle, N., and B. Fogel. 1998. "Characteristics of Nursing Homes That Are Restraint Free." *The Gerontologist* 38 (2): 181–88.

Catlin, A., C. Cowan, M. Hartman, and S. Heffler. 2008. "National Health Spending in 2006: A Year of Change for Prescription Drugs." *Health Affairs* 27 (1): 14–32.

Center for American Progress. 2007. "Public Opinion Snapshot: Universal Health Care Momentum Swells." [Online article; retrieved 4/6/09.] www.american progress.org/issues/2007/03/opinion_health_care.html.

Centers for Disease Control and Prevention. 2007. *Health, United States, 2007.* [Online report; retrieved 4/6/09.] www.cdc.gov/nchs/data/hus/hus07.pdf.

———. 2001. *Health, United States, 2001.* [Online report; retrieved 6/15/08.] www.cdc.gov/nchs/data/hus/hus01.pdf.

———. 2000. *The National Nursing Home Survey: 1997 Summary.* [Online report; retrieved 4/10/09.] www.cdc.gov/nchs/data/series/sr_13/sr13_147.pdf.

Chandra, A., and G. A. Holt. 1999. "Pharmaceutical Advertisements: How They Deceive Patients." *Journal Business Ethics* 18: 359–66.

Chassin, M. R. 2002. "Achieving and Sustaining Improved Quality: Lessons from New York State and Cardiac Surgery." *Health Affairs* 21 (4): 40–62.

Chattopadhyay, S., and D. Heffley. 1994. "Are For-Profit Nursing Homes More Efficient? Data Envelopment Analysis with a Case-Mix Constraint." *Eastern Economics Journal* 20: 173–88.

Cheng, T.-M., and U. E. Reinhardt. 2008. "Shepherding Major Health System Reforms: A Conversation with German Health Minister Ulla Schmidt." *Health Affairs* 27 (3): W204–W213.

Chernew, M. E., A. B. Rosen, and A. M. Fendrick. 2007. "Value-Based Insurance Design." *Health Affairs* 26 (2): W195–W203.

Chernew, M. E., M. R. Shah, A. Wegh, S. N. Rosenberg, I. A. Juster, A. B. Rosen, M. C. Sokol, K. Yu-Isenberg, and A. M. Fendrick. 2008. "Impact of Decreasing Copayments on Medication Adherence Within a Disease Management Environment." *Health Affairs* 27 (1): 103–12.

Chiha, Y. A., and C. R. Link. 2003. "The Shortage of Registered Nurses and Some New Estimates of the Effects of Wages on Registered Nurses Labor Supply: A Look at the Past and a Preview of the 21st Century." *Health Policy* 64: 349–75.

Cho, S., S. Ketefian, V. H. Barkauskas, and D. G. Smith. 2003. "The Effects of Nurse Staffing on Adverse Events, Morbidity, Mortality, and Medical Costs." *Nursing Research* 52 (2): 71–79.

Chren, M. M., and C. S. Landefeld. 1994. "Physicians' Behavior and Their Interactions with Drug Companies." *Journal of the American Medical Association* 271: 684–89.

Christianson, J., B. Dowd, J. Kralewski, S. Hayes, and C. Wisner. 1995. "Managed Care in the Twin Cities: What Can We Learn?" *Health Affairs* 14 (2): 114–30.

Christianson, J. B., C. S. Lessor, L. E. Felland, and S. Felt-Lisk. 2000. "Increased

Consolidation Raises Concerns." Community Report No. 2. Washington, DC: Center for Studying Health System Change.

Clarke, S. P., C. Raphael, and J. Disch. 2008. "Challenges and Directions for Nursing in the Pay-for-Performance Movement." *Policy, Politics, & Nursing Practice* 9 (2): 127–34.

Claxton, G., J. Feder, D. Shactman, and S. Altman. 1997. "Public Policy Issues in Nonprofit Conversions: An Overview." *Health Affairs* 16 (2): 9–28.

Claxton, G., J. Gabel, B. DiJulio, J. Pickreign, H. Whitmore, B. Finder, P. Jacobs, and S. Hawkins. 2007. "Health Benefits in 2007: Premium Increases Fall to an Eight-Year Low, While Offer Rates and Enrollment Remain Stable." *Health Affairs* 26 (5): 1407–16.

Claxton, G., J. R. Gabel, B. DiJulio, J. Pickreign, H. Whitmore, B. Finder, M. Jarlenski, and S. Hawkins. 2008. "Health Benefits in 2008: Premiums Moderately Higher, While Enrollment in Consumer-Directed Plans Rises in Small Firms." *Health Affairs* 27 (6): W429–W502.

Claxton, G., J. Gabel, I. Gill, J. Pickreign, H. Whitmore, B. Finder, B. DiJulio, and S. Hawkins. 2006. "Health Benefits in 2006: Premium Increases Moderate, Enrollment in Consumer-Directed Health Plans Remains Modest." *Health Affairs* 25 (6): W476–W485.

Clement, J. P. 1997–1998. "Dynamic Cost Shifting in Hospitals: Evidence from the 1980s and 1990s." *Inquiry* 34 (4): 340–50.

Coalition for Health Services Research. 2008. "Federal Funding for Health Services Research." [Online information; retrieved 4/6/09.] www.chsr.org/Coalition FundingReport08.pdf.

Coase, R. 1960. "The Problem of Social Cost." *Journal of Law and Economics* 3 (1): 1–44.

Coast, J., R. Smith, and P. Lorgelly. 2008. "Should the Capability Approach Be Applied in Health Economics?" *Health Economics* 17: 667–70.

Coburn, D. 2000. "Income Inequality, Social Cohesion and the Health Status of Populations: The Role of Neo-Liberalism." *Social Science and Medicine* 51: 135–46.

Cohen, J., and W. Spector. 1996. "The Effect of Medicaid Reimbursement on Quality of Care in Nursing Homes." *Journal of Health Economics* 15: 23–48.

Collard, D. 1978. *Altruism and Economy: A Study in Non-Selfish Economics.* Oxford: Martin Robertson.

Colombo, F. 2001. "Towards More Choice in Social Protection? Individual Choice of Insurer in Basic Mandatory Health Insurance in Switzerland." OECD Labour Market and Social Policy Occasional Papers No. 53. Paris: Organisation for Economic Co-operation and Development.

Commonwelath Department of Health and Aged Care. 2000. "The Australian Health Care System: An Outline." [Online article; retrieved 6/3/09.] www.health .gov.au/haf/ozhelath/.

———. 1999. "Public and Private—In Partnership for Australia's Health." *Occasional Papers: Health Financing Series.* Canberra: Commonwealth Department of Health and Aged Care.

Connor, R. A., R. D. Feldman, and B. E. Dowd. 1998. "The Effects of Market Concentration and Horizontal Mergers on Hospital Costs and Prices." *International Journal of the Economics of Business* 5 (2): 159–80.

Conrad, P., and V. Leiter. 2004. "Medicalization, Markets and Consumers." *Journal of Health and Social Behavior* 45 (Suppl.): 158–76.

Conrad, R. F., and R. P. Strauss. 1983. "A Multiple-Output Multiple-Input Model of the Hospital Industry in North Carolina." *Applied Economics* 15: 341–52.

Consumer Reports. 1996. "How Good Is Your Health Plan?" *Consumer Reports,* August, 40.

Cookson, R. 2005. "QALYs and the Capability Approach." *Health Economics* 14: 817–29.

Cooper, R. A. 2004. "Weighing the Evidence for Expanding Physician Supply." *Annals of Internal Medicine* 141 (9): 705–14.

Cooper, R., and L. Aiken. 2001. "Human Inputs: The Health Care Workforce and Medical Markets." *Journal of Health Politics, Policy and Law* 26 (5): 925–38.

Cooper, R. A., T. E. Getzen, H. J. McKee, and P. Laud. 2002. "Economic and Demographic Trends Signal an Impending Physician Shortage." *Health Affairs* 21 (1): 140–54.

Costich, J. F. 2002. "France." In *World Health Systems: Challenges and Perspectives,* edited by B. J. Fried and L. M. Gaydos, 153–72. Chicago: Health Administration Press.

Couffinhal, A., and V. Paris. 2003. "Cost Sharing in France." [Online working paper; retrieved 4/6/09.] www.irdes.fr/EspaceAnglais/Publications/OtherPubs/CostSharingInFrance.pdf.

———. 2001. "Utilization Fees Imposed to Public Health Care Systems Users in France." [Online presentation; retrieved 4/6/09.] www.irdes.fr/EspaceAnglais/Publications/OtherPubs/UtilisationFeesImposedFrance.pdf.

Coulam, R. F., and G. L. Gaumer. 1991. "Medicare's Prospective Payment System: A Critical Appraisal." *Health Care Financing Review* 13 (Ann. Suppl.): 45–77.

Council for Affordable Health Insurance. 1997. "Mandated Health Insurance Benefits." Alexandria, VA: Council for Affordable Health Insurance.

Council on Graduate Medical Education (COGME). 2005. *Physician Workforce Policy Guidelines for the United States, 2000–2020.* [Online report; retrieved 4/6/09.] www.cogme.gov/16.pdf.

Cramer, M., J. Nienaber, P. Helget, and S. Agrawal. 2006. "Comparative Analysis of Urban and Rural Nursing Workforce Shortages in Nebraska Hospitals." *Policy, Politics, & Nursing Practice* 7 (4): 248–60.

Cromwell, J., and J. Mitchell. 1986. "Physician-Induced Demand for Surgery." *Journal of Health Economics* 5 (3): 293–313.

Cuellar, A. E., and P. J. Gertler. 2005. "How the Expansion of Hospital Systems Has Affected Consumers." *Health Affairs* 24 (1): 213–19.

Culyer, A. J. 2001. "Equity—Some Theory and Its Policy Implications." *Journal of Medical Ethics* 27: 275–83.

———. 1993. "Health, Health Expenditures, and Equity." In *Equity in the Finance and Delivery of Health Care: An International Perspective,* edited by E. van Doorslaer, A. Wagstaff, and F. Rutten, 299–319. Oxford: Oxford Medical Publications.

———. 1989. "The Normative Economics of Health Care Finance and Provision." *Oxford Review of Economic Policy* 5 (1): 34–58.

———. 1982. "The Quest for Efficiency in the Public Sector: Economists Versus Dr. Pangloss." In *Public Finance and the Quest for Efficiency. Proceedings of the 38th Congress of the International Institute of Public Finance*, edited by H. Hanusch, 39–48. Munich, Germany: International Institute of Public Finance.

Cunningham, P. J., C. Denk, and M. Sinclair. 2001. "Do Consumers Know How Their Health Plan Works?" *Health Affairs* 20 (2): 159–66.

Cunningham, R. 2001. "Hospital Finance: Signs of 'Pushback' Amid Resurgent Cost Pressures." *Health Affairs* 20 (2): 233–40.

Currie, J., M. Farsi, and B. Macleod. 2005. "Cut to the Bone? Hospital Takeovers and Nurse Employment Contracts." *Industrial and Labor Relations Review* 58 (3): 471–93.

Cutler, D. M., M. McClellan, and J. P. Newhouse. 2000. "How Does Managed Care Do It?" *RAND Journal of Economics* 31 (3): 526–48.

Cutler, D. M., and S. J. Reber. 1998. "Paying for Health Insurance: The Trade-Off Between Competition and Adverse Selection." *Quarterly Journal of Economics* 113 (2): 433–66.

Dafny, L. 2005. "How Do Hospitals Respond to Price Changes?" *American Economic Review* 95 (5): 1525–47.

Daly, G., and F. Giertz. 1972. "Welfare Economics and Welfare Reform." *American Economic Review* 62 (1): 131–38.

Daly, M. C., G. J. Duncan, G. A. Kaplan, and J. W. Lynch. 1998. "Macro-to-Micro Links in the Relation Between Income Inequality and Mortality." *Milbank Quarterly* 76 (3): 315–39.

Dang, D., M. E. Johantgen, P. J. Pronovost, M. W. Jenckes, and E. B. Bass. 2002. "Postoperative Complications: Does Intensive Care Unit Staff Nursing Make a Difference?" *Heart and Lung* 31 (3): 219–28.

Danger, K. L. 1997. "Nonprofit Hospital Merger: What Can We Learn for Financial Markets?" *International Journal of the Economics of Business* 4 (1): 63–69.

Daniels, N. 2001. "Justice, Health, and Healthcare." *American Journal of Bioethics* 1 (2): 2–16.

———. 1985. "Health Care Needs and Distributive Justice." In *In Search of Equity: Health Needs and the Health Care System*, edited by R. Bayer, A. O. Caplan, and N. Daniels. New York: Plenum Press.

Daniels, N., B. Kennedy, and I. Kawachi. 2000. *Is Inequality Bad for Our Health?* Boston: Beacon Press.

Danzon, P. M., and M. F. Furukawa. 2003. "Prices and Availability of Pharmaceuticals: Evidence from Nine Countries." *Health Affairs* Web Exclusives (July–December, Suppl.) W3-521–W3-536.

Davies, H. T. O., A. E. Washington, and A. B. Bindman. 2002. "Health Care Report Cards: Implications for Vulnerable Patient Groups and the Organizations Providing Them Care." *Journal of Health Politics, Policy and Law* 27 (3): 379–99.

Davis, K., C. Schoen, S. C. Schoenbaum, A. J. Audet, M. M. Doty, A. L. Holmgren, and J. L. Kriss. 2006. "Mirror, Mirror on the Wall: An Update on the Quality of American Health Care Through the Patient's Lens," 4. New York: The Commonwealth Fund.

Deaton, A. 2001. "Health, Inequality, and Economic Development." NBER Working Paper No. 8318. Cambridge, MA: National Bureau of Economic Research.

Deber, R. B. 2000. "Getting What We Pay For: Myths and Realities About Financing Canada's Health Care System." Toronto: Department of Health Administration, University of Toronto.

Debrock, L., and R. J. Arnould. 1992. "Utilization Control in HMOs." *Quarterly Review of Economics & Finance* 32 (3): 31–53.

Dembe, A. E., and L. I. Boden. 2000. "Moral Hazard: A Question of Morality?" *New Solutions* 10 (3): 257–79.

Demerouti, E., A. Bakker, F. Nachreiner, and W. Schaufeli. 2000. "A Model of Burnout and Life Satisfaction Amongst Nurses." *Journal of Advanced Nursing* 32 (2): 454–64.

Department of Health, United Kingdom. 2008. "Hospital Waiting Times/List Statistics." [Online information; retrieved 4/6/09.] www.performance.doh.gov.uk/waitingtimes.

Devereaux, P. J., D. Heels-Ansdell, C. Lacchetti, T. Haines, K. E. Burns, D. J. Cook, N. Ravindran, S. D. Walter, H. McDonald, S. B. Stone, R. Patel, N. Bhandari, H. J. Schünemann, P. T. Choi, A. M. Bayoumi, J. N. Lavis, T. Sullivan, G. Stoddart, and G. H. Guyatt. 2004. "Payments for Care at Private For-Profit and Private Not-for-Profit Hospitals: A Systematic Review and Meta-Analysis." *Canadian Medical Association Journal* 170 (12): 1817–24.

Devereaux, P. J., H. J. Schünemann, D. J. Cook, M. Bhandari, N. Ravindran, B. J. B. Grant, C. Lacchetti, J. N. Lavis, D. R. S. Haslam, T. Haines, T. Sullivan, and G. H. Guyatt. 2003. "Quality of Care in Profit vs. Not-for-Profit Dialysis Centers—Reply." *Journal of the American Medical Association* 289 (23): 3089–90.

Devereaux, P. J., H. J. Schünemann, N. Ravindran, M. Bhandari, A. X. Garg, P. T.-L. Choi, B. J. B. Grant, T. Haines, C. Lacchetti, B. Weaver, J. N. Lavis, D. J. Cook, D. R. S. Haslam, T. Sullivan, and G. H. Guyatt. 2002. "Comparison of Mortality Between Private For-Profit and Private Not-for-Profit Hemodialysis Centers: A Systematic Review and Meta-Analysis." *Journal of the American Medical Association* 288 (19): 2449–57.

Devers, K. J., L. R. Brewster, and L. P. Casalino. 2003. "Changes in Hospital Competitive Strategy: A New Medical Arms Race?" *Health Services Research* 38 (1): 447–69.

Devers, K., J. B. Christianson, L. E. Felland, S. Felt-Lisk, L. Rudell, and J. L. Hargraves. 2001. "Highly Consolidated Market Poses Cost Control Challenges." Community Report No. 06. Washington, DC: Center for Studying Health System Change.

Diderichsen, F. 2000. "Sweden." *Journal of Health Politics, Policy and Law* 25 (5): 931–35.

Dimasi, J. A., R. W. Hansen, and H. G. Grabowski. 2003. "The Price of Innovation: New Estimates of Drug Development Costs." *Journal of Health Economics* 22 (2): 151–82.

———. 1991. "Cost of Innovation in the Pharmaceutical Industry." *Journal of Health Economics* 10 (2): 107–42.

Dobson, A., J. DaVanzo, and N. Sen. 2006. "The Cost-Shift Payment Hydraulic: Foundation, History, and Implications." *Health Affairs* 25 (1): 22–33.

Domino, M. E., S. C. Stearns, E. C. Norton, and W.-S. Yeh. 2008. "Why Using Current Medications to Select a Medicare Part D Plan May Lead to Higher Out-of-Pocket Payments." *Medical Care Research and Review* 65 (1): 114–26.

Donelan, K., R. J. Blendon, C. Schoen, K. Davis, and K. Binns. 1999. "The Cost of Health System Change: Public Discontent in Five Nations." *Health Affairs* 18 (3): 206–16.

Donohue, J. 2006. "A History of Drug Advertising: The Evolving Roles of Consumers and Consumer Protection." *Milbank Quarterly* 84 (4): 659–99.

Dovey, S., L. Green, R. Phillips, and G. Fryer. 2002. "The Delicate Task of Workforce Determination." *Effective Clinical Practice* 5 (2): 95–97.

Dowless, R. M. 2007. "The Health Care Cost-Shifting Debate: Could Both Sides Be Right?" *Journal of Health Care Finance* 34 (1): 64–71.

Dranove, D. 1995. "A Problem with Consumer Surplus Measures of the Cost of Practice Variations." *Journal of Health Economics* 14 (2): 243–51.

———. 1988. "Pricing by Non-Profit Institutions: The Case of Hospital Cost-Shifting." *Journal of Health Economics* 7 (1): 45–57.

Dranove, D., and R. Ludwick. 1999. "Competition and Pricing by Nonprofit Hospitals: A Reassessment of Lynk's Analysis." *Journal of Health Economics* 18 (1): 87–98.

Dranove, D., and M. A. Satterthwaite. 1992. "Monopolistic Competition When Price and Quality Are Imperfectly Observable." *RAND Journal of Economics* 23 (4): 518–34.

Dranove, D., C. J. Simon, and W. D. White. 2002. "Is Managed Care Leading to Consolidation in Health-Care Markets?" *Health Services Research* 37 (3): 573–93.

Drucker, P. F. 1989. "What Business Can Learn from Nonprofits." *Harvard Business Review* 67 (4): 88–93.

Duan, N., W. G. Manning, C. N. Morris, and J. P. Newhouse. 1984. "Choosing Between the Sample-Selection Model and the Multi-Part Model." *Journal of Business and Economic Statistics* 2 (3): 283–89.

Dubois, R. W., and B. B. Dean. 2006. "Evolution of Clinical Practice Guidelines: Evidence Supporting Expanded Use of Medicines." *Disease Management* 9 (4): 210–23.

Duesenberry, J. S. 1952. *Income, Saving and the Theory of Consumer Behavior*. Cambridge, MA: Harvard University Press.

Dunn, S., B. Wilson, and A. Esterman. 2005. "Perceptions of Working as a Nurse in an Acute Care Setting." *Journal of Nursing Management* 13: 22–31.

Dunton, N., B. Gajewski, R. L. Taunton, and J. Moore. 2004. "Nurse Staffing and Patient Falls on Acute Care Hospital Units." *Nurse Outlook* 52: 53–59.

Dussault, G., and M. C. Franceschini. 2006. "Not Enough There, Too Many Here: Understanding Geographical Imbalances in the Distribution of the Health Workforce." *Human Resources and Health* 4 (12): 1–28.

Dworkin, R. 1981. "What Is Equality? Part 2: Equality of Resources." *Philosophy & Public Affairs* 10 (4): 283–345.

Eastaugh, S. R. 2007. "Hospital Nurse Productivity Enhancement." *Journal of Health Care Finance* 33 (3): 39–47.

Easterlin, R. A. 2005. "Diminishing Marginal Utility of Income? Caveat Emptor." *Social Indicators Research* 70: 243–55.

———. 2001. "Income and Happiness: Towards a United Theory." *The Economic Journal* 111: 465–84.

———. 1995. "Will Raising the Incomes of All Increase the Happiness of All?" *Journal of Economic Behavior and Organization* 27: 35–47.

———. 1974. "Does Economic Growth Improve the Human Lot? Some Empirical Evidence." In *Nations and Households in Economic Growth: Essays in Honor of Moses Abramovitz*, edited by P. A. David and M. W. Reder, 89–125. New York: Academic Press.

Economic and Social Research Institute (Japan). 2006. *Policy Options for Health Insurance and Long-Term Care Insurance.* [Online report; retrieved 4/6/09.] www.esri.go.jp/jp/prj-2004_2005/macro/macro17/01-1-R-1.pdf.

Eggleston, K., Y. Shen, J. Lau, C. Schmid, and J. Chan. 2006. "Hospital Ownership and Quality of Care: What Explains the Different Results?" NBER Working Paper 12241. Cambridge, MA: National Bureau of Economic Research.

Ellis, R. P., and T. G. McGuire. 1993. "Supply-Side and Demand-Side Cost Sharing in Health Care." *Journal of Economic Perspectives* 7 (4): 135–51.

Elster, J. 1992. *Local Justice: How Institutions Allocate Scarce Goods and Necessary Burdens.* New York: Russell Sage Foundation.

Elting, L. S., C. Pettaway, B. N. Bekele, H. B. Grossman, C. Cooksley, E. B. C. Avritscher, K. Saldin, and C. P. N. Dinney. 2005. "Correlation Between Annual Volume of Cystectomy, Professional Staffing, and Outcomes." *Cancer* 104 (5): 975–84.

Elwell, F. 1984. "The Effects of Ownership on Institutional Services." *The Gerontologist* 24 (1): 77–83.

England, P., P. Budig, and N. Folbre. 2002. "Wages of Virtue: The Relative Pay of Care Work." *Social Problems* 49 (4): 455–73.

Enthoven, A. 2008. "A Living Model of Managed Competition: A Conversation with Dutch Health Minister Ab Klink." *Health Affairs* 27 (3): W196–W203.

———. 2003. "Employment-Based Health Insurance Is Failing: Now What?" *Health Affairs* Web Exclusives (January–June, Suppl.): W3-237–W3-249.

———. 2000. "In Pursuit of an Improving National Health Service." *Health Affairs* 19 (3): 102–19.

———. 1988. *Theory and Practice of Managed Competition in Health Care Finance.* Amsterdam: North-Holland.

———. 1980. *Health Plan: The Only Practical Solution to the Soaring Cost of Medical Care.* Reading, MA: Addison-Wesley.

———. 1978a. "Consumer-Choice Health Plan. Inflation and Inequity in Health Care Today: Alternatives for Cost Control and an Analysis of Proposals for National Health Insurance." *New England Journal of Medicine* 298 (12): 650–58.

———. 1978b. "Consumer-Choice Health Plan. A National-Health-Insurance Proposal Based on Regulated Competition in the Private Sector." *New England Journal of Medicine* 298 (13): 709–20.

Enthoven, A., and R. Kronick. 1989a. "A Consumer-Choice Health Plan for the 1990s: Universal Health Insurance in a System Designed to Promote Quality and Economy." Part 1. *New England Journal of Medicine* 320 (1): 29–37.

———. 1989b. "A Consumer-Choice Health Plan for the 1990s: Universal Health Insurance in a System Designed to Promote Quality and Economy." Part 2. *New England Journal of Medicine* 320 (2): 94–101.

Epstein, A. J. 2006. "Do Cardiac Surgery Report Cards Reduce Mortality? Assessing the Evidence." *Medical Care Research and Review* 63 (4): 403–26.

Escarce, J. J. 1993a. "Effects of Lower Surgical Fees on the Use of Physician Services Under Medicare." *Journal of the American Medical Association* 269 (19): 2513–18.

———. 1993b. "Medicare Patients' Use of Overpriced Procedures Before and After the Omnibus Budget Reconciliation Act of 1987." *American Journal of Public Health* 83 (3): 349–55.

———. 1992. "Explaining the Association Between Surgeon Supply and Utilization." *Inquiry* 29 (4): 403–15.

Escarce, J., D. Polsky, G. Wozniak, and P. Kletke. 2000. "HMO Growth and the Geographical Redistribution of Generalist and Specialist Physicians, 1987–1997." *Health Services Research* 35 (4): 825–48.

European Observatory on Health Systems and Policies. 2004. "Health Care Systems in Transition. HiT Summary: Germany, 2004." [Online information; retrieved 4/6/09.] www.euro.who.int/document/e85472sum.pdf.

———. 2000a. "Health Care Systems in Transition: Germany." Copenhagen: World Health Organization Regional Office for Europe.

———. 2000b. "Health Care Systems in Transition: Switzerland." Copenhagen: World Health Organization Regional Office for Europe.

———. 1999. "Health Care Systems in Transition: United Kingdom." Copenhagen: World Health Organization Regional Office for Europe.

Evans, R. 1974. "Supplier-Induced Demand: Some Empirical Evidence and Implications." In *The Economics of Health*, edited by M. Perlman, 162–73. New York: MacMillan.

Evans, R. G. 2000. "Canada." *Journal of Health Politics, Policy and Law* 25 (5): 889–97.

———. 1999. "What We Do—and Don't—Know About Social Inequalities in Health." In *Social Inequalities in Health: Keynote Addresses from the Annual Meeting on Health Philanthropy.* Washington, DC: Grantmakers in Health.

———. 1984. *Strained Mercy.* Toronto: Butterworth.

———. 1983. "Health Care in Canada: Patterns of Funding and Regulation." *Journal of Health Politics, Policy and Law* 8 (1): 1–43.

Evans, R. G., M. L. Barer, and G. L. Stoddart. 1993. "The Truth About User Fees." In *Policy Option.* Montreal: Institute for Research on Public Policy.

Evans, R. G., M. L. Barer, G. L. Stoddart, and V. Bhatia. 1983. "It's Not the Money, It's the Principle: Why User Charges for Some Services and Not Others?" Vancouver, BC: Centre for Health Services and Policy Research, University of British Columbia.

Evans, R. G., E. M. A. Parish, and F. Sully. 1973. "Medical Productivity, Scale Effects, and Demand Generation." *Canadian Journal of Economics* 6 (3): 376–93.

Evans, R. G., and G. L. Stoddart. 1990. "Producing Health, Consuming Health Care." *Social Science and Medicine* 31 (12): 1347–63.

Executive Office of the President, Office of National Drug Control Policy. 2004. *The Economic Costs of Drug Abuse in the United States, 1992–2002.* [Online report; retrieved 4/10/09.] www.whitehousedrugpolicy.gov/publications/economic_costs.

Ezrati, J. B. 1987. "Labor Force Participation of Registered Nurses." *Nursing Economics* 5 (2): 82–89.

Fahs, M. C. 1992. "Physician Response to the United Mine Workers' Cost-Sharing Program: The Other Side of the Coin." *Health Services Research* 27 (1): 25–45.

Families USA. 2005. "The Choice: Health Care for People or Drug Industry Profits." [Online information; retrieved 4/6/09.] http://familiesusa.org/resources/publications/reports/the-choice.html.

Farley, D. O. 1993. "Effects of Competition on Dialysis Facility Service Levels and Patient Selection." PhD diss., Pardee RAND Graduate School, Santa Monica, CA.

Feldman, R., and B. Dowd. 1993. "What Does the Demand Curve for Medical Care Measure?" *Journal of Health Economics* 12 (2): 192–200.

———. 1991. "A New Estimate of the Welfare Loss of Excess Health Insurance." *American Economic Review* 81 (1): 297–301.

Feldman, R., J. Kralewski, J. Shapiro, and H. C. Chan. 1990. "Contracts Between Hospitals and Health Maintenance Organizations." *Health Care Management Review* 15 (1): 47–60.

Feldman, R., S. T. Parente, J. Abraham, J. B. Christianson, and R. Taylor. 2005. "Health Savings Accounts: Early Estimates of National Take-Up." *Health Affairs* 24 (6): 1582–91.

Feldman, R., S. T. Parente, and J. B. Christianson. 2007. "Consumer-Directed Health Plans: New Evidence on Spending and Utilization." *Inquiry* 44: 26–40.

Feldman, R., and F. Sloan. 1988. "Competition Among Physicians, Revisited." *Journal of Health Politics, Policy and Law* 13 (2): 239–61.

Feldman, R., and D. Wholey. 2001. "Do HMOs Have Monopsony Power?" *International Journal of Health Care Finance and Economics* 1: 7–22.

Feldstein, M. S. 1973. "The Welfare Loss of Excess Health Insurance." *Journal of Political Economy* 81 (2): 251–80.

Feldstein, P. J. 1998. *Health Care Economics*, 5th ed. New York: John Wiley.

———. 1996. *The Politics of Health Legislation: An Economic Perspective.* Chicago: Health Administration Press.

———. 1988. *Health Care Economics.* New York: John Wiley.

Fendrick, A. M., and M. E. Chernew. 2006. "Value-Based Insurance Design: Aligning Incentives to Bridge the Divide Between Quality Improvement and Cost Containment." *American Journal of Managed Care* 12 (Special Issue): SP5–SP10.

Fendrick, A. M., D. G. Smith, M. Chernew, and S. N. Shah. 2001. "A Benefit-Based

Copay for Prescription Drugs: Patient Contributions Based on Total Benefits, Not Drug Acquisition Cost." *American Journal of Managed Care* 7 (9): 861–67.

Ferrante, J. M., E. C. Gonzalez, N. Pal, and R. G. Roetzheim. 2000. "Effects of Physician Supply on Early Detection of Breast Cancer." *Journal of the American Board of Family Practice* 13 (6): 408–14.

Ferris, J. M., and E. A. Graddy. 1999. "Structural Changes in the Hospital Industry, Charity Care, and the Nonprofit Role in Health Care." *Nonprofit and Voluntary Sector Quarterly* 28 (1): 18–31.

Fielding, J. E., and T. Rice. 1993. "Can Managed Care Competition Solve the Problems of Market Failure?" *Health Affairs* 12 (Suppl.): 216–28.

Finkelstein, A. 2002. "The Effect of Tax Subsidies to Employer-Provided Supplementary Health Insurance: Evidence from Canada." *Journal of Public Economics* 84: 305–39.

Finkler, S. A. 1979. "Cost-Effectiveness of Regionalization: The Heart Surgery Example." *Inquiry* 16 (3): 264–70.

Fisher, E. S. 2006. "Paying for Performance—Risks and Recommendations." *New England Journal of Medicine* 355 (18): 1845–47.

Fisher, E. S., D. E. Wennberg, T. A. Stukel, D. J. Gottlieb, F. L. Lucas, and E. L. Pinder. 2003a. "The Implications of Regional Variations in Medicare Spending. Part 1: The Content, Quality, and Accessibility of Care." *Annals of Internal Medicine* 138: 273–87.

———. 2003b. "The Implications of Regional Variations in Medicare Spending. Part 2: Health Outcomes and Satisfaction with Care." *Annals of Internal Medicine* 138: 288–98.

Fishlow, A. 1965. *American Railroads and the Transformation of the Antebellum Economy.* Cambridge, MA: Harvard University Press.

———. 1992. "Technical Efficiency of For-Profit and Non-Profit Nursing Homes." *Managerial and Decision Economics* 13 (5): 429–39.

Flegal, K. M, M. D. Carroll, C. L. Ogden, and C. L. Johnson. 2002. "Prevalence and Trends in Obesity Among U.S. Adults, 1999–2000." *Journal of the American Medical Association* 288 (14): 1723–27.

Flynn, L., and L. H. Aiken. 2002. "Does International Nurse Recruitment Influence Practice Values in U.S. Hospitals?" *Journal of Nursing Scholarship* 34 (1): 65–71.

Fogel, R. A. 1964. *Railroads and American Economic Growth: Essays in Econometric History.* Baltimore, MD: Johns Hopkins University Press.

Forrest, C. B. 2006. "Strengthening Primary Care to Bolster the Health Care Safety Net." *Journal of the American Medical Association* 295 (9): 1062–64.

Fortney, J., K. Rost, M. Zhang, and J. Pyne. 2001. "The Relationship Between Quality and Outcomes in Routine Depression Care." *Psychiatric Services* 52: 56–62.

Fottler, M., H. Smith, and W. James. 1981. "Profits and Patient Care Quality in Nursing Homes: Are They Compatible?" *The Gerontologist* 21 (5): 532–38.

Fottler, M. D., and L. S. Widra. 1995. "Intention of Inactive Registered Nurses to Return to Nursing." *Medical Care Research and Review* 52 (4): 492–517.

Foubister, T., S. Thomson, E. Mossialos, and A. McGuire. 2006. *Private Medical Insurance in the United Kingdom.* Copenhagen: World Health Organization, on behalf of the European Observatory on Health Systems and Policies.

Fox, D. M., and H. M. Leichter. 1993. "The Ups and Downs of Oregon's Rationing Plan." *Health Affairs* 12 (2): 66–70.

Frank, R., and K. Lamiraud. 2008. *Choice, Price Competition and Complexity in Markets for Health Insurance.* NBER Working Paper No. 13817. Cambridge, MA: National Bureau of Economic Research.

Frank, R. G., and D. S. Salkever. 1994. "Nonprofit Organizations in the Health Sector." *Journal of Economic Perspectives* 8 (4): 120–44.

Frank, R. G., D. S. Salkever, and F. Mullan. 1990. "Hospital Ownership and the Care of Uninsured and Medicaid Patients: Findings from the National Hospital Discharge Survey, 1979–1984." *Health Policy* 14 (1): 1–11.

Frank, R. H. 1999. *Luxury Fever.* New York: Free Press.

———. 1985. *Choosing the Right Pond: Human Behavior and the Quest for Status.* New York: Oxford University Press.

Franks, P., and K. Fiscella. 1998. "Primary Care Physicians and Specialists as Personal Physicians: Health Care Expenditures and Mortality Experience." *Journal of Family Practice* 47: 105–9.

Freebairn, J. 2001. "Evaluation of the Supplier-Induced Demand for Medical Care Model." *Australian Economic Review* 34 (3): 353–55.

Freeman, J., R. L. Ferrer, and K. A. Greiner. 2007. "Developing a Physician Workforce for America's Disadvantaged." *Academic Medicine* 82 (2): 133–38.

Freund, C. M., and J. Mitchell. 1985. "Multi-institutional Systems: The New Arrangement." *Nursing Economics* 3 (1): 24–32.

Frey, R. 2007. "Ambulatory Surgery Centers." [Online information; retrieved 4/6/09.] www.surgeryencyclopedia.com/A-Ce/Ambulatory-Surgery-Centers .html.

Friedman, E. 2008. "Surf, Turf and the Future of Primary Care." [Online article; retrieved 4/6/09. www.hhnmag.com/hhnmag_app/jsp/printer_friendly.jsp ?dcrPath=HHNMAG/Article/data/06JUN2008/080603HHN_Online_ Friedman&domain=HHNMAG.

Friedman, M. 1962. *Price Theory.* Chicago: Aldine Press.

Friedman, M., and L. J. Savage. 1948. "The Utility Analysis of Choices Involving Risk." *Journal of Political Economy* 56 (40): 279–304.

Fronstin, P., and S. Collins. 2008. "Findings from the 2007 ERBI/Commonwealth Fund Consumerism in Health Survey." Issue Brief No. 315. Washington, DC: Employee Benefit Research Institute.

Fuchs, V. 1983. *Who Shall Live?* New York: Basic.

———. 1978. "The Supply of Surgeons and the Demand for Operations." *Journal of Human Resources* 12 (Suppl.): 35–56.

Fuchs, V. R., and J. S. Hahn. 1990. "How Does Canada Do It? A Comparison of Expenditures for Physicians' Services in the United States and Canada." *New England Journal of Medicine* 323 (13): 884–90.

Gabel, J., L. Levitt, J. Pickreign, H. Whitmore, E. Holve, D. Rowland, K. Dhont, and S. Hawkins S. 2001. "Job-Based Health Insurance in 2001: Inflation Hits Double Digits, Managed Care Retreats." *Health Affairs* 20 (5): 180–86.

Gabel, J. R., and G. A. Jensen. 1989. "The Price of State Mandated Benefits." *Inquiry* 26 (3): 419–31.

Gabel, J. R., and T. H. Rice. 1985. "Reducing Public Expenditures for Physician Services: The Price of Paying Less." *Journal of Health Politics, Policy and Law* 9 (4): 595–609.

Gabel, J. R., H. Whitmore, T. Rice, and A. T. Lo Sasso. 2004. "Employers' Contradictory Views About Consumer-Driven Health Care: Results from a National Survey." *Health Affairs* Web Exclusives (January–June, Suppl.): W4-210–W4-218.

Garber, A. M., and H. C. Sox. 2004. "The U.S. Physician Workforce: Serious Questions Raised, Answers Needed." *Annals of Internal Medicine* 141 (9): 732–34.

Garg, P., and K. Frick. 2000. "Ownership of Dialysis Facilities and Patients' Survival—Author Reply." *New England Journal of Medicine* 342 (14): 1056.

Garg, P., K. Frick, M. Diener-West, and N. Powe. 1999. "Effect of the Ownership of Dialysis Facilities on Patients' Survival and Referral for Transplantation." *New England Journal of Medicine* 341 (22): 1653–60.

Garg, P. P., and N. R. Powe. 2001. "Profit-Making in the Treatment of Chronic Kidney Disease: Truth and Consequences." *Seminars in Dialysis* 14 (3): 153–56.

Gaskin, D. J., and J. Hadley. 1997. "The Impact of HMO Penetration on the Rate of Hospital Cost Inflation. 1985–1993." *Inquiry* 34: 205–16.

Gaynor, M., and D. Haas-Wilson. 1999. "Change, Consolidation, and Competition in Health Care Markets." *Journal of Economic Perspectives* 13 (1): 141–64.

Geiger-Brown, J., A. M. Trinkoff, K. Nielsen, S. Lirtmunlikaporn, B. Brady, and E. I. Vasquez. 2004. "Nurses' Perception of Their Work Environment, Health, and Well-Being: A Qualitative Perspective." *AAOHN Journal* 52 (1): 16–22.

Gerteis, M., J. S. Gerteis, D. Newman, and C. Koepke. 2007. "Testing Consumers' Comprehension of Quality Measures Using Alternative Reporting Formats." *Health Care Financing Review* 28 (3): 31–45.

Giaimo, S., and P. Manow. 1997. "Institutions and Ideas into Politics: Health Care Reform in Britain and Germany." In *Health Policy Reform, National Variations and Globalization*, edited by C. Altenstetter and J. Warner Björkman. New York: St. Martins Press.

Gift, T. L., R. Arnould, and L. Debrock. 2002. "Is Healthy Competition Healthy? New Evidence of the Impact of Hospital Competition." *Inquiry* 39 (1): 45–55.

Gilmer, T., and R. Kronick. 2005. "It's the Premiums, Stupid: Projections of the Uninsured Through 2013." *Health Affairs* Web Exclusives (January–June, Suppl.): W5-143–W5-151.

Ginn, G., and C. Moseley. 2004. "Community Health Orientation, Community-Based Quality Improvement, and Health Promotion Services in Hospitals." *Journal of Healthcare Management* 49 (5): 293–306.

Ginsburg, P. B. 2005. "Competition in Health Care: Its Evolution over the Past Decade." *Health Affairs* 24 (6): 1513–22.

———. 2003a. "Can Hospitals and Physicians Shift the Effects of Cuts in Medicare Reimbursement to Private Payers?" *Health Affairs* Web Exclusives (July–December, Suppl.): W3-472–W3-479.

———. 2003b. "Payment and the Future of Primary Care." *Annals of Internal Medicine* 138: 233–34.

Ginsburg, P. B., L. B. LeRoy, and G. T. Hammons. 1990. "Medicare Physician Payment Reform." *Health Affairs* 9 (1): 178–88.

Gintis, H. 1970. *Neo-Classical Welfare Economics and Individual Development*. Cambridge, MA: Union for Radical Political Economists.

Glandon, G. L., K. W. Colbert, and M. Thomasma. 1989. "Nursing Delivery Models and RN Mix: Cost Implications." *Nursing Management* 20 (5): 30–33.

Glascock, S. 2008. "In Oregon, Healthcare for the Lucky." *Los Angeles Times*, March 10.

Glaser, W. A. 1991. *Health Insurance in Practice: International Variations in Financing, Benefits, and Problems*. San Francisco: Jossey-Bass.

Glenngård, A. H., F. Hjalte, M. Svensson, A. Anell, and V. Bankauskaite. 2005. *Health Systems in Transition: Sweden*. Copenhagen: World Health Organization Regional Office for Europe.

Goldman, D. P., G. F. Joyce, J. J. Escarce, J. E. Pace, M. D. Solomon, M. Laouri, P. B. Landsman, and S. M. Teutsch. 2004. "Pharmacy Benefits and the Use of Drugs by the Chronically Ill." *Journal of the American Medical Association* 291 (19): 2344–50.

Goldman, D. P., G. F. Joyce, G. Lawless, W. H. Crown, and V. Willey. 2006. "Benefit Design and Specialty Drug Use." *Health Affairs* 25 (5): 1319–31.

Goldsmith, L. J. 2002. "Canada." In *World Health Systems: Challenges and Perspectives*, edited by B. J. Fried and L. M. Gaydos, 227–48. Chicago: Health Administration Press.

Goode, C. J., D. J. Tanaka, M. Krugman, P. A. O'Connor, C. Bailey, M. Deutchman, and N. M. Stolpman. 2000. "Outcomes from Use of an Evidence-Based Practice Guideline." *Nursing Economics* 18 (4): 202–7.

Goodman, B. 2001. "Do Drug Company Promotions Influence Physician Behavior?" *Western Journal of Medicine* 174 (4): 232–33.

Goodman, D., and E. Fisher. 2008. "Physician Workforce Crisis? Wrong Diagnosis, Wrong Prescription." *New England Journal of Medicine* 358 (16): 1658–61.

Goodman, D. C., E. S. Fisher, G. A Little, T. A. Stukel, and C. Chang. 2001. "Are Neonatal Intensive Care Resources Located According to Need? Regional Variation in Neonatologists, Beds, and Low Birth Weight Newborns." *Pediatrics* 108 (2): 426–31.

Goodman, D. C., E. S. Fisher, G. A. Little, T. A. Stukel, C. Chang, and K. S. Schoendorf. 2002. "The Relation Between the Availability of Neonatal Intensive Care and Neonatal Mortality." *New England Journal of Medicine* 346 (20): 1538–44.

Goodman, D. C., and K. Grumbach. 2008. "Does Having More Physicians Lead to Better Health System Performance?" *Journal of the American Medical Association* 299 (3): 335–37.

Goyal, M., R. L. Mehta, L. J. Schneiderman, and A. R. Sehgal. 2002. "Economics and Health Consequences of Selling a Kidney in India." *Journal of the American Medical Association* 288 (13): 1589–93.

Graaff, J. V. 1971. *Theoretical Welfare Economics*. London: Cambridge University Press.

Graber, D. R., and P. D. Sloane. 1995. "Nursing Home Survey Deficiencies for Physical Restraint Use." *Medical Care* 33 (10): 1051–63.

Grabowski, D. C. 2001. "Medicaid Reimbursement and the Quality of Nursing Home Care." *Journal of Health Economics* 20: 549–69.

Gravelle, H. 1998. "How Much of the Relation Between Population Mortality and Unequal Distribution of Income Is a Statistical Artifact?" *British Medical Journal* 316: 382–85.

Gray, B. 1997. "Conversion of HMOs and Hospitals: What's at Stake?" *Health Affairs* 16 (2): 29–47.

Gray, B., ed. 1986. *For-Profit Enterprise in Health Care*. Washington, DC: National Academies Press.

Gray, G. 1996. "Reform and Reaction in Australian Health Policy." *Journal of Health Politics, Policy and Law* 21 (3): 587–615.

Green, D. P., and I. Shapiro. 1994. *Pathologies of Rational Choice Theory*. New Haven, CT: Yale University Press.

Green, R. M. 1976. "Health Care and Justice in Contract Theory Perspective." In *Ethics and Health Policy*, edited by R. M. Veatch and R. Branson. Cambridge, MA: Ballinger.

Greenberg, L., and J. Cultice. 1997. "Forecasting the Need for Physicians in the United States: The Health Resources and Services Administration's Physician Requirements Model." *Health Services Research* 31 (6): 723–37.

Greene, J. 1998. "Blue Skies or Black Eyes? HEDIS Puts Not-for-Profit Plans on Top." *Hospitals and Health Networks* 72 (8): 26–30.

Greene, J., J. Hibbard, J. F. Murray, S. M. Teutsch, and M. L. Berger. 2008. "The Impact of Consumer-Directed Health Plans on Prescription Drug Use." *Health Affairs* 27 (4): 1111–31.

Griffiths, R., N. Powe, D. Gaskin, G. de Anderson, G. Lissovoy, and P. Whelton. 1994. "The Production of Dialysis by For-Profit Versus Not-for-Profit Freestanding Renal Dialysis Facilities." *Health Service Research* 29: 473–87.

Grossman, M. 2004. "The Demand for Health, 30 Years Later: A Very Personal Retrospective and Prospective Reflection." *Journal of Health Economics* 23 (4): 629–36.

———. 1972a. "On the Concept of Health Capital and the Demand for Health." *Journal of Political Economy* 80 (2): 223–55.

———. 1972b. *The Demand for Health: A Theoretical and Empirical Investigation*. New York: National Bureau of Economic Research.

Grossman, S., and O. Hart. 1986. "The Costs and Benefits of Ownership: A Theory of Vertical and Lateral Integration." *Journal of Political Economy* 98: 1119–58.

Gruber, J., and M. Lettau. 2004. "How Elastic Is the Firm's Demand for Health Insurance?" *Journal of Public Economics* 88: 1273–93.

Gruber, J., and J. Poterba. 1994. "Tax Incentives and the Decision to Purchase Health Insurance: Evidence from the Self-Employed." *Quarterly Journal of Economics* 109 (3): 701–33.

Grumbach, K., and R. Mendoza. 2008. "Disparities in Human Resources: Addressing the Lack of Diversity in the Health Professions." *Health Affairs* 27 (2): 413–22.

Grytten, J., F. Carlsen, and I. Skaus. 2001. "The Income Effect and Supplier Induced Demand. Evidence from Primary Physician Services in Norway." *Applied Economics* 33: 1455–67.

Grytten, J., and R. Sorensen. 2001. "Type of Contract and Supplier-Induced Demand for Primary Care Physicians in Norway." *Journal of Health Economics* 20: 379–93.

Gulley, O. D., and R. E. Santerre. 2007. "Market Structure Elements: The Case of California Nursing Homes." *Journal of Health Care Finance* 33 (4): 1–16.

Guterman, S. 2006. "Specialty Hospitals: A Problem or a Symptom? The Problems Surrounding Specialty Hospitals Indicate Broader Problems with the U.S. Payment and Health Care Financing Systems." *Health Affairs* 25 (1): 95–105.

Hadley, J., J. Holahan, and W. Scanlon. 1979. "Can Fee-for-Service Reimbursement Coexist with Demand Creation?" *Inquiry* 16 (3): 247–58.

Hadley, J., S. Zuckerman, and L. Iezzoni. 1996. "Financial Pressure and Competition: Changes in Hospital Efficiency and Cost-Sharing Behavior." *Medical Care* 34 (3): 205–19.

Hahnel, R., and M. Albert. 1990. *Quiet Revolution in Welfare Economics.* Princeton, NJ: Princeton University Press.

Hall, J. 1999. "Incremental Change in the Australian Health Care System." *Health Affairs* 18 (3): 95–113.

Hall, M. A. 2005. "The Death of Managed Care: A Regulated Autopsy." *Journal of Health Politics, Policy and Law* 30 (3): 427–52.

Hannan, E. L., H. Kilburn Jr., H. Bernard, J. F. O'Donnell, G. Lukacik, and E. P. Shields. 1991. "Coronary Artery Bypass Surgery: The Relationship Between In-Hospital Mortality Rate and Surgical Volume After Controlling for Clinical Risk Factors." *Medical Care* 29 (11): 1094–1107.

Hanning, M. 2001. "Waiting Lists Initiatives in Sweden." Paper presented at the session, "Incentives for Reduced Waiting Times in Health Systems: A Comparison of Experiences in Different Countries," International Health Economics Association Third International Conference. York, UK, July 23.

Hanoch, Y., S. Wood, T. Rice, B. Tanius, and J. Cummings. 2008. "Does Too Much Choice Reduce the Quality of Older Adults' Decisions? An Experiment with Prescription Drug Plans." Presented at the AcademyHealth annual meetings, Washington, DC, June 8.

Hansmann, H. 1980. "The Role of Non-Profit Enterprise." *Yale Law Journal* 90 (November): 835–90.

Hardin, G. 1968. "The Tragedy of the Commons." *Science* 162: 1243–48.

Harrington, C., H. Carrillo, and B. W. Blank. 2007. *Nursing Facilities, Staffing, Residents and Facility Deficiencies, 2000 Through 2006.* [Online report; retrieved 4/7/09.] www.nccnhr.org/uploads/HarringtonOSCARcomplete2006.pdf.

Harrington, C., S. Woolhandler, J. Mullan, H. Carrillo, and D. Himmelstein. 2001. "Does Investor Ownership of Nursing Homes Compromise the Quality of Care?" *American Journal of Public Health* 91 (9): 1452–55.

Harrington, C., D. Zimmerman, S. Karon, J. Robinson, and P. Beutel. 2000. "Nursing Home Staffing and Its Relationship to Deficiencies." *Journal of Gerontology* 55B (5): S278–S287.

Harrison, J. P., and C. Sexton. 2004. "The Paradox of the Not-for-Profit Hospital." *The Health Care Manager* 23 (3): 192–204.

Hausman, D. M., and M. S. McPherson. 1993. "Taking Ethics Seriously: Economics and Contemporary Moral Philosophy." *Journal of Economic Literature* 31 (2): 671–731.

Hay, J., and M. J. Leahy. 1982. "Physician-Induced Demand: An Empirical Analysis of the Consumer Information Gap." *Journal of Health Economics* 1 (3): 231–44.

Hay, J. W., and R. J. Olsen. 1984. "Let Them Eat Cake: A Note on Comparing Alternative Models of the Demand for Medical Care." *Journal of Business and Economic Statistics* 2 (3): 279–82.

Hayek, F. A. 1945. "The Use of Knowledge by Society." *American Economic Review* 35 (4): 519–34.

Health Canada. 2008a. "Federal Support for Health Care: The Facts." [Online information; retrieved 4/7/09.] www.hc-sc.gc.ca/hcs-sss/delivery-prestation/fptcollab/2004-fmm-rpm/fs-if_16-eng.php.

———. 2008b. "Canada Health Act: Overview." [Online information; retrieved 4/6/09.] www.hc-sc.gc.ca/hcs-sss/medi-assur/cha-lcs/overview-apercu-eng.php.

Healthcare Commission, United Kingdom. 2008. *State of Healthcare 2008*. London: Stationery Office.

Healy, J., E. Sharman, and B. Lokuge. 2006. "Australia: Health System Review." *Health Systems in Transition* 8 (5): 1–158.

Heidenreich, P. A., and M. McClellan. 2001. "Trends in Treatment and Outcomes for Acute Myocardial Infarction: 1975–1995." *American Journal of Medicine* 110 (3): 165–74.

Held, P. J., N. W. Levin, R. R. Bovbjerg, M. V. Pauly, and L. H. Diamond. 1991. "Mortality and Duration of Hemodialysis Treatment." *Journal of the American Medical Association* 265: 871–75.

Hemenway, D., and D. Fallon. 1985. "Testing for Physician-Induced Demand with Hypothetical Cases." *Medical Care* 23 (4): 344–49.

Henderson, J. M., and R. E. Quandt. 1980. *Microeconomic Theory: A Mathematical Approach*. New York: McGraw-Hill.

Hendrix, T. J., and S. E. Foreman. 2001. "Optimal Long-Term Care Nurse-Staffing Levels." *Nursing Economics* 19 (4): 164–75.

Hennessy-Fiske, M., and D. Zahniser. 2008. "Council Bans New Fast-Food Outlets." *Los Angeles Times*, July 30.

Hertzman, C. 2001. "Population Health and Child Development: A View from Canada." In *Income, Socioeconomic Status, and Health: Exploring the Relationships*, edited by J. A. Auerbach and B. K. Krimgold. Washington, DC: National Policy Association.

Hester, J., and I. Leveson. 1974. "The Health Insurance Study: A Critical Appraisal." *Inquiry* 11 (1): 53–60.

Heymann, J., C. Hertzman, M. L. Barer, and R. G. Evans, eds. 2006. *Healthier Societies: From Analysis to Action*. Oxford, UK: Oxford University Press.

Hibbard, J. H., J. Greene, and M. Tusler. 2008. "Does Enrollment in a CDHP Stimulate Cost-Effective Utilization?" *Medical Care Research and Review* 65 (4): 437–49.

Hibbard, J. H., L. Harris-Kojetin, P. Mullin, J. Lubalin, and S. Garfinkel. 2000. "Increasing the Impact of Health Plan Report Cards by Addressing Consumers' Concerns." *Health Affairs* 19 (5): 138–43.

Hibbard, J. H., and J. J. Jewett. 1997. "Will Quality Report Cards Help Consumers?" *Health Affairs* 16 (3): 218–28.

Hibbard, J. H., S. Sofaer, and J. J. Jewett. 1996. "Condition-Specific Performance Information: Assessing Salience, Comprehension, and Approaches for Communicating Quality." *Health Care Financing Review* 18 (1): 95–109.

Hibbard, J. H., and E. C. Weeks. 1989a. "The Dissemination of Physician Fee Information: Impact on Consumer Knowledge, Attitudes, and Behaviors." *Journal of Health & Social Policy* 1 (1): 75–87.

———. 1989b. "Does the Dissemination of Comparative Data on Physician Fees Affect Consumer Use of Services?" *Medical Care* 27 (12): 1167–74.

Hicks, J. R. 2008. "Fast-Food Moratorium Is Meddling." [Online article; retrieved 4/7/09.] www.latimes.com/news/opinion/commentary/la-oe-hicks31-2008jul31,0,4488779.story.

High, J. 1991. *Regulation: Economic Theory and History*. Ann Arbor, MI: University of Michigan Press.

High Committee on Public Health. 1998. *Health in France*. Montrogue, France: Editions John Libbey Eurotext.

Hillman, A. 1987. "Financial Incentives for Physicians in HMOs." *New England Journal of Medicine* 317 (27): 1743–48.

Hillman, A. L., M. V. Pauly, and J. J. Kerstein. 1989. "How Do Financial Incentives Affect Physicians' Clinical Decisions and the Financial Performance of Health Maintenance Organizations?" *New England Journal of Medicine* 321 (1): 86–92.

Himmelstein, D., S. Woolhandler, I. Hellander, and S. Wolfe. 1999. "Quality of Care in Investor-Owned vs. Not-for-Profit HMOs." *Journal of the American Medical Association* 282 (2): 159.

Hirsch, B. T., and E. J. Schumacher. 1995. "Monopsony Power and Relative Wages in the Labor Market for Nurses." *Journal of Health Economics* 14: 443–76.

Ho, V., and B. H. Hamilton. 2000. "Hospital Mergers and Acquisitions: Does Market Consolidation Harm Patients?" *Journal of Health Economics* 19: 767–91.

Hoerger, T. J., and L. Z. Howard. 1995. "Search Behavior and Choice of Physician in the Market for Prenatal Care." *Medical Care* 33 (4): 332–49.

Hoffman, C., and A. Schlobohm. 2000. *Uninsured in America: A Chart Book*. Washington, DC: Kaiser Family Foundation.

Holahan, J., and W. Scanlon. 1979. "Physician Pricing in California: Price Controls, Physician Fees, and Physician Incomes from Medicare and Medicaid." Grants and Contracts Report, Pub. No. 03006. Washington, DC: Centers for Medicare & Medicaid Services.

Hollingsworth, J. R., and E. J. Hollingsworth. 1987. *Controversy About American Hospitals: Funding, Ownership, and Performance*. Washington, DC: American Enterprise Institute.

Hollon, M. F. 1999. "Direct-to-Consumer Marketing of Prescription Drugs: Creating Consumer Demand." *Journal of the American Medical Association* 281 (4): 382–84.

Holmer, A. F. 2002. "Direct-to-Consumer Advertising—Strengthening Our Health Care System." *New England Journal of Medicine* 346 (7): 526–28.

———. 1999. "Direct-to-Consumer Prescription Drug Advertising Builds Bridges Between Patients and Physician." *Journal of the American Medical Association* 281 (4): 380–82.

Hoogervorst, H. 2007. "Health Reform in the Netherlands: A Model for Hungary?" [Online speech; retrieved 4/8/09.] www.minvws.nl/en/speeches/z/2007/health-reform-in-the-netherlands-a-model-for-hungary.asp.

Horwitz, J. R. 2005. "Making Profits and Providing Care: Comparing Nonprofit, For-Profit, and Government Hospitals." *Health Affairs* 24 (3): 790–801.

House, J. S., K. R. Landis, and D. Umberson. 1999. "Social Relationships and Health." In *Income Inequality and Health*, edited by I. Kawachi, B. P. Kennedy, and R. G. Wilkinson. New York: New Press.

Howard, D. H., and B. Kaplan. 2006. "Do Report Cards Influence Hospital Choice? The Case of Kidney Transplantation." *Inquiry* 43 (Summer): 150–59.

Hsiao, W. C. 1992. "Comparing Health Care Systems: What Nations Can Learn from One Another." *Journal of Health Politics, Policy and Law* 17 (4): 613–36.

Hsiao, W. C., P. Braun, D. Yntema, and E. R. Becker. 1988. "Estimating Physicians' Work for a Resource-Based Relative Value Scale." *New England Journal of Medicine* 319 (13): 835–41.

Hurd, R. W. 1973. "Equilibrium Vacancies in a Labor Market Dominated by Non-Profit Firms: The "Shortage" of Nurses." *Review of Economics and Statistics* 55 (2): 234–40.

Hurley, J. 2008. Personal communication, December 8.

Hurley, J., and R. Labelle. 1995. "Relative Fees and the Utilization of Physicians' Services in Canada." *Health Economics* 4 (6): 419–38.

Hurley, J., R. Labelle, and T. Rice. 1990. "The Relationship Between Physician Fees and the Utilization of Medical Services in Ontario." *Advances in Health Economics and Health Services Research* 11: 49–78.

Hurst, J., and L. Siciliani. 2003. "Tackling Excessive Waiting Times for Elective Surgery: A Comparison of Policies in Twelve OECD Countries." OECD Health Working Papers, No. 6. Paris: OECD Publishing.

Hyman, D. A., and W. E. Kovacic. 2004. "Monopoly, Monopsony, and Market Definition: An Antitrust Perspective on Market Concentration Among Health Insurers." *Health Affairs* 23 (6): 25–28.

Iglehart, J. K. 2008. "Grassroots Activism and the Pursuit of an Expanded Physician Supply." *New England Journal of Medicine* 358 (16): 1741–49.

Iglehart, J. K. 2000. "Restoring the Status of an Icon: A Talk with Canada's Minister of Health." *Health Affairs* 19 (3): 132–40.

Ikegami, N., and J. C. Campbell. 2008. "Dealing with the Medical Axis-of-Power: The Case of Japan." *Health Economics, Policy and Law* 3 (2): 107–13.

———. 2004. "Japan's Health Care System: Containing Costs and Attempting Reform." *Health Affairs* 23 (3): 26–36.

———. 1999. "Health Care Reform in Japan: The Virtues of Muddling Through." *Health Affairs* 18 (3): 56–75.

Imai, Y. 2002. "Health Care Reform in Japan." OECD Economics Department Working Papers, No. 321. Paris: OECD.

Imai, Y., S. Jacobzone, and P. Lenain. 2000. "The Changing Health System in France." OECD Economics Department Working Papers, No. 269. Paris: OECD.

Inglehart, R., R. Foa, C. Peterson, and C. Welzel. 2008. "Development, Freedom, and Rising Happiness: A Global Perspective." *Perspectives on Psychological Science* 3 (4): 264–85.

Institute of Medicine (IOM). 2001. *Coverage Matters: Insurance and Health Care.* Washington, DC: National Academies Press.

Ipsos. 2008. *Consumer Survey: Informed Financial Consent 2007.* Melbourne: Ipsos Australia Pty Ltd.

Isaacs, S. L. 1996. "Consumers' Information Needs: Results of a National Survey." *Health Affairs* 15 (4): 31–41.

Iversen, T. 2004. "The Effects of a Patient Shortage on General Practitioners' Future Income and List of Patients." *Journal of Health Economics* 23: 673–94.

Iyengar, S. S., and M. R. Lepper. 2000. "When Choice Is Demotivating: Can One Desire Too Much of a Good Thing?" *Journal of Personality and Social Psychology* 76: 995–1006.

Jackson, T. 2007. "Health Technology Assessment in Australia: Challenges Ahead." *Medical Journal of Australia* 187 (5): 262–64.

Jamison, D. T., and M. E. Sandbu. 2001. "WHO Rankings of Health System Performance." *Science* 293: 1595–96.

Jeffers, J. R., M. F. Bognanno, and J. C. Bartlett. 1971. "On the Demand Versus Need for Medical Services and the Concept of 'Shortage.'" *American Journal of Public Health* 61 (1): 46–63.

Jensen, G. A., and M. A. Morrisey. 1999. "Employer-Sponsored Health Insurance and Mandated Benefit Laws." *Milbank Quarterly* 77 (4): 425–59.

Jensen, G. A., M. A. Morrisey, S. Gaffney, and D. K. Liston. 1997. "The New Dominance of Managed Care: Insurance Trends in the 1990s." *Health Affairs* 16 (1): 125–36.

Jewett, J. J., and J. H. Hibbard. 1996. "Comprehension of Quality Indicators: Differences Among Privately Insured, Publicly Insured, and Uninsured." *Health Care Financing Review* 18 (1): 75–94.

Jiang, H. J., B. Friedman, and J. W. Begun. 2006a. "Factors Associated with High-Quality/Low-Cost Hospital Performance." *Journal of Health Care Finance* 32 (3): 39–52.

———. 2006b. "Sustaining and Improving Hospital Performance: The Effects of Organizational and Market Factors." *Health Care Management Review* 31 (3): 188–96.

Jin, G. Z., and A. T. Sorensen. 2006. "Information and Consumer Choice: The Value of Publicized Health Plan Ratings." *Journal of Health Economics* 25: 248–75.

Johnson-Pawlson, J., and D. Infeld. 1996. "Nurse Staffing and Quality of Care in Nursing Facilities." *Journal of Gerontological Nursing* 22 (8): 36–45.

Jones, C. B. 2008. "Revisiting Nurse Turnover Costs: Adjusting for Inflation." *Journal of Nursing Administration* 38 (1): 11–18.

Jonsson, B. 1989. "What Can Americans Learn from Europeans?" *Health Care Financing Review* 11 (Suppl.): 79–109.

Jordan, W. J. 2001. "An Early View of the Impact of Deregulation and Managed Care on Hospital Profitability and Net Worth." *Journal of Healthcare Management* 46 (3): 161–72.

Judge, K. 1995. "Income Distribution and Life Expectancy: A Critical Appraisal." *British Medical Journal* 311: 1285–87.

Kahn, K. L., E. B. Keeler, M. J. Sherwood, W. H. Rogers, D. Draper, S. S. Bentow, E. J. Reinisch, L. V. Rubenstein, J. Kosecoff, and R. H. Brook. 1990. "Comparing Outcomes of Care Before and After Implementation of the DRG-Based Prospective Payment System." *Journal of the American Medical Association* 264 (15): 1984–88.

Kaiser Commission on Medicaid and the Uninsured. 2008. "Medicaid Facts." [Online information; retrieved 4/8/09.]www.kff.org/medicaid/upload/7235_03-2.pdf.

Kaiser Family Foundation (KFF). n.d. *State Health Facts.* [Online information; retrieved 4/8/09.] www.statehealthfacts.org/comparebar.jsp?ind=412&cat=8.

———. 2008a. "Medicare Advantage." [Online fact sheet; retrieved 4/8/09.] www.kff.org/medicare/upload/2052-11.pdf.

———. 2008b. "The Medicare Prescription Drug Benefit." [Online fact sheet; retrieved 4/8/09.] www.kff.org/medicare/upload/7044_08.pdf.

———. 2007a. "Prescription Drug Trends." [Online information; retrieved 4/8/09.] www.kff.org/rxdrugs/upload/3057_06.pdf.

———. 2007b. *Trends and Indicators in the Changing Health Care Marketplace.* [Online report; retrieved 4/8/09.] www.kff.org/insurance/7031/index.cfm.

———. 2006. "Medicare: CMS Proposes Rule to Increase Acute Care Hospital Reimbursements by 3.4% in FY 2007." [Online information; retrieved 4/8/09.] www.kaisernetwork.org/daily_reports/rep_index.cfm?hint=3&DR_ID=36611.

Kaiser Family Foundation and Harvard School of Public Health. 2006. "Topline: The Public's Health Care Agenda for the New Congress and the Presidential Campaign." [Online information; retrieved 4/8/09.] www.kff.org/kaiser polls/upload/7598.pdf.

Kanda, K., and M. Mezey. 1991. "Registered Nurse Staffing in Pennsylvania Nursing Homes: Comparison Before and After Implementation of Medicare's Prospective Payment System." *The Gerontologist* 31 (3): 318–24.

Kane, R. L., T. Shamliyan, C. Mueller, S. Duval, and T. J. Wilt. 2007. "The Association of Registered Nurse Staffing Levels and Patient Outcomes: Systematic Review and Meta-Analysis." *Medical Care* 45 (12): 1195–1204.

Kaplan, G. A., E. R. Pamuk, J. W. Lynch, R. D. Cohen, and J. L. Balfour. 1996. "Inequality in Income and Mortality in the United States: Analysis of Mortality and Potential Pathways." *British Medical Journal* 312 (7037): 999–1003.

Kassirer, J. P. 2007. "Review of Leonard J. Weber, *Profits Before People? Ethical Standards and the Marketing of Prescription Drugs.*" *American Journal of Bioethics* 7 (3): 54–55.

Kaveny, M. C. 1999. "Commodifying the Polyvalent Good of Health Care." *Journal of Medicine and Philosophy* 24 (3): 207–23.

Kawachi, I. 2000. "Income Inequality and Health." In *Income Inequality and Health,* edited by L. F. Berman and I. Kawachi. New York: Oxford University Press.

Kawachi, I., and B. P. Kennedy. 2001. "How Income Inequality Affects Health: Evidence from Research in the United States." In *Income, Socioeconomic Status, and Health: Exploring the Relationships*, edited by J. A. Auerbach and B. K. Krimgold. Washington, DC: National Policy Association.

———. 1999. "Health and Social Cohesion: Why Care About Income Inequality?" In *Income Inequality and Health*, edited by I. Kawachi, B. P. Kennedy, and R. G. Wilkinson. New York: New Press.

Kawachi, I., B. P. Kennedy, and R. G. Wilkinson. 1999. *Income Inequality and Health*. New York: New Press.

Keeler, E. B., R. H. Brook, G. A. Goldberg, C. J. Kamberg, and J. P. Newhouse. 1985. "How Free Care Reduced Hypertension in the Health Insurance Experiment." *Journal of the American Medical Association* 254 (14): 1926–31.

Keeler, E. B., G. Melnick, and J. Zwanziger. 1999. "The Changing Effects of Competition on Non-Profit and For-Profit Hospital Pricing Behavior." *Journal of Health Economics* 18: 69–86.

Keeler, E. B., and J. E. Rolph. 1983. "How Cost Sharing Reduced Medical Spending of Participants in the Health Insurance Experiment." *Journal of the American Medical Association* 249 (16): 2220–22.

Keepnews, D. M. 2007. "Evaluating Nurse Staffing Regulation." *Policy, Politics, & Nursing Practice* 8 (4): 236–37.

Kennedy, B. P., I. Kawachi, and D. Prothrow-Stith. 1996. "Income Distribution and Mortality: Cross-Sectional Ecological Study of the Robin Hood Index in the United States." *British Medical Journal* 312: 1004–7.

Kessel, R. 1958. "Price Discrimination in Medicine." *Journal of Law and Economics* 1 (October): 20–53.

Kessler, D. P., and M. B. McClellan. 2000. "Is Hospital Competition Socially Wasteful?" *Quarterly Journal of Economics* 115 (2): 577–615.

Khandker, R., and W. Manning. 1992. "The Impact of Utilization Review on Costs and Utilization." In *Health Economics Worldwide*, edited by P. Zweifel and H. Frech III, 47–62. Developments in Health Economics and Public Policy series, vol. 1. New York: Springer.

Khowaja, K., R. J. Merchant, and D. Hirani. 2005. "Registered Nurses Perception of Work Satisfaction at a Tertiary Care University Hospital." *Journal of Nursing Management* 13: 32–39.

Kirch, D., and D. Vernon. 2008. "Confronting the Complexity of the Physician Workforce Equation." *Journal of the American Medical Association* 299 (22): 2680–82.

Kitchener, M., J. O'Meara, A. Brody, H. Y. Lee, and C. Harrington. 2007. "Shareholder Value and the Performance of a Large Nursing Home Chain." *Health Services Research* 43 (3): 1062–84.

Knottnerus, J. A., and G. H. ten Velden. 2007. "Dutch Doctors and Their Patients—Effects of Health Care Reform in the Netherlands." *New England Journal of Medicine* 357 (24): 2424–26.

Knox, K. J., E. C. Blankmeyer, and J. R. Stutzman. 2001. "The Efficiency of Nursing Home Chains and the Implications of Nonprofit Status: A Comment." *Journal of Real Estate Portfolio Management* 7 (2): 177–82.

———. 1999. "Relative Economic Efficiency in Texas Nursing Facilities: A Profit Function Analysis." *Journal of Economics and Finance* 23 (3): 199–213.

Koen, V. 2000. "Public Expenditure Reform: The Health Care Sector in the United Kingdom." OECD Economics Department Working Papers, No. 256. Paris: OECD.

Kopelman, P. G. 2000. "Obesity as a Medical Problem." *Nature* 404: 635–43.

Kopit, W. G. 2004. "Is There Evidence That Recent Consolidation in the Health Insurance Industry Has Adversely Affected Premiums?" *Health Affairs* 23 (6): 29–31.

Kosecoff, J., K. L. Kahn, W. H. Rogers, E. J. Reinisch, M. J. Sherwood, L. V. Rubenstein, D. Draper, C. P. Roth, C. Chew, and R. H. Brook. 1990. "Prospective Payment System and Impairment at Discharge: The 'Quicker-and-Sicker' Story Revisited." *Journal of the American Medical Association* 264 (15): 1980–83.

Kovner, C., C. Jones, C. Zhan, P. Gergen, and J. Basu. 2002. "Nurse Staffing and Post Surgical Adverse Events: An Analysis of Administrative Data from a Sample of U.S. Hospitals, 1990–1996." *Health Services Research* 37 (3): 611–29.

Kozak, L. J., E. McCarthy, and R. Pokras. 1999. "Changing Patterns of Surgical Care in the U.S., 1980–1995." *Health Care Financing Review* 21 (1): 31–49.

Krauss, C. 2006. "Canada's Private Clinics Surge as Public System Falters." [Online article; retrieved 4/8/09.] www.nytimes.com/2006/02/28/international/americas/28canada.html.

Krauss, M. J., B. Evanoff, E. Hitcho, K. E. Ngugi, W. C. Dunagan, I. Fischer, S. Birge, S. Johnson, E. Costantinou, and V. J. Fraser. 2005. "A Case Control Study of Patient, Medication, and Care-Related Risk Factors for Inpatient Falls." *Journal of General Internal Medicine* 20: 116–22.

Krishnan, R. 2001. "Market Restructuring and Pricing in the Hospital Industry." *Journal of Health Economics* 20 (2): 213–37.

Kronick. R., and T. Gilmer. 1999. "Explaining the Decline in Health Insurance Coverage, 1979–1995." *Health Affairs* 18 (2): 30–47.

Kuttner, R. 2008. "Market-Based Failure—A Second Opinion on U.S. Health Care Costs." *New England Journal of Medicine* 358 (6): 549–51.

———. 1999. "The American Health Care System: Wall Street and Health Care." *New England Journal of Medicine* 340 (8): 664–68.

———. 1997. *Everything for Sale: The Virtue and Limits of Markets.* New York: Alfred A. Knopf.

———. 1996. "Columbia/HCA and the Resurgence of the For-Profit Hospital Business." *New England Journal of Medicine* 335 (5): 362–68.

———. 1984. *The Economic Illusion: False Choices Between Prosperity and Social Justice.* Boston: Houghton Mifflin.

Labelle, R., G. Stoddart, and T. Rice. 1994. "A Re-examination of the Meaning and Importance of Supplier-Induced Demand." *Journal of Health Economics* 13 (3): 347–68.

Laeven, L. 2001. "Incentives and Waiting Lists: Interventions on Waiting Lists and Their Impact on Demand." Paper presented at the session, "Incentives for Reduced Waiting Times in Health Systems: A Comparison of Experiences in

Different Countries." International Health Economics Association Third International Conference, York, UK, July 23.

Laing, G. P., and A. W. Rademaker. 1990. "Married Registered Nurses' Labor Force Participation." *Canadian Journal of Nursing Research* 22 (1): 21–38.

Lancry, P. J., and S. Sandier. 1999. "Rationing Health Care in France." *Health Policy* 50 (1): 23–38.

Landon, B. E., J. Reschovsky, and D. Blumenthal. 2003. "Changes in Career Satisfaction Among Primary Care and Specialist Physicians, 1997–2001." *Journal of the American Medical Association* 289 (4): 442–49.

Landon, B. E., A. M. Zaslavsky, N. D. Beaulieu, J. A. Shaul, and P. D. Cleary. 2001. "Health Plan Characteristics and Consumers' Assessments of Quality." *Health Affairs* 20 (2): 274–86.

Larrabee, J. H., M. A. Janney, C. L. Ostrow, M. L. Withrow, G. R. Hobbs Jr., and C. Burant. 2003. "Predicting Registered Nurse Job Satisfaction and Intent to Leave." *Journal of Nursing Administration* 33 (5): 271–83.

Latham, S. R. 2003. "Pharmaceutical Costs." *Journal of Legal Medicine* 24 (2): 141–73.

Leape, L. 1989. "Unnecessary Surgery." *Health Services Research* 24 (3): 351–407.

Lee, J. S., R. A. Berenson, R. Mayes, and A. K. Gauthier. 2003. "Medicare Payment Policy: Does Cost Shifting Matter?" [Online article; retrieved 4/8/09.] http://content.healthaffairs.org/cgi/content/short/hlthaff.w3.480v1.

Lee, P. R., and J. Herzstein. 1986. "International Drug Regulation." *Annual Review of Public Health* 7: 217–35.

Le Grand, J. 1999. "Competition, Cooperation, or Control? Tales from the British National Health Service." *Health Affairs* 18 (3): 27–39.

———. 1992. "The Theory of Government Failure." *British Journal of Political Science* 21 (4): 423–42.

Leibenstein, H. 1976. *Beyond Economic Man: Feminist Theory and Economics.* Cambridge, MA: Harvard University Press.

Lemke, S., and R. Moos. 1989. "Ownership and Quality of Care in Residential Facilities for the Elderly." *The Gerontologist* 29 (2): 209–15.

Lesser, C. S., P. B. Ginsburg, and K. J. Devers. 2003. "The End of an Era: What Became of the 'Managed Care Revolution' in 2001?" *Health Services Research* 38 (1, Pt. 2): 337–55.

Lessler, D., and T. Wickizer. 2000. "The Impact of Utilization Management on Readmissions Among Patients with Cardiovascular Disease." *Health Services Research* 34 (6): 1315–36.

Levi, J., L. M. Segal, and C. Juliano. 2008. *Prevention for a Healthier America.* [Online report; retrieved 4/8/09.] www.rwjf.org/publichealth/product.jsp?id=32711.

Levit, K. R., H. Lazenby, D. R. Waldo, and L. M. Davidoff. 1985. "National Health Expenditures, 1984." *Health Care Financing Review* 7 (1): 1–35.

Lexchin, J. 2006. "Do Manufacturers of Brand-Name Drugs Engage in Price Competition? An Analysis of Introductory Prices." *Canadian Medical Association Journal* 174 (8): 1120–21.

Lien, H. M., C. T. Albert Ma, and T. G. McGuire. 2004. "Provider-Client Interactions and Quantity of Health Care Use." *Journal of Health Economics* 23 (6): 1261–83.

Light, D. W. 2008. Reply to DiMasi, Hansen, and Grabowski. *Journal of Health Politics, Policy and Law* 33 (2): 325–27.

———. 2007. "Misleading Congress About Drug Development." *Journal of Health Politics, Policy and Law* 32 (5): 895–913.

———. 2001a. "Managed Competition, Governmentality and Institutional Response in the United Kingdom." *Social Science and Medicine* 52 (8): 1167–81.

———. 2001b. "Comparative Institutional Response to Economic Policy, Managed Competition and Governmentality." *Social Science and Medicine* 52 (8): 1151–66.

———. 1995. "*Homo Economicus*: Escaping the Traps of Managed Competition." *European Journal of Public Health* 5 (3): 145–54.

Light, D. W., and J. Lexchin. 2005. "Foreign Free Riders and the High Price of U.S. Medicines." *British Medical Journal* 331: 958–60.

Light, D. W., and R. N. Warburton. 2005. "Extraordinary Claims Require Extraordinary Evidence." *Journal of Health Economics* 24: 1030–33.

Lindrooth, R. C., G. J. Bazzoli, J. Needleman, and R. Hasnain-Wynia. 2006. "The Effects of Changes in Hospital Reimbursement on Nurse Staffing Decisions at Safety Net and Nonsafety Net Hospitals." *Health Services Research* 41 (3): 701–11.

Link, C. R. 1992. "Labor Supply Behavior of Registered Nurses: Female Labor Supply in the Future?" *Research in Labor Economics* 13: 287–320.

Link, C. R., and J. H. Landon. 1975. "Monopsony and Union Power in the Market for Nurses." *Southern Economic Journal* 41 (4): 649–59.

Link, C. R., and R. F. Settle. 1985. "Labor Supply Responses of Licensed Practical Nurses: A Partial Solution to a Nurse Shortage." *Journal of Economics and Business* 37: 49–57.

———. 1981. "Wage Incentives and Married Professional Nurses: A Case of Backward-Bending Supply?" *Economic Inquiry* 19: 144–56.

Lipsey, R. G., and K. Lancaster. 1956–1957. "The General Theory of the Second Best." *Review of Economic Studies* 24 (1): 11–32.

Little, I. M. D. 1957. *A Critique of Welfare Economics*. London: Oxford at the Clarendon Press, Oxford University Press.

Lleras-Muney, A. 2005. "The Relationship Between Education and Adult Mortality in the United States." *Review of Economic Studies* 72: 189–221.

Lohr, K. N., R. H. Brook, C. J. Kamberg, G. Goldberg, A. Leibowitz, J. Keesey, D. Reboussin, and J. P. Newhouse. 1986. "Effect of Cost Sharing on Use of Medically Effective and Less Effective Care." *Medical Care* 24 (9, Suppl.): S31–S38.

Lorgelly, P. K., and J. Lindley. 2008. "What Is the Relationship Between Income Inequality and Health? Evidence from BHPS." *Health Economics* 17: 249–65.

Lo Sasso, A. T., T. Rice, J. R. Gabel, and H. Whitmore. 2004. "Tales from the New Frontier: Pioneers' Experiences with Consumer-Driven Health Care." *Health Services Research* 39 (2, Pt. II): 1071–89.

Luft, H. S. 1999. "Why Are Physicians So Upset About Managed Care?" *Journal of Health Politics, Policy and Law* 24 (5): 957–66.

Luft, H. S., J. P. Bunker, and A. C. Enthoven. 1979. "Should Operations Be Regionalized? The Empirical Relation Between Surgical Volume and Mortality." *New England Journal of Medicine* 301 (25): 1364–69.

Lurie, P. P. 2005. "Testimony Before the Senate Special Committee on Aging on the Impact of DTC Drug Advertising on Seniors' Health and Health Care Costs." [Online information; retrieved 4/8/09.] www.citizen.org/publications/release.cfm?ID=7402.

Lynch, J., G. D. Smith, S. Harper, M. Hillemeier, N. Ross, G. A. Kaplan, and M. Wolfson. 2004. "Is Income Inequality a Determinant of Population Health? Part 1. A Systematic Review." *Milbank Quarterly* 82 (1): 5–99.

Lynk, W. J. 1995a. "Nonprofit Hospital Mergers and the Exercise of Market Power." *Journal of Law and Economics* 38 (2): 437–61.

———. 1995b. "The Creation of Economic Efficiencies in Hospital Mergers." *Journal of Health Economics* 14: 507–30.

Macinko, J., and B. Starfield. 2001. "The Utility of Social Capital in Research on Health Determinants." *Milbank Quarterly* 79 (3): 387–427.

Macinko, J. A., L. Shi, B. Starfield, and J. T. Wulu. 2003. "Income Inequality and Health: A Critical Review of the Literature." *Medical Care Research and Review* 60 (4): 407–52.

Manning, W. G., J. P. Newhouse, N. Duan, E. B. Keeler, A. Leibowitz, and M. S. Marquis. 1987. "Health Insurance and the Demand for Medical Care: Evidence from a Randomized Experiment." *American Economic Review* 77 (3): 251–77.

Margolis, H. 1982. *Selfishness, Altruism, and Rationality.* Cambridge, UK: Cambridge University Press.

Mark, B. A., and D. W. Harless. 2007. "Nurse Staffing, Mortality, and Length of Stay in For-Profit and Not-for-Profit Hospitals." *Inquiry* 44: 167–86.

Mark, B. A., D. W. Harless, M. McCue, and Y. Xu. 2004. "A Longitudinal Examination of Hospital Registered Nurse Staffing and Quality of Care." *Health Services Research* 39 (2): 279–99.

Mark, T. 1999. "Analysis of the Rationale for, and Consequences of, Nonprofit and For-Profit Ownership Conversions." *Health Services Research* 34 (1): 83–101.

Marmor, T. R., and A. Dunham. 1983. "Political Science and Health Services Administration." In *Political Analysis and American Medical Care: Essays*, edited by T. R. Marmor, 3–44. London: Cambridge University Press.

Marmot, M. G., H. Bosma, H. Hemingway, E. Brunner, and S. Stansfeld. 1997. "Contribution of Job Control and Other Risk Factors to Social Variations in Coronary Heart Disease Incidence." *Lancet* (350): 235–39.

Marquis, M. S., and G. F. Kominski. 1994. "Alternative Volume Performance Standards for Medicare Physicians' Services." *Milbank Quarterly* 72 (2): 329–57.

Marshall, A. 1920. *Principles of Economics.* London: Macmillan.

Marsteller, J. A., R. R. Bovbjerg, and L. M. Nichols. 1998. "Nonprofit Conversion: Theory, Evidence, and State Policy Options." *Health Services Research* 33 (5): 1495–1517.

Martens, J. D., R. A. Winkens, T. van der Weijden, D. de Bruyn, and J. L. Severens.

2006. "Does a Joint Development and Dissemination of Multidisciplinary Guidelines Improve Prescribing Behaviour: A Pre/Post Study with Concurrent Control Group and a Randomised Trial." *BMC Health Services Research* 6: 145.

Maryland Statewide Commission on the Crisis in Nursing. 2005. *Nursing Faculty Shortage: Causes, Effects, and Suggestions for Resolution.* [Online report; retrieved 4/8/09.] www.mbon.org/commission/nsg_faculty_shortage.pdf.

Maynard, A. 2006. "Medical Workforce Planning: Some Forecasting Challenges." *Australian Economic Review* 39 (3): 323–29.

———. 2005. "European Health Policy Challenges." *Health Economics* 14: S255–S263.

McCarberg, B. 2004. "Impact of Guidelines on Healthcare from the Patient and Payor Perspective." *Disease Management and Health Outcomes* 12 (2): 73–79.

McCarthy, T. R. 1985. "The Competitive Nature of the Primary Care Physician Services Market." *Journal of Health Economics* 4 (2): 93–117.

McClellan, M., and D. Kessler for the TECH Investigators. 1999. "A Global Analysis of Technological Change in Health Care: The Case of Heart Attacks." *Health Affairs* 18 (3): 250–55.

McCormack, L. A., S. A. Garfinkel, J. H. Hibbard, E. C. Norton, and U. J. Bayen. 2001. "Health Plan Decision Making with New Medicare Information Materials." *Health Services Research* 36 (3): 531–54.

McCue, M., and R. Furst. 1986. "Financial Characteristics of Hospitals Purchased by Investor-Owned Chains." *Health Services Research* 23 (4): 515–27.

McGreevy, P. 2008. "Schwarzenegger Signs Law Banning Trans Fats in Restaurants." [Online article; retrieved 4/8/09.] www.latimes.com/news/local/la-me-transfat26-2008jul26,0,2161554.story.

McGregor, M. J., M. Cohen, K. McGrail, A. M. Broemeling, R. N. Adler, M. Schulzer, L. Ronald, Y. Cvitkovich, and M. Beck. 2005. "Staffing Levels in Not-for-Profit and For-Profit Long-Term Care Facilities: Does Type of Ownership Matter?" *Canadian Medical Association Journal* 172 (5): 645–49.

McGuire, T. G., and M. Pauly. 1991. "Physician Response to Fee Changes with Multiple Payers." *Journal of Health Economics* 10 (4): 385–410.

McKay, N. 1994. "The Prisoner's Dilemma: An Obstacle to Cooperation in Health Care Markets." *Medical Care Review* 51 (2): 179–204.

McKay, N. L., and M. E. Deily. 2005. "Comparing High- and Low-Performing Hospitals Using Risk-Adjusted Excess Mortality and Cost Inefficiency." *Health Care Management Review* 30 (4): 347–60.

McKie, J., and J. Richardson. 2003. "The Rule of Rescue." *Social Science & Medicine* 56: 2407–19.

McNutt, D. 1981. "GMENAC: Its Manpower Forecasting Framework." *American Journal of Public Health* 71 (10): 1116–24.

Mechanic, D. 2003. "Physician Discontent: Challenges and Opportunities." *Journal of the American Medical Association* 290 (7): 941–46.

———. 1990. "The Role of Sociology in Health Affairs." *Health Affairs* 9 (1): 85–97.

———. 1979. *Future Issues in Health Care.* New York: Free Press.

Medicare Payment Advisory Commission (MedPAC). 2005. *Report to the Congress:*

Physician-Owned Specialty Hospitals. Washington, DC: Medicare Payment Advisory Commission.

———. 2000. "Health Plans' Selection and Payment of Health Care Providers, 1999." Washington, DC: Medicare Payment Advisory Commission.

Mellor, J. M., and J. Milyo. 2001. "Reexamining the Evidence of an Ecological Association Between Income Inequality and Health." *Journal of Health Politics, Policy and Law* 26 (3): 487–521.

Melnick, G., E. Keeler, and J. Zwanziger. 1999. "Market Power and Hospital Pricing: Are Nonprofits Different?" *Health Affairs* 18 (3): 167–73.

Melnick, G. A., and J. Zwanziger. 1988. "Hospital Behavior Under Competition and Cost-Containment Policies." *Journal of the American Medical Association* 260 (18): 2669–75.

Menke, T. J. 1997. "The Effect of Chain Membership on Hospital Costs." *Health Services Research* 32 (2): 177–96.

Menke, T. J., and N. P. Wray. 1999. "Cost Implications of Regionalizing Open Heart Surgery Units." *Inquiry* 36: 57–67.

Milgram, S. 1963. "Behavioral Study of Obedience." *Journal of Abnormal and Social Psychology* 67 (4): 371–78.

Miller, D. 1992. "Distributive Justice." *Ethics* 102 (April): 555–93.

Miller, M. E., W. P. Welch, and E. Englert. 1995. "Physicians Practicing in Hospitals: Implications for a Medical Staff Policy." *Inquiry* 32 (2): 204–10.

Miller, R. H. 1996. "Competition in the Health System: Good News and Bad News." *Health Affairs* 15 (2): 107–20.

Miller, R. H., and R. R. Bovbjerg. 2002. "Efforts to Improve Patient Safety in Large, Capitated Medical Groups: Description and Conceptual Model." *Journal of Health Politics, Policy and Law* 27 (3): 402–40.

Miller, R. H., and H. S. Luft. 2002. "HMO Plan Performance Update: An Analysis of the Literature, 1997–2001." *Health Affairs* 21 (4): 63–86.

———. 1997. "Does Managed Care Lead to Better or Worse Quality of Care?" *Health Affairs* 16 (5): 7–25.

———. 1994. "Managed Care Plan Performances Since 1980." *Journal of the American Medical Association* 271 (19): 1512–19.

Ministry of Health, Labour, and Welfare (Japan). 2008. "Physician Statistics." (In Japanese.) [Online information; retrieved 4/8/09.] www.mhlw.go.jp/shingi/2005/03/s0311-5a4.html.

Ministry of Health and Social Affairs, Government Offices of Sweden. 2003. The Health and Medical Service Act (1982:763). [Online information; retrieved 4/8/09.] www.regeringen.se/content/1/c6/02/31/25/a7ea8ee1.pdf.

Ministry of Health, Welfare, and Sport (the Netherlands). 2008. "Risk Adjustment Under the Health Insurance Act in the Netherlands." [Online information; retrieved 4/8/09.] www.minvws.nl/en/reports/z/2008/risk-adjustment-under-the-health-insurance-act-in-the-netherlands.asp.

Mintzes, B. 2002. "Direct-to-Consumer Advertising Is Medicalising Normal Human Experience." *British Medical Journal* 324 (April 13): 908–9.

Mishan, E. J. 1969a. *Welfare Economics: Ten Introductory Essays.* New York: Random House.

———. 1969b. *Welfare Economics: An Assessment.* Amsterdam: North-Holland.

Mitchell, J. B., and F. Bentley. 2000. "Impact of Oregon's Priority List on Medicaid Beneficiaries." *Medical Care Research and Review* 57 (2): 216–34.

Mitchell, J. B., G. Wedig, and J. Cromwell. 1989. "The Medicare Physician Fee Freeze: What Really Happened?" *Health Affairs* 8 (1): 21–33.

Mitchell, J. M. 2007. "Utilization Changes Following Market Entry by Physician-Owned Specialty Hospitals." *Medical Care Research and Review* 64 (4): 395–415.

Mitchell, J. M., J. Hadley, and D. J. Gaskin. 2000. "Physicians' Response to Medicare Fee Schedule Reductions." *Medical Care* 38 (10): 1029–39.

Mobley, L. R., and W. D. Bradford. 1997. "Behavioral Differences Among Hospitals: Is It Ownership, or Location?" *Applied Economics* 29 (9): 1125–38.

Mobley, L. R., and J. Magnussen. 2002. "The Impact of Managed Care Penetration and Hospital Quality on Efficiency in Hospital Staffing." *Journal of Health Care Finance* 28 (4): 24–42.

Mooney, G. 1996a. "And Now for Vertical Equity? Some Concerns Arising from Aboriginal Health in Australia." *Health Economics* 5 (2): 99–103.

———. 1996b. "A Communitarian Critique of Health (Care) Economics." Presented at the inaugural meetings of the International Health Economics Association, Vancouver, British Columbia, May 21, 1996.

———. 1994. *Key Issues in Health Economics.* New York: Harvester Wheatsheaf.

Mooney, G., J. Hall, C. Donaldson, and K. Gerard. 1991. "Utilisation as a Measure of Equity: Weighing Heat?" *Journal of Health Economics* 10 (4): 475–80.

Mooney, G., and V. Wiseman. 2000. "World Health Report: Challenging a World View." *Journal of Health Services Research and Policy* 5 (4): 198–99.

Moore, F. C. 1877. *Fires: Their Causes, Prevention, and Extinction.* New York: F. C. Moore.

Morbidity and Mortality Weekly Report. 2002. "Annual Smoking-Attributable Mortality, Years of Potential Life Lost, and Economic Costs—United States, 1995–1999. *Morbidity and Mortality Weekly Report* 51 (14): 300–303.

Morone, J. A. 2000. "Citizens or Shoppers? Solidarity Under Siege." *Journal of Health Politics, Policy and Law* 25 (5): 959–68.

Morrisey, M. A. 2006. "Not-for-Profit Survival in a Competitive World." *Frontiers of Health Services Management* 22 (4): 35–38.

———. 2003. "Cost Shifting: New Myths, Old Confusion, and Enduring Reality." *Health Affairs* Web Exclusives (July–December, Suppl.): W3-489–W3-491.

———. 1994. *Cost-Shifting in Health Care: Separating Evidence from Rhetoric.* Washington, DC: AEI Press.

Morrisey, M. A., and J. Cawley. 2008. "Health Economists' View of Health Policy." *Journal of Health Politics, Policy and Law* 33 (4): 707–24.

Morrisey, M., G. Wedig, and M. Hassan. 1996. "Do Nonprofit Hospitals Pay Their Way?" *Health Affairs* 15 (4): 132–44.

Mueller, D. C. 1989. *Public Choice II.* Cambridge, UK: Cambridge University Press.

Munroe, D. 1990. "The Influence of Registered Nurse Staffing on the Quality of Nursing Home Care." *Research in Nursing and Health* 13: 263–70.

Murer, C. G. 2006. "Definitive New Guidelines." [Online information; retrieved 4/9/09.] www.rehabpub.com/issues/articles/2006-10_10.asp.

Musgrave, R. A., and P. B. Musgrave. 1989. *Public Finance in Theory and Practice*, 5th ed. New York: McGraw-Hill.

Nath, S. K. 1969. *A Reappraisal of Welfare Economics*. London: Routledge & Kegan Paul.

National Association for Home Care. 2001. "Basic Statistics About Home Care." [Online information; retrieved 4/9/09.] www.nahc.org/Consumer/hcstats.html.

National Health Policy Forum. 1995. *Consolidation in the Health Care Marketplace and Antitrust Policy*. Washington, DC: George Washington University.

National Institute for Health and Clinical Excellence. 2008. Home page. [Online information; retrieved 4/9/09.] www.nice.org.uk.

Needleman, J. 2008. "Is What's Good for the Patient Good for the Hospital? Aligning Incentives and the Business Case for Nursing." *Policy, Politics, and Nursing Practice* 9 (2): 80–87.

———. 2001. "The Role of Nonprofits in Health Care." *Journal of Health Politics, Policy and Law* 26 (5): 1113–30.

Needleman, J., P. Buerhaus, S. Mattke, M. Stewart, and K. Zelevinsky. 2002. "Nurse-Staffing Levels and the Quality of Care in Hospitals." *New England Journal of Medicine* 346 (22): 1715–22.

Needleman, J., P. I. Buerhaus, M. Stewart, K. Zelevinsky, and S. Mattke. 2006. "Nurse-Staffing in Hospitals: Is There a Business Case for Quality?" *Health Affairs* 25 (1): 204–11.

Needleman, J., J. Lamphere, and D. Chollet. 1999. "Uncompensated Care and Hospital Conversion in Florida." *Health Affairs* 18 (4): 125–33.

Neuman, P., M. K. Strollo, S. Guterman, W. H. Rogers, A. Li, A. M. Rodday, and D. G. Safran. 2007. "Medicare Prescription Drug Benefit Progress Report: Findings from a 2006 National Survey of Seniors." *Health Affairs* 26 (5): W630–W643.

Newhouse, J. P. 1993a. *Free for All? Lessons from the RAND Health Insurance Experiment*. Cambridge, MA: Harvard University Press.

———. 1993b. "An Iconoclastic View of Health Cost Containment." *Health Affairs* 12 (Suppl.): 152–71.

———. 1978. *The Economics of Medical Care*. Reading, MA: Addison-Wesley.

———. 1974. "The Health Insurance Study: Response to Hester and Leveson." *Inquiry* 11 (3): 236–41.

———. 1970. "Toward a Theory of Nonprofit Institutions: An Economic Model of a Hospital." *American Economic Review* 55 (1): 64–74.

Newhouse, J. P., G. Anderson, and L. L. Roos. 1988. "Hospital Spending in the United States and Canada: A Comparison." *Health Affairs* 7 (3): 6–24.

Newhouse, J. P., R. H. Brook, N. Duan, E. B. Keeler, A. Leibowitz, W. G. Manning, M. S. Marquis, C. N. Morris, C. E. Phelps, and J. E. Rolph. 2008. "Attrition in the RAND Health Insurance Experiment: A Response to Nyman." *Journal of Health Politics, Policy and Law* 33 (2): 295–308.

Newhouse, J. P., W. G. Manning, N. Duan, C. N. Morris, E. B. Keeler, A. Leibowitz, M. S. Marquis, W. H. Rogers, A. R. Davies, K. N. Lohr, et al. 1987. "The Findings of the RAND Health Insurance Experiment—A Response to Welch et al." *Medical Care* 25 (2): 157–79.

Ng, Y.-K. 1979. *Welfare Economics*. London: Macmillan.

Nguyen, N. X., and F. W. Derrick. 1994. "Hospital Markets and Competition: Implications for Antitrust Policy." *Health Care Management Review* 19 (1): 34–43.

Norman, L. D., K. Donelan, P. I. Buerhaus, G. Willis, M. Williams, B. Ulrich, and R. Dittus. 2005. "The Older Nurse in the Workplace: Does Age Matter?" *Nursing Economics* 23 (6): 282–89.

Norton, E., and D. Staiger. 1994. "How Hospital Ownership Affects Access to Care for the Uninsured." *RAND Journal of Economics* 25 (1): 171–85.

Nowak, M. J., and A. C. Preston. 2001. "Can Human Capital Theory Explain Why Nurses Are So Poorly Paid?" *Australian Economic Paper* 40 (2): 232–45.

Nozick, R. 1974. *Anarchy, State, and Utopia.* New York: Basic.

Nussbaum, M. C. 2003. "Capabilities as Fundamental Entitlements: Sen and Social Justice." *Feminist Economics* 9: 33–59.

Nyman, J. A. 2007. "American Health Policy: Cracks in the Foundation." *Journal of Health Politics, Policy and Law* 32 (5): 759–83.

———. 2002. *The Theory of the Demand for Health Insurance.* Stanford, CA: Stanford University Press.

———. 1999a. "The Economics of Moral Hazard Revisited." *Journal of Health Economics* 18: 811–24.

———. 1999b. "The Value of Health Insurance: The Access Motive." *Journal of Health Economics* 18: 141–52.

Nyman, J. A., and D. L. Bricker. 1989. "Profit Incentives and Technical Efficiency in the Production of Nursing Home Care." *Review of Economics and Statistics* 171 (4): 586–94.

Nyman, J. A., D. L. Bricker, and D. Link. 1990. "Technical Efficiency in Nursing Homes." *Medical Care* 28 (6): 541–51.

Oberlander, J. 2006. "Health Reform Interrupted: The Unraveling of the Oregon Health Plan." *Health Affairs* 26 (1): W96–W105.

Office of the Assistant Secretary for Planning and Evaluation (ASPE), U.S. Department of Health and Human Services. 2007. "Overview of the Uninsured in the United States: An Analysis of the 2007 Current Population Survey." [Online information; retrieved 4/9/09.] http://aspe.hhs.gov/health/reports/07/uninsured/index.htm.

Okamoto, E. 2008. *Public Health of Japan*, edited by K. Tatara. Tokyo: Japan Public Health Association.

O'Kane, M. 2006. "Redefining Value in Health Care: A New Imperative." *Healthcare Financial Management* 60 (8): 64–68.

Oliver, A. 2005. "The English National Health Service: 1979–2005." *Health Economics* 14: S75–S99.

Olson, M. 1965. *The Logic of Collective Action.* Cambridge, MA: Harvard University Press.

O'Neil, C., C. Harrington, M. Kitchener, and D. Saliba. 2003. "Quality of Care in Nursing Homes: An Analysis of Relationships Among Profit, Quality, and Ownership." *Medical Care* 41 (12): 1318–30.

Organisation for Economic Co-operation and Development (OECD). 2008. "OECD Health Data 2008: Statistics and Indicators for 30 Countries." Paris: OECD.

———. 2006. *OECD Reviews of Health Systems.* Paris: OECD.

———. 2001. "OECD Health Data 2001: A Comparative Analysis of 30 Countries." [CD-ROM.] Paris: OECD.

Pahor, M., B. M. Psaty, M. H. Alderman, W. B. Applegate, J. D. Williamson, C. Cavazzini, and C. D. Furberg. 2000. "Health Outcomes Associated with Calcium Antagonists Compared with Other First-Line Antihypertensive Therapies: A Meta-Analysis of Randomised Controlled Trials." *Lancet* 356: 1949–54.

Palangkaraya, A., and J. Yong. 2005. "Effects of Recent Carrot-and-Stick Policy Initiatives on Private Health Insurance Coverage in Australia." *Economic Record* 81 (254): 262–72.

Parker, C. D., and B. D. Rickman. 1996. "The Labor Force Re-entry Decision of Registered Nurses." *Journal of Economics* 22 (1): 73–79.

Parkin, M. 2007. *Microeconomics*, 8th ed. Reading, MA: Addison-Wesley.

Paul-Shaheen, P., J. D. Clark, and D. Williams. 1987. "Small Area Analysis: A Review and Analysis of the North American Literature." *Journal of Health Politics, Policy and Law* 12 (4): 741–809.

Pauly, M. V. 1997. "Who Was That Straw Man Anyway? A Comment on Evans and Rice." *Journal of Health Politics, Policy and Law* 22 (2): 467–73.

———. 1987. "Nonprofit Firms in Medical Markets." *American Economic Review* 77 (2): 257–62.

———. 1978. "Is Medical Care Different?" In *Competition in the Health Care Sector: Past, Present, and Future*, edited by W. Greenberg, 19–48. Washington, DC: Bureau of Economics, Federal Trade Commission.

———. 1968. "The Economics of Moral Hazard: Comment." *American Economic Review* 58 (3, Pt. I): 531–37.

Pauly, M. V., and M. Redisch. 1973. "The Not-for-Profit Hospital as a Physician's Cooperative." *American Economic Review* 63: 87–99.

Pauly, M. V., and M. Satterthwaite. 1981. "The Pricing of Primary Care Physicians' Services: A Test of the Role of Consumer Information." *Bell Journal of Economics* 12 (2): 488–506.

Pearce, N., and G. D. Smith. 2003. "Is Social Capital the Key to Inequalities in Health?" *American Journal of Public Health* 93 (1): 122–29.

Peltzman, S. 1976. "Toward a More General Theory of Regulation." *Journal of Law & Economics* 19 (2): 211–40.

Pender, D. R., and M. H. Meier. 2005. *Overview of FTC Antitrust Actions in Health Care Services and Products.* [Online report; retrieved 4/9/09.] www.ftc.gov/bc/0608hcupdate.pdf.

Person, S. D., J. J. Allison, C. I. Kiefe, M. T. Weaver, O. D. Williams, R. M. Centor, and N. W. Weissman. 2004. "Nurse Staffing and Mortality for Medicare Patients with Acute Myocardial Infarction." *Medical Care* 42 (1): 4–12.

Pescosolido, B. 2006. "Professional Dominance and the Limits of Erosion." *Society* 43 (6): 21–29.

Petersen, L. A., L. D. Woodard, T. Urech, C. Daw, and S. Sookanan. 2006. "Does Pay-for-Performance Improve the Quality of Health Care?" *Annals of Internal Medicine* 145 (4): 265–72.

Pfaff, M., and D. Wassener. 2000. "Germany." *Journal of Health Politics, Policy and Law* 25 (5): 907–13.

Pharmaceutical Health and Rational Use of Medicines (PHARM) Committee. 2004. "Direct to Consumer Advertising (DTCA) of Prescription Medicines and the Quality Use of Medicines (QUM)." [Online article; retrieved 4/9/09.] www.health.gov.au/internet/main/publishing.nsf/Content/43A536 BA7ABC1DA5CA256F9D00168F17/$File/dtca.pdf.

Pharmaceutical Researchers and Manufacturers of America. 2004. *Pharmaceutical Industry Profile 2004.* Washington, DC: Pharmaceutical Researchers and Manufacturers of America.

Phelps, C. E. 1997. *Health Economics.* New York: HarperCollins.

———. 1995. "Welfare Loss from Variations: Further Considerations." *Journal of Health Economics* 14 (2): 253–60.

Phelps, C. E., and C. Mooney. 1992. "Correction and Update on Priority Setting in Medical Technology Assessment in Medical Care." *Medical Care* 30 (8): 744–51.

Phelps, C. E., and S. T. Parente. 1990. "Priority Setting in Medical Technology and Medical Practice Assessment." *Medical Care* 29 (8): 703–23.

Philips, V. L. 1995. "Nurses' Labor Supply: Participation, Hours of Work, and Discontinuities in the Supply Function." *Journal of Health Economics* 14: 567–82.

Phillips, J. 1999. "Do Managerial Efficiency and Social Responsibility Drive Long-Term Financial Performance of Not-for-Profit Hospitals?" *Journal of Health Care Finance* 25: 67–76.

Physician Payment Review Commission (PPRC). 1993. *Annual Report to Congress.* Washington, DC: PPRC.

Pigou, A. C. 1932. *The Economics of Welfare*, 4th ed. London: Macmillan.

Pindus, N., J. Tilly, and S. Weinstein. 2002. *Skill Shortages and Mismatches in Nursing Related Health Care Employment.* Report to the U.S. Department of Labor, Employment and Training Administration. Washington, DC: The Urban Institute.

Poisal, J. A., C. Truffer, S. Smith, A. Sisko, C. Cowan, S. Keehan, and B. Dickensheets. 2007. "Health Spending Projections Through 2016: Modest Changes Obscure Part D's Impact." *Health Affairs* 26 (2): W242–W253.

Pollack, D. A., B. H. McFarland, R. A. George, and R. H. Angell. 1994. "Prioritization of Mental Health Services in Oregon." *Milbank Quarterly* 72 (3): 515–50.

Pollack, R. A. 1978. "Endogenous Tastes in Demand and Welfare Analysis." *American Economic Review* 68 (2): 374–79.

Porell, F., F. Caro, A. Silva, and M. Monane. 1998. "A Longitudinal Analysis of Nursing Home Outcomes." *Health Services Research* 33 (4): 835–65.

Port, F. K., R. A. Wolfe, and P. J. Held. 2000. "Ownership of Dialysis Facilities and Patients' Survival." *New England Journal of Medicine* 342 (14): 1053–56.

Poullier, J. P., and S. Sandier. 2000. "France." *Journal of Health Politics, Policy and Law* 25 (5): 899–905.

Preker, A. S., and A. Harding. 2007. "Political Economy of Strategic Purchasing." In *Public Ends, Private Means: Strategic Purchasing of Health Services*, edited by A. S. Preker, X. Liu, E. V. Velenyi, and E. Barris. Washington, DC: The World Bank.

Preker, A. S., A. Harding, and P. Travis. 2000. "'Make or Buy' Decisions in the Production of Health Care Goods and Services: New Insights from Institutional Economics and Organizational Theory." *Bulletin of the World Health Organization* 78 (6): 779–90.

Private Health Insurance Administration Council (Australia). 2008. "Membership Statistics." [Online information; retrieved 4/9/09.] www.phiac.gov.au/statistics/membershipcoverage/table1.htm.

Prospective Payment Assessment Commission (ProPAC). 1994. "Enrollment and Disenrollment Experience in the Medicare Risk Program." Washington, DC: ProPAC.

Public Citizen. 2001. "Tufts Drug Study Sample Is Skewed: True Figure of R&D Costs Likely Is 75 Percent Lower." [Online article; retrieved 4/9/09.] www.citizen.org/pressroom/release.cfm?ID=954.

Quaglini, S., A. Cavallini, S. Gerzeli, and G. Micieli. 2004. "Economic Benefit from Clinical Practice Guideline Compliance in Stroke Patient Management." *Health Policy* 69: 305–15.

Rabinowitz, H. K., J. J. Diamond, F. W. Markham, and J. R. Wortman. 2008. "Medical School Programs to Increase the Rural Physician Supply: A Systematic Review and Projected Impact of Widespread Replication." *Academic Medicine* 83 (3): 235–43.

Rantz, M. J., L. Popejoy, D. R. Mehr, M. Zwygart-Stauffacher, L. Hicks, V. Grando, V. S. Conn, R. Porter, J. Scott, and M. Maas. 1997. "Verifying Nursing Home Care Quality Using Minimum Data Set Quality Indicators and Other Quality Measures." *Journal of Nursing Care Quality* 12 (2): 54–62.

Rapoport, J., S. Gehlbach, S. Lemeshow, and D. Teres. 1992. "Resource Utilization Among Intensive Care Patients." *Archives of Internal Medicine* 152: 2207–12.

Rawls, J. 1971. *A Theory of Justice.* Cambridge, MA: Belknap Press.

Reinhardt, U. E. 2002. "Analyzing Cause and Effect in the U.S. Physician Workforce." *Health Affairs* 21 (1): 165–66.

———. 2001a. "Can Efficiency in Health Care Be Left to the Market?" *Journal of Health Politics, Policy and Law* 26 (5): 967–92.

———. 2001b. "Perspectives on the Pharmaceutical Industry." *Health Affairs* 20 (5): 136–49.

———. 2000. "The Economics of For-Profit and Not-for-Profit Hospitals." *Health Affairs* 19 (6): 178–86.

———. 1998. "Abstracting from Distributional Effects, This Policy Is Efficient." In *Health, Health Care and Health Economics: Perspectives on Distribution*, edited by M. L. Barer, T. E. Getzen, and G. L. Stoddart. New York: John Wiley.

———. 1994. "Germany's Health Care System: It's Not the American Way." *Health Affairs* 13 (4): 22–24.

———. 1992. "Reflections on the Meaning of Efficiency: Can Efficiency Be Separated from Equity?" *Yale Law & Policy Review* 10: 302–15.

———. 1989. "Economists in Health Care: Saviors, or Elephants in a Porcelain Shop?" *American Economic Review Papers and Proceedings* 79 (2): 337–42.

———. 1985. "The Theory of Physician-Induced Demand: Reflections After a Decade." *Journal of Health Economics* 4 (2): 187–93.

———. 1978. "Comment on Paper by Frank A. Sloan and Roger Feldman." In

Competition in the Health Care Sector: Past, Present, and Future, edited by W. Greenberg, 156–90. Washington, DC: Bureau of Economics, Federal Trade Commission.

Remler, D. K., and S. A. Glied. 2006. "How Much More Cost Sharing Will Health Savings Accounts Bring? *Health Affairs* 25 (4): 1070–78.

Rettig, R., and N. Levinsky. 1991. *Kidney Failure and the Federal Government*. Washington, DC: National Academies Press.

Rice, N., and P. Smith. 2001. "Capitation and Risk Adjustment in Health Care Financing: An International Progress Report." *Milbank Quarterly* 79 (1): 81–113.

Rice, T. H. 2001. "Should Consumer Choice Be Encouraged in Health Care?" In *Social Economics and Health Care*, edited by J. B. Davis. London: Routledge.

———. 1998. "The Case for Universal Coverage." In *The Future of the U.S. Healthcare System: Who Will Care for the Poor and Uninsured?* edited by S. H. Altman, U. E. Reinhardt, and A. E. Shields, 387–404. Chicago: Health Administration Press.

———. 1992. "An Alternative Framework for Evaluating Welfare Losses in the Health Care Market." *Journal of Health Economics* 11 (1): 88–92.

———. 1984. "Physician-Induced Demand for Medical Care: New Evidence from the Medicare Program." *Advances in Health Economics and Health Services Research* 5: 129–60.

———. 1983. "The Impact of Changing Medicare Reimbursement Rates on Physician-Induced Demand." *Medical Care* 21 (8): 803–15.

Rice, T., and J. Bernstein. 1990. "Volume Performance Standards: Can They Control Growth in Medicare Services?" *Milbank Quarterly* 68: 295–319.

Rice, T., B. Biles, E. R. Brown, F. Diderichsen, and H. Kuehn. 2000. "Reconsidering the Role of Competition in Health Care Markets." *Journal of Health Politics, Policy and Law* 25 (5): 863–73.

Rice, T., E. R. Brown, and R. Wyn. 1993. "Holes in the Jackson Hole Approach to Health Care Reform." *Journal of the American Medical Association* 270 (11): 1357–62.

Rice, T., J. Cummings, and D. Kao. 2008. "Reducing the Number of Drug Plans for Seniors: A Proposal and Analysis of Three Case Studies." Presented at the AcademyHealth annual meetings, Washington, DC, June 9.

Rice, T., and K. A. Desmond. 2004. "The Distributional Consequences of a Medicare 'Premium Support' Proposal." *Journal of Health Politics, Policy and Law* 29 (6): 1187–1226.

Rice, T., and Y. Hanoch. 2008. "Can Consumers Have Too Much Choice?" *Expert Review of Pharmacoeconomics & Outcomes Research* 8 (4): 3256–3327.

Rice, T., and K. R. Morrison. 1994. "Patient Cost Sharing for Medical Services: A Review of the Literature and Implications for Health Care Reform." *Medical Care Review* 51 (3): 235–87.

Rice, T., S. Stearns, S. DesHarnais, D. Pathman, M. Tai-Seale, and M. Brasure. 1996. "Do Physicians Cost Shift?" *Health Affairs* 15 (3): 215–25.

Rice, T. H., and G. F. Kominski. 2007. "Containing Health Care Costs." In *Changing the U.S. Health Care System*, edited by R. M. Anderson, T. H. Rice, and G. F. Kominski, 135–54. San Francisco: Jossey-Bass.

Rice, T. H., and R. J. Labelle. 1989. "Do Physicians Induce Demand for Medical Services?" *Journal of Health Politics, Policy and Law* 14 (3): 587–600.

Rice, T. H., and K. Y. Matsuoka. 2004. "The Impact of Cost Sharing on Appropriate Utilization and Health Status: A Review of the Literature on Seniors." *Medical Care Research and Review* 61 (4): 415–52.

Richardson, J., and J. McKie. 2005. "Empiricism, Ethics and Orthodox Economic Theory: What Is the Appropriate Basis for Decision-Making in the Health Sector?" *Social Science & Medicine* 60: 265–75.

Richardson, J. R. J., S. J. Peacock, and D. Mortimer. 2006. "Does an Increase in the Doctor Supply Reduce Medical Fees? An Econometric Analysis of Medical Fees Across Australia." *Applied Economics* 38: 253–66.

Ringel, J. S., S. D. Hosek, B. A. Vollaard, and S. Mahnovski. 2002. *The Elasticity of Demand for Health Care: A Review of the Literature and Its Application to the Military Health System.* Santa Monica, CA: RAND Corporation.

Rivers, P. A., and S. Bae. 1999. "Hospital Competition in Major U.S. Metropolitan Areas: An Empirical Evidence." *Journal of Socio-Economics* 28 (5): 597–608.

Rivers, P. A., and M. D. Fottler. 2004. "Do HMO Penetration and Hospital Competition Impact Quality of Hospital Care?" *Health Services Management Research* 17 (4): 237–48.

Rizzo, J. A., and D. Blumenthal. 1996. "Is the Target Income Hypothesis an Economic Heresy?" *Medical Care Research and Review* 53 (3): 243–66.

Robbins, A. 2001. "WHO Ranking of Health Systems." [Letter to the editor.] *Science* 294: 1832–33.

Robbins, L. 1984. "Economics and Political Economy." In *An Essay on the Nature and Significance of Economic Science*, 3rd ed., xi–xxxiii. London: Macmillan.

Robert Wood Johnson Foundation. 2008. "Robert Wood Johnson Foundation Nurse Faculty Scholars: Developing the Next Generation of Leaders in Academic Nursing." [Online article; retrieved 4/9/09.] www.rwjf.org/human capital/product.jsp?id=25191.

Robeyns, I. 2006. "The Capability Approach in Practice." *Journal of Political Philosophy* 14 (3): 351–76.

Robinson, J. 1962. *Economic Philosophy.* Chicago: Aldine.

Robinson, J. C. 2004. "Consolidation and the Transformation of Competition in Health Insurance." *Health Affairs* 23 (6): 11–24.

———. 2001. "The End of Managed Care." *Journal of the American Medical Association* 285: 2622–26.

———. 1996. "Decline in Hospital Utilization and Cost Inflation Under Managed Care in California." *Journal of the American Medical Association* 276 (13): 1060–64.

———. 1993. "Payment Mechanisms, Nonprice Incentives, and Organizational Innovation in Health Care." *Inquiry* 30 (3): 328–33.

———. 1991. "HMO Market Penetration and Hospital Cost in California." *Journal of the American Medical Association* 266 (19): 2719–23.

———. 1988a. "Market Structure, Employment, and Skill Mix in the Hospital Industry." *Southern Economic Journal* 55 (2): 315–25.

———. 1988b. "Hospital Competition and Hospital Nursing." *Nursing Economics* 6 (3): 116–24.

Robinson R. 2000. "Managed Care in the United States: A Dilemma for Evidence-Based Policy?" *Health Economics* 9: 1–7.

Rochaix, L., and D. Wilsford. 2005. "State Autonomy, Policy Paralysis: Paradoxes of Institutions and Culture in the French Health Care System." *Journal of Health Politics, Policy and Law* 30 (1–2): 97–119.

Rodgers, G. B. 1979. "Income and Inequality as Determinants of Mortality: An International Cross-Section Analysis." *Population Studies* 33: 343–51.

Rodwin, M. A. 2001. "Consumer Voice and Representation in Managed Healthcare." *Journal of Health Law* 34 (2): 233–76.

———. 1996. "Consumer Protection and Managed Care: The Need for Organized Consumers." *Health Affairs* 15 (3): 110–21.

Rodwin, V. G., and C. Le Pen. 2004. "Health Care Reform in France—The Birth of State-Led Managed Care." *New England Journal of Medicine* 351 (22): 2259–62.

Roemer, J. E. 1995. "Equality and Responsibility." *Boston Review* 20 (2): 3–7.

———. 1994. *Egalitarian Perspectives.* Cambridge, MA: Cambridge University Press.

Roemer, M. I. 1991. *National Health Systems of the World: Volume One, The Countries.* New York: Oxford University Press.

Roetzheim, R. G., P. Naazneen, E. C. Gonzalez, J. M. Ferrante, D. J. Van Durme, J. Z. Ayanian, and J. P. Krischer. 1999. "The Effects of Physician Supply on the Early Detection of Colorectal Cancer." *Journal of Family Practice* 48 (11): 850–58.

Rogowski, J., A. K. Jain, and J. J. Escarce. 2007. "Hospital Competition, Managed Care, and Mortality After Hospitalization for Medical Conditions in California." *Health Services Research* 42 (2): 682–705.

Roos, L. L., E. S. Fisher, R. Brazauskas, S. M. Sharp, and E. Shapiro. 1992. "Health and Surgical Outcomes in Canada and the United States." *Health Affairs* 11 (2): 56–72.

Roos, L. L., E. S. Fisher, S. M. Sharp, J. P. Newhouse, G. Anderson, and T. A. Bubolz. 1990. "Postsurgical Mortality in Manitoba and New England." *Journal of the American Medical Association* 263 (18): 2453–58.

Rose-Ackerman, S. 1996. "Altruism, Nonprofits, and Economic Theory." *Journal of Economic Literature* 34 (2): 701–28.

Rosenau, P. V. 2003. "Performance Evaluations of For-Profit and Nonprofit U.S. Hospitals Since 1980." *Nonprofit Management & Leadership* 13 (4): 401–23.

Rosenblatt, R., C. Andrilla, T. Curtinand, and L. Hart. 2006. "Shortages of Medical Personnel at Community Health Centers." *Journal of the American Medical Association* 295 (9): 1042–49.

Rosenthal, M., C. Hsuan, and A. Milstein. 2005. "A Report Card on the Freshman Class of Consumer-Directed Health Plans." *Health Affairs* 24 (6): 1592–1600.

Rosenthal, M. B., R. Fernandopulle, H. R. Song, and B. Landon. 2004. "Paying for Quality: Providers' Incentives for Quality Improvement." *Health Affairs* 23 (2): 127–41.

Rosenthal, M. B., and R. G. Frank. 2006. "What Is the Empirical Basis for Paying for Quality in Health Care?" *Medical Care Research and Review* 63 (2): 135–57.

Rosenthal, M. B., B. E. Landon, S. T. Normand, R. G. Frank, and A. M. Epstein. 2006. "Pay for Performance in Commercial HMOs." *New England Journal of Medicine* 355 (18): 1895–1902.

Rosenthal, M. B., A. Zaslavsky, and J. P. Newhouse. 2005. "The Geographic Distribution of Physicians Revisited." *Health Services Research* 40 (6, Pt. I): 1931–52.

Rosko, M. D., J. A. Chilingerian, J. S. Zinn, and W. E. Aaronson. 1995. "The Effects of Ownership, Operating Environment, and Strategic Choices on Nursing Home Efficiency." *Medical Care* 33 (10): 1001–21.

Ross, L., and R. E. Nisbett. 1991. *The Person and the Situation: Perspectives of Social Psychology*. Philadelphia, PA: Temple University Press.

Ross, L. D. 1988. "Situational Perspectives on the Obedience Experiments." *Contemporary Psychology* 33 (2): 101–4.

Rosser, W. W. 1996. "Approach to Diagnosis by Primary Care Clinicians and Specialists: Is There a Difference?" *Journal of Family Practice* 42: 139–44.

Rotarius, T., A. Trujillo, A. Liberman, and B. Ramirez. 2005. "Not-for-Profit Versus For-Profit Health Care Providers—Part I: Comparing and Contrasting Their Records." *Health Care Manager* 24 (4): 296–310.

Rothberg, M. B., I. Abraham, P. K. Lindenauer, and D. N. Rose. 2005. "Improving Nurse-to-Patient Staffing Ratios as a Cost-Effective Safety Intervention." *Medical Care* 43 (8): 785–91.

Rourke, J. 2008. "Increasing the Number of Rural Physicians." *Canadian Medical Association Journal* 178 (3): 322–25.

Rowley, C. K., and A. T. Peacock. 1975. *Welfare Economics: A Liberal Restatement*. New York: John Wiley.

Russell, B. 2007. "Budget Plan Funds Nursing Buildings, Skimps on Faculty." [Online article; retrieved 4/9/09.] www.teamiha.org/Documents/IHANews/0124%20Nursing%20bill.pdf.

Sagoff, M. 1986. "Values and Preferences." *Ethics* 96 (January): 301–16.

Salkeld, G., M. Ryan, and L. Short. 2000. "The Veil of Experience: Do Consumers Prefer What They Know Best?" *Health Economics* 9: 267–70.

Saltman, R. B., and S.-E. Bergman. 2005. "Renovating the Commons: Swedish Health Care Reforms in Perspective." *Journal of Health Politics, Policy and Law* 30 (1–2): 253–75.

Saltman, R. B., and J. Figueras. 1998. "Analyzing the Evidence on European Health Care Reforms." *Health Affairs* 17 (2): 85–108.

Samuelson, P. A. 1947. *Foundations of Economic Analysis*. New York: Atheneum.

———. 1938. "A Note on the Pure Theory of Consumer Behavior." *Economica* 5 (17): 61–71.

Sandier, S., V. Paris, and D. Polton. 2004. *Health Care Systems in Transition: France*. Copenhagen: WHO Regional Office for Europe on behalf of the European Observatory on Health Systems and Policies.

Sanofi-aventis. 2006. *Managed Care Digest Series® 2006*. [Online report; retrieved 4/9/09.] www.managedcaredigest.com/resources/hmo2006/2006hmo.pdf.

Sapolsky, R. M., S. C. Alberts, and J. Altmann. 1997. "Hypercortisolism Associated with Social Subordinance or Social Isolation Among Wild Baboons." *Archives of General Psychiatry* 54 (12): 1137–43.

Satterthwaite, M. 1979. "Consumer Information, Equilibrium Industry Price, and the Number of Sellers." *Bell Journal of Economics* 10 (2): 483–502.

Schlesinger, M., J. Bentkover, D. Blumenthal, R. Musacchio, and J. Willer. 1987. "The Privatization of Health Care and Physicians' Perceptions of Access to Hospital Services." *Milbank Quarterly* 65 (1): 25–28.

Schlesinger, M., and B. H. Gray. 2006. "How Nonprofits Matter in American Medicine, and What to Do About It." *Health Affairs* 25 (4): 287–303.

Schoen, C., R. Osborn, M. M. Doty, M. Bishop, J. Peugh, and N. Murukutla. 2007. "Toward Higher-Performance Health Systems: Adults' Health Care Experiences in Seven Countries, 2007." *Health Affairs* 26 (6): W717–W734.

Schoen, C., R. Osborn, S. K. H. How, M. M. Doty, and J. Peugh. 2008. "In Chronic Condition: Experiences of Patients with Complex Health Care Needs, in Eight Countries, 2008." *Health Affairs* 28 (1): W1–W16.

Schoen, C., R. Osborn, P. T. Huynh, M. M. Doty, K. Zapert, J. Peugh, and K. Davis. 2005. "Taking the Pulse of Health Care Systems: Experiences of Patients with Health Problems in Six Countries." *Health Affairs* Web Exclusives (July–December, Suppl.): W5-509–W5-525.

Schroeder, S. A. 1984. "Western European Responses to Physician Oversupply: Lessons for the United States." *Journal of the American Medical Association* 252: 373–84.

Schumacher, E. J. 1997. "Relative Wages and Exit Behavior Among Registered Nurses." *Journal of Labor Research* 18 (4): 581–92.

Schuster, M. A., E. A. McGlynn, and R. H. Brook. 1998. "How Good Is the Quality of Health Care in the United States?" *Milbank Quarterly* 76 (4): 517–63.

Schut, F. T. 1995. "Health Care Reform in the Netherlands: Balancing Corporatism, Etatism, and Market Mechanisms." *Journal of Health Politics, Policy and Law* 20 (3): 615–52.

Schut, F. T., and W. P. M. M. Van de Ven. 2005. "Rationing and Competition in the Dutch Health-Care System." *Health Economics* 14: S59–S74.

Schwartz, B. 2004. *The Paradox of Choice: Why More Is Less.* New York: HarperCollins.

Schweitzer, M., J. C. Hershey, and D. A. Asch. 1996. "Individual Choice in Spending Accounts: Can We Rely on Employees to Choose Well?" *Medical Care* 34 (6): 583–93.

Scitovsky, T. 1976. *The Joyless Economy.* New York: Oxford University Press.

Seago, J., M. Ash, J. Spetz, J. Coffman, and K. Grumbach. 2001. "Hospital Registered Nurse Shortages: Environmental, Patient, and Institutional Predictors." *Health Services Research* 36 (5): 831–54.

Seago, J. A., J. Spetz, and S. Mitchell. 2004. "Nurse Staffing and Hospital Ownership in California." *Journal of Nursing Administration* 34 (5): 228–37.

Secretary of State for Health (England). 2000. *The NHS Plan.* London: Her Majesty's Stationery Office.

Sen, A. K. 2002. "Why Health Equity?" *Health Economics* 11 (8): 659–66.

———. 1992. *Inequality Revisited.* Cambridge, MA: Harvard University Press.

———. 1987. *On Ethics and Economics.* Oxford, UK: Basil Blackwell.

———. 1982. *Choice, Welfare, and Measurement.* Oxford, UK: Basil Blackwell.

———. 1970. *Collective Choice and Social Welfare.* San Francisco: Holden-Day.

Serow, W., M. Cowart, Y. Chen, and D. Speake. 1993. "Health Care Corporatization and the Employment Conditions of Nurses." *Nursing Economics* 11 (5): 279–91.

Sethi-Iyengar, S. G., W. Huberman, and W. Jiang. 2004. "How Much Choice Is Too Much? Contributions to 401(k) Retirement Plans." In *Pension Design and Structure: New Lessons from Behavioral Finance*, edited by O. S. Mitchell and S. Utkus, 83–95. Oxford, UK: Oxford University Press.

Sexton, T. R., A. M. Leiken, S. Sleeper, and A. F. Coburn. 1989. "The Impact of Prospective Reimbursement on Nursing Home Efficiency." *Medical Care* 27 (2): 154–63.

Shain, M., and M. I. Roemer. 1959. "Hospital Costs Relate to the Supply of Beds." *Modern Hospital* (April): 71–73, 168.

Shapiro, C. 1983. "Premiums for High Quality Products as Returns to Reputations." *Quarterly Journal of Economics* 98 (November): 659–79.

Shapiro, M. F., J. E. Ware Jr., and C. D. Sherbourne. 1986. "Effects of Cost Sharing on Seeking Care for Serious and Minor Symptoms." *Annals of Internal Medicine* 104 (2): 246–51.

Shaver, K. H., and L. M. Lacey. 2003. "Job and Career Satisfaction Among Staff Nurses." *Journal of Nursing Administration* 33 (3): 166–72.

Shen, Y., K. Eggleston, J. Lau, and C. Schmid. 2007. "Hospital Ownership and Financial Performance: What Explains the Different Findings in the Empirical Literature?" *Inquiry* 44 (1): 41–68.

Sheward, L., J. Hunt, S. Hagen, M. Macleod, and J. Ball. 2005. "The Relationship Between UK Hospital Nurse Staffing and Emotional Exhaustion and Job Dissatisfaction." *Journal of Nursing Management* 13 (1): 51–60.

Shi, L. 1994. "Primary Care, Specialty Care, and Life Changes." *International Journal of Health Services* 24 (3): 431–58.

Shi, L., J. Macinko, B. Starfield, J. Wulu, J. Regan, and R. Politzer. 2003a. "The Relationship Between Primary Care, Income Inequality, and Mortality in the United States, 1980–1995." *Journal of the American Board of Family Practice* 16: 412–22.

Shi, L., J. Macinko, B. Starfield, J. Xu, and R. Politzer. 2003b. "Primary Care, Income Inequality, and Stroke Mortality in the United States: A Longitudinal Analysis, 1985–1995." *Stroke* 34: 1958–64.

Shi, L., J. Macinko, B. Starfield, J. Xu, J. Regan, R. Politzer, and J. Wulu. 2004. "Primary Care, Infant Mortality, and Low Birth Weight in the States of the USA." *Journal of Epidemiology and Community Health* 58: 374–80.

Shipman, S. A., J. D. Lurie, and D. C. Goodman. 2004. "The General Pediatrician: Projecting Future Workforce Supply and Requirements." *Pediatrics* 113: 435–42.

Shively, C. A., and T. B. Clarkson. 1994. "Social Status and Coronary Artery Atherosclerosis in Female Monkeys." *Arteriosclerosis and Thrombosis* 14: 721–26.

Shukla, R. K., J. Pestian, and J. Clement. 1997. "A Comparative Analysis of Revenue and Cost-Management Strategies of Not-for-Profit and For-Profit Hospitals." *Hospital & Health Services Administration* 42 (1): 117–34.

Sidgwick, H. 1887. *Principles of Political Economy*. London: Macmillan.

Simon, H. A. 1955. "A Behavioral Model of Rational Choice." *Quarterly Journal of Economics* 69: 99–118.

Simpson, J., and R. Shin. 1998. "Do Non-Profit Hospitals Exercise Market Power?" *International Journal of the Economics of Business* 5 (2): 141–58.

Siu, A. L., F. A. Sonnenberg, W. G. Manning, G. A. Goldberg, E. S. Bloomfield, J. P. Newhouse, and R. H. Brook. 1986. "Inappropriate Use of Hospitals in a Randomized Trial of Health Insurance Plans." *New England Journal of Medicine* 315 (20): 1259–66.

Skatun, D., E. Antonazzo, A. Scott, and R. F. Elliott. 2005. "The Supply of Qualified Nurses: A Classical Model of Labour Supply." *Applied Economics* 37: 57–65.

Sloan, F. A. 1998. "Commercialism in Nonprofit Hospitals." *Journal of Policy Analysis and Management* 17 (2): 234–52.

Sloan, F. A., and R. Feldman. 1978. "Competition Among Physicians." In *Competition in the Health Care Sector: Past, Present, and Future*, edited by W. Greenberg. Washington, DC: Bureau of Economics, Federal Trade Commission.

Smee, C. 2000. "United Kingdom." *Journal of Health Politics, Policy and Law* 25 (5): 945–51.

Smith, A. 1776 [1994]. *Wealth of Nations: An Inquiry into the Nature and Causes.* New York: Modern Library.

Smith, D. 1997. "The Effects of Preferred Provider Organizations on Health Care Use and Costs." *Inquiry* 34 (Winter): 278–87.

Smith, J., and K. Walshe. 2004. "Big Business: The Corporatization of Primary Care in the UK and the USA." *Public Money & Management* 24 (2): 87–96.

Spang, H. R., G. J. Bazzoli, and R. J. Arnould. 2001. "Hospital Mergers and Savings for Consumers: Exploring New Evidence." *Health Affairs* 20 (4): 150–58.

Spector, W. D., T. M. Selden, and J. W. Cohen. 1998. "The Impact of Ownership Type on Nursing Home Outcomes." *Health Economics* 7 (7): 639–53.

Spector, W. D., and H. A. Takada. 1991. "Characteristics of Nursing Homes That Affect Resident Outcomes." *Journal of Aging and Health* 3 (4): 427–54.

Spence, A. M. 1977. "Consumer Misperceptions, Product Failure and Product Liability." *Review of Economic Studies* 44 (3): 561–72.

Spence-Laschinger, H. K., J. Shamian, and D. Thomson. 2001. "Impact of Magnet Hospital Characteristics on Nurses' Perceptions of Trust, Burnout, Quality of Care, and Work Satisfaction." *Nursing Economics* 19 (5): 209–19.

Spetz, J. 1999. "The Effects of Managed Care and Prospective Payment on the Demand for Hospital Nurses: Evidence from California." *Health Services Research* 34 (5): 993–1009.

Spetz, J., W. T. Dyer, S. Chapman, and J. A. Seago. 2006. "Hospital Demand for Licensed Practical Nurses." *Western Journal of Nursing Research* 28 (6): 726–39.

Spetz, J., and R. Given. 2003. "The Future of the Nurse Shortage: Will Wage Increases Close the Gap?" *Health Affairs* 22 (6): 199–206.

Stafford, R. S. 1991. "The Impact of Nonclinical Factors on Repeat Cesarean Section." *Journal of the American Medical Association* 265 (1): 59–63.

Staiger, D., J. Spetz, and C. Phibbs. 1999. "Is There Monopsony in the Labor Market? Evidence from a Natural Experiment." [Online article; retrieved 4/10/09.] www.nber.org/papers/w7258.

Stanbury, W. T. 1986. *Business-Government Relations in Canada*. Toronto: Methuen.

Stano, M. 1985. "An Analysis of the Evidence on Competition in the Physician Services Market." *Journal of Health Economics* 4 (3): 197–211.

Starfield, B., L. Shi, A. Glover, and J. Macinko. 2005. "The Effects of Specialist Supply on Populations' Health: Assessing the Evidence." *Health Affairs* Web Exclusives (January–June, Suppl.) W5-97–W5-107.

Starfield, B., L. Shi, and J. Macinko. 2005. "Contribution of Primary Care to Health Systems and Health." *Milbank Quarterly* 83 (3): 457–502.

Starr, P. 1982. *The Social Transformation of American Medicine*. New York: Basic.

Statistisches Bundesamt (Federal Statistical Office). 2008a. "Health Expenditure Accounts" (in German). [Online article; retrieved 4/10/09.] www.gbe-bund.de/gbe10/trecherche.prc_them_rech?tk=19200&tk2=19300&p_uid=gast&p_aid=48523624&p_sprache=E&cnt_ut=10&ut=19310.

———. 2008b. "Co-payments of Private Households by Field of Service in the Statutory Health Insurance in Expenditures, Costs and Financing." The Information System of the Federal Health Monitoring. [Online information; retrieved 5/1/09.] www.gbe-bund.de.

Statistics Bureau of Japan. 2008. *Statistical Handbook of Japan 2008*. Tokyo: Statistics Bureau.

Stearns, S., B. Wolfe, and D. Kindig. 1992. "Physician Responses to Fee-for-Service and Capitation Payment." *Inquiry* 29 (4): 416–25.

Steffen, T., and P. Nystrom. 1997. "Organizational Determinants of Service Quality in Nursing Homes." *Hospital & Health Services Administration* 42 (2): 179–91.

Steinbrook, R. 2006. "Private Health Care in Canada." *New England Journal of Medicine* 354 (16): 1661–64.

Stevens, S. 2004. "Reform Strategies for the English NHS." *Health Affairs* 23 (3): 37–44.

Stigler, G. J. 1971. "The Theory of Economic Regulation." *Bell Journal of Economics and Management Science* 2: 3–21.

Stigler, G. J., and G. S. Becker. 1977. "*De Gustibus Non Est Disputandum*." *American Economic Review* 67 (2): 76–90.

Stone, D. A. 2001. *Policy Paradox: The Art of Political Decision-Making*. New York: Norton.

Stone, P. W., E. L. Larson, C. Mooney-Kane, J. Smolowitz, S. X. Lin, and A. W. Dick. 2006. "Organizational Climate and Intensive Care Unit Nurses' Intention to Leave." *Critical Care Medicine* 34 (7): 1907–12.

Subramanian, S. V., and I. Kawachi. 2004. "Income Inequality and Health: What Have We Learned So Far?" *Epidemiologic Reviews* 26: 78–91.

Sugden, R. 1993. "Welfare, Resources, and Capabilities: A Review of Inequality Reeexamined by Amartya Sen." *Journal of Economic Literature* 31: 1947–62.

Swedish Federation of County Councils. 2001. *Publicly Financed Ambulatory Care 2000*. Offentligt Finansierad Privat Öppen vård 2000 2001-11-15. [Online article.] www.lf.se/sek/tankstatistik.htm.

Synderman, R., G. F. Sheldon, and T. A. Bischoff. 2002. "Gauging Supply and De-

mand: The Challenging Quest to Predict the Future Physician Workforce."
Health Affairs 21 (1): 167–69.

Szczech, L. A., P. S. Klassen, B. Chua, S. S. Hedayati, M. Flanigan, W. M. McClellan, D. N. Reddan, R. A. Rettig, D. L. Frankenfield, and W. F. Owen Jr. 2006. "Associations Between CMS's Clinical Performance Measures Project Benchmarks, Profit Structure, and Mortality in Dialysis Units." *Kidney International* 69: 2094–2100.

Tai-Seale, M., T. H. Rice, and S. C. Stearns. 1998. "Volume Response to Medicare Payment Reductions with Multiple Payers: A Test of the McGuire-Pauly Model." *Health Economics* 7: 199–219.

Tanio, C. 1989. *Unnecessary Cesarean Sections, a Rapidly Growing National Epidemic.* Washington, DC: Public Citizen Health Research Group.

Taylor, D., D. Whellan, and F. Sloan. 1999. "Effects of Admission to a Teaching Hospital on the Cost and Quality of Care for Medicare Beneficiaries." *New England Journal of Medicine* 340 (4): 293–99.

Technological Change in Health Care (TECH) Research Network. 2001. "Technological Change Around the World: Evidence from Heart Attack Care." *Health Affairs* 20 (3): 25–42.

Thaler, R. H. 1992. *The Winner's Curse: Paradoxes and Anomalies of Economic Life.* New York: Free Press.

Thaler, R. H., and C. R. Sunstein. 2008. *Nudge: Improving Decisions About Health, Wealth, and Happiness.* New Haven, CT: Yale University Press.

Thiebaud, P., B. V. Patel, and M. B. Nichol. 2008. "The Demand for Statin: The Effect of Copay on Utilization and Compliance." *Health Economics* 17: 83–97.

Thorpe, K. E., C. S. Florence, D. H. Howard, and P. Joski. 2004. "The Impact of Obesity on Rising Medical Spending." *Health Affairs* Web Exclusive (July–December, Suppl.): W4-480–W4-486.

Thurow, L. C. 1983. *Dangerous Currents: The State of Economics.* New York: Random House.

———. 1980. *The Zero-Sum Society.* New York: Penguin.

———. 1977. "Government Expenditures: Cash or In-Kind Aid?" In *Markets and Morals,* edited by G. Dworkin, G. Bermant, and P. G. Brow. Washington, DC: Hemisphere.

Tomal, A. 1998. "The Relationship Between Hospital Mortality Rates, and Hospital, Market and Patient Characteristics." *Applied Economics* 30: 717–25.

Town, R. 2001. "The Welfare Impact of HMO Mergers." *Journal of Health Economics* 20: 967–90.

Town, R. J., D. Wholey, R. Feldman, and L. R. Burns. 2007. "Revisiting the Relationship Between Managed Care and Hospital Consolidation." *Health Services Research* 42 (1): 219–38.

Trivedi, A. N., W. Rakowski, and J. Z. Ayanian. 2008. "Effect of Cost Sharing on Screening Mammography in Medicare Health Plans." *New England Journal of Medicine* 358 (4): 375–83.

Trovey, E. J., and A. E. Adams. 1999. "The Changing Nature of Nurses' Job Satisfaction: An Exploration of Sources of Satisfaction in the 1990s." *Journal of Advanced Nursing* 30 (1): 150–58.

Tsai, P. F., and C. M. Molinero. 2002. "A Variable Returns to Scale Data Envelopment Analysis Model for the Joint Determination of Efficiencies with an Example of the UK Health Service." *European Journal of Operational Research* 141: 21–38.

Tu, J. V., C. L. Pashos, C. D. Naylor, E. Chen, S. L. Normand, J. P. Newhouse, and B. J. McNeil. 1997. "Use of Cardiac Procedures and Outcomes in Elderly Patients with Myocardial Infarction in the United States and Canada." *New England Journal of Medicine* 336 (21): 1500–5.

Tullock, G. 1979. "Objectives of Income Redistribution." In *Sociological Economics*, edited by L. Levy-Garboua. Beverly Hills, CA: Sage.

Tuohy, C. H. 1999. *Accidental Logics: The Dynamics of Change in the Health Care Arena in the United States, Britain, and Canada.* New York: Oxford University Press.

Tuohy, C. H., C. M. Flood, and M. Stabile. 2004. "How Does Private Finance Affect Public Health Care Systems? Marshaling the Evidence from OECD Nations." *Journal of Health Politics, Policy and Law* 29 (3): 359–96.

Tussing, A. D., and M. A. Wojtowycz. 1986. "Physician-Induced Demand by Irish GPs." *Social Science and Medicine* 23 (9): 851–60.

Tversky, A., and D. Kahneman. 1981. "The Framing of Decisions and the Psychology of Choice." *Science* 211 (January 30): 453–58.

University of California. 2001. *Getting the Most from Your Benefits Plan.* [Online report.] www.ucop.edu/bencom/hw/ygip/ygip2001.pdf.

Unruh, L. 2008. "Nurse Staffing and Patient, Nurse, and Financial Outcomes." *American Journal of Nursing* 108 (1): 62–71.

———. 2003. "Licensed Nurse Staffing and Adverse Events in Hospitals." *Medical Care* 41 (1): 142–52.

———. 2002. "Nursing Staff Reductions in Pennsylvania Hospitals: Exploring the Discrepancy Between Perceptions and Data." *Medical Care Research and Review* 59 (2): 197–214.

Unruh, L., and M. Fottler. 2006. "Patient Turnover and Nursing Staff Adequacy." *Health Services Research* 41 (2): 599–612.

———. 2005. "Projections and Trends in Nursing Supply: What Do They Tell Us About the Nursing Shortage?" *Policy, Politics and Nursing Practice* 6 (3): 171–82.

Unruh, L., N. J. Zhang, and T. H. Wan. 2006. "The Impact of Medicare Reimbursement Changes on Staffing and the Quality of Care in Nursing Homes." *International Journal of Public Policy* 1 (4): 421–34.

United States Renal Data System. 2006. *Annual Report: Atlas of End-Stage Renal Disease in the United States.* [Online report; retrieved 4/10/09.] www.usrds.org/adr_2006.htm.

———. 1997. *Annual Report: Atlas of End-Stage Renal Disease in the United States.* [Online report; retrieved 4/10/09.] http://www.usrds.org/adr_1997.htm.

U.S. Census Bureau. 2006. *Statistical Abstract of the United States.* Washington, DC: Government Printing Office.

U.S. Food and Drug Administration (FDA), Center for Drug Evaluation and Research. 2008. "Information About the Products We Regulate." [Online information; retrieved 4/10/09.] www.fda.gov/CDER/drug/default.htm.

U.S. Government Accountability Office (GAO). 1994. *Cancer Survival: An International Comparison of Outcomes*. Washington, DC: GAO.

UVaToday. 2007. "Virginia Gov. Timothy Kaine Announces 10 Percent Increase in Nursing Faculty Salaries." [Online article; retrieved 4/10/09.] www.virginia.edu/uvatoday/newsRelease.php?id=1595.

Vaiana, M. E., and E. A. McGlynn. 2002. "What Cognitive Science Tells Us About the Design of Reports for Consumers." *Medical Care Research and Review* 59 (1): 3–35.

Valdez, R. B., R. H. Brook, W. H. Rogers, J. E. Ware Jr., E. B. Keeler, C. A. Sherbourne, K. N. Lohr, G. A. Goldberg, P. Camp, and J. P. Newhouse. 1985. "Consequences of Cost-Sharing for Children's Health." *Pediatrics* 75 (5): 952–61.

Valdez, R. O. 1986. *The Effects of Cost Sharing on the Health of Children*. Santa Monica, CA: RAND Corp.

Van de Ven, W. P. M. M., and F. T. Schut. 2008. "Universal Mandatory Health Insurance in the Netherlands: A Model for the U.S.?" *Health Affairs* 27 (3): 771–81.

van de Werd, P. 2008. "Health Insurance Reform in the Netherlands." [Online slide presentation; retrieved 4/10/09.] www.cea.eu/uploads/DocumentsLibrary/documents/1223568815_pim-revised.ppt.

van Doorslaer, E., and F. T. Schut. 2000. "Belgium and the Netherlands Revisited." *Journal of Health Politics, Policy and Law* 25 (5): 875–87.

van Doorslaer, E., A. Wagstaff, and F. Rutten. 1993. *Equity in the Finance and Delivery of Health Care: An International Perspective*. Oxford, UK: Oxford Medical Publications.

van Doorslaer, E., A. Wagstaff, H. van der Burg, T. Christiansen, G. Citoni, R. Di Biase, U. G. Gerdtham, M. Gerfin, L. Gross, U. Häkkinen, J. John, P. Johnson, J. Klavus, C. Lachaud, J. Lauritsen, R. Leu, B. Nolan, J. Pereira, C. Propper, F. Puffer, L. Rochaix, M. Schellhorn, G. Sundberg, and O. Winkelhake. 1999. "The Redistributive Effect of Health Care Finance in Twelve OECD Countries." *Journal of Health Economics* 18 (3): 291–313.

van Doorslaer, E., A. Wagstaff, H. van de Burg, T. Christiansen, D. De Graeve, I. Duchesne, U. G. Gerdtham, M. Gerfin, J. Geurts, L. Gross, U. Häkkinen, J. John, J. Klavus, R. E. Leu, B. Nolan, O. O'Donnell, C. Propper, F. Puffer, M. Schellhorn, G. Sundberg, and O. Winkelhake. 2000. "Equity in the Delivery of Health Care in Europe and the U.S." *Journal of Health Economics* 19 (5): 553–83.

Verrilli, D. K., R. Berenson, and S. J. Katz. 1998. "A Comparison of Cardiovascular Procedure Use Between the United States and Canada." *Health Services Research* 33 (3, Pt. I): 467–87.

Vining, A. R., and D. L. Weimer. 1990. "Government Supply and Government Production Failure: A Framework Based on Contestability." *Journal of Public Policy* 10 (1): 1–22.

Vita, M., and D. Sacher. 2001. "The Competitive Effects of Not-for-Profit Hospital Mergers: A Case Study." *Journal of Industrial Economics* 49 (1): 63–84.

Vladeck, B. C. 1990. *Simple, Elegant, and Wrong*. New York: United Hospital Fund.

Voltaire, F.-M. A. 1759. *Candide*, translated by L. Bair. New York: Bantam.

Wagstaff, A., and E. van Doorslaer. 2000. "Income Inequality and Health: What Does the Literature Tell Us?" *Annual Review of Public Health* 21: 543–67.

———. 1993. "Equity in Finance and Delivery of Health Care: Concepts and Definitions." In *Equity in the Finance and Delivery of Health Care: An International Perspective*, edited by E. van Doorslaer, A. Wagstaff, and F. Rutten, 7–19. Oxford, UK: Oxford Medical Publications.

Wagstaff, A., E. van Doorslaer, S. Calonge, T. Christiansen, M. Gerfin, P. Gottschalk, R. Janssen, C. Lachaud, R. E. Leu, B. Nolan B, et al. 1992. "Equity in the Finance of Health Care: Some International Comparisons." *Journal of Health Economics* 11 (4): 361–87.

Wagstaff, A., E. van Doorslaer, H. van der Burg, S. Calonge, T. Christiansen, G. Citoni, U. G. Gerdtham, M. Gerfin, L. Gross, U. Häkkinen, P. Johnson, J. John, J. Klavus, C. Lachaud, J. Lauritsen, R. Leu, B. Nolan, E. Perán, J. Pereira, C. Propper, F. Puffer, L. Rochaix, M. Rodríguez, M. Schellhorn, O. Winkelhake, et al. 1999. "Equity in the Finance of Health Care: Some Further International Comparisons." *Journal of Health Economics* 18 (3): 263–90.

Wan, T., N. Zhang, and L. Unruh. 2006. "Predictors of Resident Outcome Improvement in Nursing Homes." *Western Journal of Nursing Research* 28 (8): 974–93.

Wazana, A. 2000. "Physicians and the Pharmaceutical Industry: Is a Gift Ever Just a Gift?" *Journal of the American Medical Association* 282 (3): 373–80.

Weaver, R. K., and B. A. Rockman. 1993. "When and How Do Institutions Matter?" In *Do Institutions Matter?* edited by R. K. Weaver and B. A. Rockman. Washington, DC: Brookings Institution.

Wedig, G., J. B. Mitchell, and J. Cromwell. 1989. "Can Price Controls Induce Optimal Physician Behavior?" *Journal of Health Politics, Policy and Law* 14 (3): 601–20.

Weeks, W. B., and A. E. Wallace. 2002. "The More Things Change: Revisiting a Comparison of Educational Costs and Incomes of Physicians and Other Professionals." *Academic Medicine* 77 (4): 312–19.

Weiner, J. 2007. "Expanding the US Medical Workforce: Global Perspectives and Parallels." *British Medical Journal* 335 (7613): 236–38.

Weisbrod, B. A. 1991. "The Health Care Quadrilemma: An Essay on Technological Change, Insurance, Quality of Care, and Cost Containment." *Journal of Economic Literature* 29 (2): 523–52.

———. 1988. *The Nonprofit Economy*. Cambridge, MA: Harvard University Press.

———. 1978. "Comment on Paper by Mark Pauly." In *Competition in the Health Care Sector: Past, Present, and Future*, edited by W. Greenberg, 49–56. Washington, DC: Bureau of Economics, Federal Trade Commission.

Welch, B. L., J. W. Hay, D. S. Miller, R. J. Olsen, R. M. Rippey, and A. S. Welch. 1987. "The RAND Health Insurance Study: A Summary Critique." *Medical Care* 25 (2): 148–56.

Wennberg, D. 2000. *Dartmouth Atlas of Cardiovascular Health Care*. Chicago: American Hospital Association.

Wennberg, J., and A. Gittlesohn. 1982. "Variations in Medical Care Among Small Areas." *Scientific American* 246 (4): 120–34.

Wheeler, J., and T. Wickizer. 1990. "Relating Health Care Market Characteristics to the Effectiveness of Utilization Review Programs." *Inquiry* 27 (Winter): 344–51.

Whitcomb, M. E. 2006. "The Shortage of Physicians and the Future Role of Nurses." *Academic Medicine* 81 (9): 779–80.

White, C. 2005. "Medicare's Prospective Payment System for Skilled Nursing Facilities: Effects on Staffing and Quality of Care." *Inquiry* 42: 351–66.

White, J. 1995. *Competing Solutions: American Health Care Proposals and International Experience.* Washington, DC: Brookings Institution.

Whitman, G. R., Y. Kim, L. J. Davidson, G. A. Wolf, and S. L. Wang. 2002. "The Impact of Staffing on Patient Outcomes Across Specialty Units." *Journal of Nursing Administration* 32 (12): 633–39.

Whittle, J., C. J. Lin, J. R. Lave, M. J. Fine, K. M. Delaney, D. Z. Joyce, W. W. Young, and W. N. Kapoor. 1998. "Relationship of Provider Characteristics to Outcomes, Process, and Costs of Care for Community-Acquired Pneumonia." *Medical Care* 36: 977–87.

Wholey, D., R. Feldman, and J. B. Christianson. 1995. "The Effect of Market Structure on HMO Premiums." *Journal of Health Economics* 14 (1): 61–105.

Wickizer, T. 1992. "The Effects of Utilization Review on Hospital Use and Expenditures: A Covariance Analysis." *Health Services Research* 27 (1): 103–21.

Wickizer, T. M., R. C. Wheeler, and P. J. Feldstein. 1989. "Does Utilization Review Reduce Unnecessary Hospital Care and Contain Costs?" *Medical Care* 27 (6): 632–47.

Wilensky, G. R., and L. F. Rossiter. 1983. "The Relative Importance of Physician-Induced Demand in the Demand for Medical Care." *Milbank Memorial Fund Quarterly* 61 (2): 252–77.

Wilhelm-Schwartz, F., and R. Busse. 1997. "Germany." In *Health Care Reform: Learning From International Experience*, edited by C. Ham. Philadelphia, PA: Open University Press.

Wilkinson, R. G. 1999. "Income Inequality, Social Cohesion, and Health: Clarifying the Theory—A Reply to Muntaner and Lynch." *International Journal of Health Services* 29 (3): 525–43.

Willcox, S. 2001. "Promoting Private Health Insurance in Australia." *Health Affairs* 20 (3): 152–61.

Williams, A. 1997. "Intergenerational Equity: An Exploration of the 'Fair Innings' Argument." *Health Economics* 6 (2): 117–32.

Williams, B. 1962. "The Idea of Equality." In *Philosophy, Politics, and Society*, 2nd ed., edited by P. Laslett and W. G. Runciman. Oxford, UK: Blackwell.

Williams, C. H., W. B. Vogt, and R. Town. 2006. "How Has Hospital Consolidation Affected the Price and Quality of Hospital Care?" [Online article; retrieved 4/13/09.] www.rwjf.org/pr/synthesis/reports_and_briefs/pdf/no9_policy brief.pdf.

Wilson, J. 2005. "U.S. Needs More Physicians Soon, but How Many More Is Debatable." *Annals of Internal Medicine* 143 (6): 469–72.

Wilson, P. W., and K. Carey. 2004. "Nonparametric Analysis of Returns to Scale in the U.S. Hospital Industry." *Journal of Applied Economics* 19: 505–24.

Wolf, C., Jr. 1993. *Markets or Governments: Choosing Between Imperfect Alternatives.* Cambridge, MA: MIT Press.

———. 1979. "A Theory of Nonmarket Failure: Framework for Implementation Analysis." *Journal of Law and Economics* 22 (1): 107–39.

Wolfe, P. R., and D. W. Moran. 1993. "Global Budgeting in the OECD Countries." *Health Care Financing Review* 14 (3): 55–76.

Wong, M. D., R. Andersen, C. D. Sherbourne, R. D. Hays, and M. F. Shapiro. 2001. "Effects of Cost Sharing on Care Seeking and Health Status: Results from the Medical Outcomes Study." *American Journal of Public Health* 91 (11): 1889–94.

Woolhandler, S., and D. U. Himmelstein. 1997. "Costs of Care and Administration at For-Profit and Other Hospitals in the United States." *New England Journal of Medicine* 336 (11): 769–74.

Woolhandler, S., D. U. Himmelstein, I. Hellander, and S. M. Wolfe. 2002. "HMO Profits and Quality." *Health Affairs* 20 (5): 302–3.

World Health Organization (WHO). 2001. *Highlights on Health in Switzerland.* Copenhagen: WHO Regional Office for Europe.

———. 2000. *Health Systems: Improving Performance.* Geneva: WHO.

———. 1997. *Highlights on Health in France.* Copenhagen: WHO Regional Office for Europe.

Worz, M., and R. Busse. 2005. "Analysing the Impact of Health-Care System Change in the EU Member States—Germany." *Health Economics* 14: S133–S149.

WWAMI. 2006. "Registered Nurse Vacancies in Federally Funded Health Centers." [Online article; retrieved 4/13/09.] depts.washington.edu/uwrhrc/pdfs/RHRC%20RNHCs%202Pgr%202-5-07.pdf.

Yang, Y. 2008. "Social Inequalities in Happiness in the United States, 1972 to 2004: An Age-Period-Cohort Analysis." *American Sociological Review* 73: 204–26.

Yip, W. C. 1998. "Physician Response to Medicare Fee Reductions: Changes in the Volume of Coronary Artery Bypass Graft (CABG) Surgeries in the Medicare and Private Sectors." *Journal of Health Economics* 17 (6): 675–99.

Yip, W. C., and W. C. Hsiao. 1997. "Medical Savings Accounts: Lessons from China." *Health Affairs* 16 (6): 244–51.

Yordy, K. D. 2006. "The Nursing Faculty Shortage: A Crisis for Healthcare." [Online article; retrieved 4/13/09.] http://www.rwjf.org/files/publications/other/NursingFacultyShortage071006.pdf.

Yoshikawa, A., and J. Bhattacharya. 2002. "Japan." In *World Health Systems: Challenges and Perspectives,* edited by B. J. Fried and L. M. Gaydos, 249–66. Chicago: Health Administration Press.

Young, G. J., J. F. Burgess Jr., K. R. Desai, and D. Valley. 2002. "The Financial Experience of Hospitals with HMO Contracts: Evidence from Florida." *Inquiry* 39: 67–75.

Young, G. J., K. R. Desai, and F. J. Hellinger. 2000. "Community Control and Pricing Patterns of Nonprofit Hospitals: An Antitrust Analysis." *Journal of Health Politics, Policy and Law* 25 (6): 1051–81.

Young, H. P. 1994. *Equity in Theory and Practice.* Princeton, NJ: Princeton University Press.

Zhang, N. J., L. Unruh, R. Liu, and T. T. Wan. 2006. "Minimum Nurse Staffing Ratios for Nursing Homes." *Nursing Economics* 24 (2): 78–85, 93.

Zhang, N. J., L. Unruh, and T. T. Wan. 2008. "Has the Medicare Prospective Payment System Led to Increased Nursing Home Efficiency?" *Health Services Research* 43 (3): 1043–61.

Zigmond, J. 2007. "Remote Possibilities." *Modern Healthcare* 37 (15): 26–28.

Zinn, J., W. Aaronson, and M. Rosko. 1993. "Variations in the Outcomes of Care Provided in Pennsylvania Nursing Homes." *Medical Care* 31 (6): 475–87.

Zuger, A. 2004. "Dissatisfaction with Medical Practice." *New England Journal of Medicine* 350 (1): 69–75.

Zwanziger, J., and A. Bamezai. 2006. "Evidence of Cost Shifting in California Hospitals." *Health Affairs* 25 (1): 197–203.

Zwanziger, J., and G. Melnick. 2000. "Can Cost Shifting Continue in a Price Competitive Environment?" *Health Economics* 9 (3): 211–25.

———. 1996. "Can Managed Care Plans Control Health Care Costs?" *Health Affairs* 15 (2): 185–99.

Zweifel, P. 2000. "Switzerland." *Journal of Health Politics, Policy and Law* 25 (5): 937–44.

INDEX

ABOUT THE AUTHORS

Thomas Rice, PhD, is a professor in the Department of Health Services at the UCLA School of Public Health. At the time of this writing, he also serves as vice chancellor, Academic Personnel, for UCLA. Dr. Rice received his doctorate in economics at the University of California at Berkeley in 1982. He served on the faculty at the University of North Carolina School of Public Health from 1983 until 1991, when he joined UCLA. Dr. Rice has published widely on issues such as competition and regulation in health services, physicians' economic behavior, cost containment, health insurance, and the Medicare program. He is an elected member of the Institute of Medicine, National Academy of Sciences. Previously, he served as editor of the journal *Medical Care Research and Review* and was chair of the board of directors of AcademyHealth. In 1998, Dr. Rice received the Article of the Year Award from the Association for Health Services Research and Health Policy (now AcademyHealth) for a piece published in the *Journal of Health Politics, Policy and Law* that formed the basis of chapters 4 and 5 of this book.

Lynn Unruh, PhD, RN, is an associate professor in the Department of Health Management and Informatics at the University of Central Florida. Dr. Unruh received her bachelor of science in nursing from the University of Illinois and her doctorate in economics from the University of Notre Dame. She has published extensively in areas such as nurse staffing and quality in hospitals and nursing homes, the nursing workforce, the work environment in hospitals and nursing homes, and the organizational responses of hospitals and nursing homes to reimbursement and regulatory and market forces. Dr. Unruh works closely with state nursing workforce centers, such as the Florida Center for Nursing, and is a member of the Research Council of the American Nurses Credentialing Center. She received the Academy of Management Best Paper Award in 2005 and 2008 and the AcademyHealth Most Outstanding Abstracts Award in 2005. From 2006 to 2007, Dr. Unruh was a Fellow in Nursing Policy and Philanthropy at the Robert Wood Johnson Foundation.